T0358940

Orthodontics for the Oral and Maxillofacial Surgery Patient

Editors

MICHAEL R. MARKIEWICZ
VEERASATHPURUSH ALLAREDDY
MICHAEL MILORO

ORAL AND MAXILLOFACIAL SURGERY CLINICS OF NORTH AMERICA

www.oralmaxsurgery.theclinics.com

Consulting Editor
RUI P. FERNANDES

February 2020 • Volume 32 • Number 1

ELSEVIER

1600 John F. Kennedy Boulevard • Suite 1800 • Philadelphia, Pennsylvania, 19103-2899

http://www.oralmaxsurgery.theclinics.com

ORAL AND MAXILLOFACIAL SURGERY CLINICS OF NORTH AMERICA Volume 32, Number 1 February 2020 ISSN 1042-3699, ISBN-13: 978-0-323-75426-2

Editor: John Vassallo; j.vassallo@elsevier.com
Developmental Editor: Laura Fisher

Oral and Maxillofacial Surgery Clinics of North America (ISSN 1042-3699) is published quarterly by Elsevier Inc., 360 Park Avenue South, New York, NY 10010-1710. Months of issue are February, May, August, and November. Business and Editorial Offices: 1600 John F. Kennedy Blvd., Suite 1800, Philadelphia, PA 19103-2899. Periodicals postage paid at New York, NY and additional mailing offices. Subscription prices are $401.00 per year for US individuals, $756.00 per year for US institutions, $100.00 per year for US students/residents, $474.00 per year for Canadian individuals, $906.00 per year for Canadian institutions, $100.00 per year for Canadian students/residents, $525.00 per year for international individuals, $906.00 per year for international institutions and $235.00 per year for international students/residents. To receive student/resident rate, orders must be accompanied by name or affiliated institution, date of term, and the *signature* of program/residency coordinator on institution letterhead. Orders will be billed at individual rate until proof of status is received. Foreign air speed delivery is included in all *Clinics* subscription prices. All prices are subject to change without notice. **POSTMASTER:** Send address changes to *Oral and Maxillofacial Surgery Clinics of North America,* Elsevier Periodicals **Customer Service, 11830 Westline Industrial Drive, St. Louis, MO 63146. Tel: 1-800-654-2452 (U.S. and Canada); 314-447-8871 (outside U.S. and Canada). Fax: 314-447-8029. E-mail: journalscustomerservice-usa@elsevier.com (for print support); journalsonlinesupport-usa@elsevier.com (for online support).**

Reprints. For copies of 100 or more, of articles in this publication, please contact the Commercial Reprints Department, Elsevier Inc., 360 Park Avenue South, New York, NY 10010-1710. Tel.: 212-633-3874; Fax: 212-633-3820; Email: reprints@elsevier.com.

Oral and Maxillofacial Surgery Clinics of North America is covered in *MEDLINE/PubMed* (*Index Medicus*), *Science Citation Index Expanded (SciSearch®)*, *Journal Citation Reports/Science Edition*, and *Current Contents®/Clinical Medicine*.

Contributors

CONSULTING EDITOR

RUI P. FERNANDES, MD, DMD, FACS, FRCS(Ed)
Clinical Professor and Chief, Division of Head and Neck Surgery, Departments of Oral and Maxillofacial Surgery, Neurosurgery, and Orthopaedic Surgery and Rehabilitation, University of Florida Health Science Center, University of Florida College of Medicine, Jacksonville, Florida, USA

EDITORS

MICHAEL R. MARKIEWICZ, DDS, MPH, MD, FACS
Professor and Chair, Department of Oral and Maxillofacial Surgery, William M. Feagans Endowed Chair, Associate Dean for Hospital Affairs, School of Dental Medicine, Clinical Professor, Department of Neurosurgery, Division of Pediatric Surgery, Department of Surgery, Jacobs School of Medicine and Biomedical Sciences, University at Buffalo, Co-Director, Craniofacial Center of Western New York, John R. Oishei Children's Hospital, Buffalo, New York, USA

VEERASATHPURUSH ALLAREDDY, BDS, PhD
Brodie Craniofacial Endowed Chair, Professor and Head, Department of Orthodontics, College of Dentistry, The University of Illinois at Chicago, Chicago, Illinois, USA

MICHAEL MILORO, DMD, MD, FACS
Professor and Head, Department of Oral and Maxillofacial Surgery, College of Dentistry, The University of Illinois at Chicago, Chicago, Illinois, USA

AUTHORS

SHELLY ABRAMOWICZ, DMD, MPH, FACS
Associate Professor, Oral and Maxillofacial Surgery and Pediatrics, Department of Surgery, Division of Oral and Maxillofacial Surgery, Emory University School of Medicine, Associate Chief of Oral and Maxillofacial Surgery, Children's Healthcare of Atlanta, Emory University, Atlanta, Georgia, USA

VEERASATHPURUSH ALLAREDDY, BDS, PhD
Brodie Craniofacial Endowed Chair, Professor and Head, Department of Orthodontics, College of Dentistry, The University of Illinois at Chicago, Chicago, Illinois, USA

SHARON ARONOVICH, DMD, FRCD(C)
Department of Oral and Maxillofacial Surgery, University of Michigan, Ann Arbor, Michigan, USA

JENNIFER CAPLIN, DMD, MS
Associate Director, Post-Graduate Orthodontics, Assistant Professor, Department of Orthodontics, College of Dentistry, The University of Illinois at Chicago, Chicago, Illinois, USA

RICHARD SCOTT CONLEY, DMD
Private Practice of Orthodontics, Washington, Pennsylvania, USA

MOHAMMED H. ELNAGAR, DDS, MS, PhD
Department of Orthodontics, College of Dentistry, The University of Illinois at Chicago, Chicago, Illinois, USA

BRIAN FARRELL, DDS, MD, FACS
Private Practitioner, Carolina Center for Oral and Facial Surgery, Charlotte, North Carolina, USA; Clinical Assistant Professor, Department of Oral and Maxillofacial Surgery, Louisiana State University, School of Dentistry, New Orleans, Louisiana, USA

MICHAEL D. HAN, DDS
Assistant Professor, Department of Oral and Maxillofacial Surgery, The University of Illinois at Chicago, Chicago, Illinois, USA

CHESTER S. HANDELMAN, DMD
Clinical Professor, Department of Orthodontics, College of Dentistry, The University of Illinois at Chicago, Chicago, Illinois, USA

JASON P. JONES, DDS, MD
Department of Oral and Maxillofacial Surgery, UT Health San Antonio, San Antonio, Texas, USA

LEONARD B. KABAN, DMD, MD
Walter C. Guralnick Distinguished Professor of Oral and Maxillofacial Surgery, Chief Emeritus, Department of Oral and Maxillofacial Surgery, Massachusetts General Hospital, Harvard School of Dental Medicine, Boston, Massachusetts, USA

KATHERINE P. KLEIN, DMD, MS
Director, Orthodontics and Dentofacial Orthopedics, Massachusetts General Hospital, Instructor in Oral and Maxillofacial Surgery, Harvard School of Dental Medicine, Boston, Massachusetts, USA

BUDI KUSNOTO, DDS, MS
Department of Orthodontics, College of Dentistry, The University of Illinois at Chicago, Chicago, Illinois, USA

MICHAEL R. MARKIEWICZ, DDS, MPH, MD, FACS
Professor and Chair, Department of Oral and Maxillofacial Surgery, William M. Feagans Endowed Chair, Associate Dean for Hospital Affairs, School of Dental Medicine, Clinical Professor, Department of Neurosurgery, Division of Pediatric Surgery, Department of Surgery, Jacobs School of Medicine and Biomedical Sciences, University at Buffalo, Co-Director, Craniofacial Center of Western New York, John R. Oishei Children's Hospital, Buffalo, New York, USA

MOHAMED I. MASOUD, BDS, DMSc
Director, Advanced Graduate Orthodontics, Assistant Professor of Developmental Biology, Harvard School of Dental Medicine, Boston, Massachusetts, USA

DANIEL J. MEARA, MS, MD, DMD, MHCDS, FACS
Chair, Department of Oral and Maxillofacial Surgery and Hospital Dentistry, Christiana Care Health System, Wilmington, Delaware, USA; Affiliate Faculty, Department of Physical Therapy, University of Delaware, Newark, Delaware, USA

LOUIS G. MERCURI, DDS, MS
Visiting Professor, Department of Orthopaedic Surgery, Rush University Medical Center, Chicago, Illinois, USA; Clinical Consultant, TMJ Concepts, Ventura, California, USA

MICHAEL MILORO, DMD, MD, FACS
Professor and Head, Department of Oral and Maxillofacial Surgery, College of Dentistry, The University of Illinois at Chicago, Chicago, Illinois, USA

SVEN ERIK NØRHOLT, DDS, PhD
Department of Oral and Maxillofacial Surgery, Aarhus University Hospital, Clinical Professor, Section of Oral Maxillofacial Surgery, Aarhus University, Aarhus, Denmark

PETRA OLIVIERI, MD, DMD
Resident, Department of Oral and Maxillofacial Surgery, Case Western Reserve University, Cleveland, Ohio, USA

THOMAS KLIT PEDERSEN, DDS, PhD
Clinical Professor, Section of Orthodontics, Aarhus University, Department of Oral and Maxillofacial Surgery, Aarhus University Hospital, Aarhus, Denmark

DANIEL E. PEREZ, DDS
Department of Oral and Maxillofacial Surgery, UT Health San Antonio, San Antonio, Texas, USA

FAISAL A. QUERESHY, MD, DDS, FACS
Professor, Department of Oral and Maxillofacial Surgery, Director, Residency Program, Department of Oral and Maxillofacial Surgery, Case Western Reserve University, University Hospitals Cleveland Medical Center, Cleveland, Ohio, USA

CORY M. RESNICK, DMD, MD, FACS
Assistant Professor, Department of Plastic and Oral Surgery, Boston Children's Hospital, Oral and Maxillofacial Surgery, Harvard School of Dental Medicine, Harvard Medical School, Boston, Massachusetts, USA

JOHAN P. REYNEKE, MChD, FCOMFS (SA), PhD
Private Practice, Director of the Center for Orthognathic Surgery, Mediclinic; Extraordinary Professor, Department of Oral and Maxillofacial Surgery, Faculty of Health Sciences, University of the Western Cape, Cape Town, South Africa; Clinical Professor, Department of Oral and Maxillofacial Surgery, University of Oklahoma, Oklahoma City, Oklahoma, USA; Associate Professor, Department of Oral and Maxillofacial Surgery, VNAI Faculty of Dentistry, Universidad Nacional Autonoma de Mexico, San Salvador, Mexico

PETER STOUSTRUP, DDS, PhD
Associate Professor, Section of Orthodontics, Aarhus University, Aarhus, Denmark

FLAVIO A. URIBE, DDS, MDentSc
Charles Burstone Professor, Program Director and Interim Chair, Associate Professor, Division of Orthodontics, Department of Craniofacial Sciences, University of Connecticut, UConn Health, Farmington, Connecticut, USA

LARRY M. WOLFORD, DMD
Clinical Professor, Departments of Oral and Maxillofacial Surgery and Orthodontics, Texas A&M University College of Dentistry, Baylor University Medical Center – Private Practice, Dallas, Texas, USA

SUMIT YADAV, MDS, PhD
Associate Professor, Department of Craniofacial Sciences, University of Connecticut School of Dental Medicine, Farmington, Connecticut, USA

Contents

Preface: Orthodontics for the Oral and Maxillofacial Surgery Patient **xiii**

Michael R. Markiewicz, Veerasathpurush Allareddy, and Michael Miloro

Digital Workflow for Combined Orthodontics and Orthognathic Surgery **1**

Mohammed H. Elnagar, Sharon Aronovich, and Budi Kusnoto

This article provides an overview of the digital workflow process for Combined orthodontics and Orthognathic surgery treatment starting from data acquisition (3-dimensional scanning, cone-beam computed tomography), data preparation, processing and Creation of a three-dimensional virtual augmented model of the head. Establishing a Proper Diagnosis and Quantification of the Dentofacial Deformity using 3D diagnostic model. Furthermore, performance of 3-dimensional Virtual orthognathic surgical treatment, and the construction of a surgical splint (via 3-dimensional printing) to allow transfer of the treatment plan to the actual patient during surgery.

Orthodontic and Surgical Considerations for Treating Impacted Teeth **15**

Veerasathpurush Allareddy, Jennifer Caplin, Michael R. Markiewicz, and Daniel J. Meara

Impacted teeth occur in a significant number of patients. Their management requires coordinated efforts of orthodontists and oral and maxillofacial surgeons. Specifically, optimal results require a prompt orthodontic diagnosis and treatment plan with execution of either closed or open exposure of impacted teeth by the oral and maxillofacial surgeon. Failure to consider orthodontic mechanics and proper surgical technique can lead to suboptimal results. Thus, orthodontist/oral and maxillofacial surgeon communication is essential for success and patient education and shared decision-making is mandatory before initiating treatment.

Temporary Skeletal Anchorage Techniques **27**

Jason P. Jones, Mohammed H. Elnagar, and Daniel E. Perez

As orthodontic treatment has advanced in complexity and in frequency, more recent techniques, using temporary skeletal anchorage, were developed to help correct more severe occlusal and dentofacial discrepancies that were treated with orthognathic surgery alone previously. These techniques have allowed the orthodontist to move teeth against a rigid fixation, allowing for more focused movements of teeth and for orthopedic growth modification. These types of treatments using rigid fixation have allowed for greater interaction between the orthodontist and the oral and maxillofacial surgeon, and have vastly enhanced the treatment planning for the orthodontist in today's society.

Interceptive Dentofacial Orthopedics (Growth Modification) **39**

Jennifer Caplin, Michael D. Han, Michael Miloro, Veerasathpurush Allareddy, and Michael R. Markiewicz

Although all dentofacial deformities involve deviation of skeletal and dental units that require correction, the timing and method of treatment can vary considerably.

Growth is a key consideration when managing dentofacial deformities, because it has a direct impact on the timing and method of management. Some deformities may be intercepted and managed during growth, whereas others can only be definitively managed after cessation of growth. This article focuses on clinical considerations of growth in managing dentofacial deformities, and discusses methods of growth evaluation and interceptive orthodontic management strategies in different types of dentofacial deformities.

Surgical/Orthodontic Correction of Transverse Maxillary Discrepancies **53**

Johan P. Reyneke and Richard Scott Conley

The transverse dimension is a critical component of comprehensive treatment in orthognathic surgery. Several treatment approaches exist and the team must consider the patient's needs, desires, and limitations when working to correct the malocclusion. Treatment approaches may include only orthodontic expansion or rapid palatal orthodontic expansion; however, in adults, the orthodontist may require surgical assistance to expand the bony maxilla. Segmental maxillary expansion may be indicated in severe transverse deficiencies of the maxillary arch or dentofacial deformity patients also requiring vertical and sagittal corrections. The various treatment options, advantages, and disadvantages, and indications for each surgical approach are discussed.

Orthognathic Surgery and Orthodontics: Inadequate Planning Leading to Complications or Unfavorable Results **71**

Katherine P. Klein, Leonard B. Kaban, and Mohamed I. Masoud

Complications in orthognathic surgery are commonly a result of inadequate preoperative planning and communication between the surgeon and orthodontist. Unfavorable outcomes can often be avoided when overall treatment goals along with a surgical and orthodontic plan are developed and agreed upon by the orthodontist, surgeon, and patient before the start of active tooth movement or any surgical procedures. Continuous evaluation of the patient's progress throughout treatment and subsequent communication between the surgeon and orthodontist are recommended to prevent frequent errors, such as inadequate dental decompensation, poor appliance selection or management, and occasional contraindicated orthodontic elastic traction or tooth movements.

Dentoalveolar Distraction Osteogenesis for Rapid Maxillary Canine Retraction: An Overview of Technique, Treatment, and Outcomes **83**

Sumit Yadav, Michael R. Markiewicz, and Veerasathpurush Allareddy

Patients and orthodontists seek to reduce treatment time in braces. Rapid canine retraction through dentoalveolar distraction osteogenesis is one of several treatment approaches to reduce treatment in braces. This article provides an overview of technique of dentoalveolar distraction osteogenesis to accomplish rapid canine retraction and associated outcomes. When this treatment protocol is implemented well, rapid canine retraction is achieved predictably with minimal side effects. Although current evidence suggests that adverse sequelae, such as root resorptions and pulp devitalization, are rare, prospective clinical studies that are adequately powered and documenting long-term follow-up of these outcomes are lacking.

Surgery-First Approach in the Orthognathic Patient 89

Flavio A. Uribe and Brian Farrell

The surgery-first approach (SFA) has become a recent alternative to the conventional 3-stage approach to orthognathic surgery. Skeletal anchorage in orthodontics has facilitated the resurgence of this treatment sequence. By eliminating the presurgical phase of orthodontic treatment, patients have immediate resolution to their facial deformity. Treatment duration has been shown to be reduced; the difference with the conventional approach being approximately 5 months. Patient satisfaction with this approach is very high as measured by quality-of-life surveys. This article describes the indications and step-by-step approach of this technique in conjunction with virtual surgical planning.

Idiopathic Condylar Resorption: What Should We Do? 105

Louis G. Mercuri and Chester S. Handelman

Idiopathic condylar resorption (ICR), alternatively called progressive condylar resorption, is an uncommon aggressive form of degenerative disease of the temporomandibular joint seen mostly in adolescent and young women. ICR occurring before the completion of growth results in a shorter mandibular condyloid process, ramus and body, compensatory growth at the gonial angle and coronoid process, as well as an increase in anterior facial vertical dimension. Management options discussed include oral appliances, orthodontics, medical management, orthognathic surgery with and without disc repositioning, and alloplastic temporomandibular joint replacement.

Interdisciplinary Management of Dentofacial Deformity in Juvenile Idiopathic Arthritis 117

Peter Stoustrup, Thomas Klit Pedersen, Sven Erik Nørholt, Cory M. Resnick, and Shelly Abramowicz

Temporomandibular joint (TMJ) arthritis impacts mandibular growth and development. This can result in skeletal deformity, such as facial asymmetry and/or malocclusion asymmetry. This article reviews the unique properties of TMJ and dentofacial growth and development in the setting of juvenile idiopathic arthritis (JIA). Specific orthopedic/orthodontic and surgical management of children with JIA and TMJ arthritis is discussed. The importance of interdisciplinary collaboration is highlighted.

Comprehensive Post Orthognathic Surgery Orthodontics: Complications, Misconceptions, and Management 135

Larry M. Wolford

Post orthognathic surgery patient management is critical for high-quality and predictable outcomes. Surgeons and orthodontists must have the knowledge and ability to implement postsurgical management protocols and strategies to provide the best care and outcomes possible. This article presents basic concepts, philosophies, treatment protocols, risks, and potential complications associated with postsurgical patient management. Postsurgical orthodontic goals are to maximize the occlusal fit and provide predictable means to retain the occlusion. Aggressive orthodontic mechanics may be required to provide the best occlusal fit. Complications can occur, but early recognition of complications and implementation of corrective tactics should minimize adverse outcomes.

Aesthetic Facial Surgery and Orthodontics: Common Goals **153**

Petra Olivieri, Flavio A. Uribe, and Faisal A. Quereshy

Many of the aesthetic facial procedures can be performed simultaneously at the time of initial orthognathic surgery. Correction of any residual deformities after surgery, such as mandibular notching, malar asymmetry, labiomental crease, and any camouflage treatment, should be performed as a delayed procedure, when the outcome is more predictable. Additionally, these procedures could be used to enhance the orthodontic result, without the need of osteotomies to reposition the bones.

ORAL AND MAXILLOFACIAL SURGERY CLINICS OF NORTH AMERICA

FORTHCOMING ISSUES

May 2020
Orthodontics for the Craniofacial Surgery Patient
Michael R. Markiewicz, Veerasathpurush Allareddy, and Michael Miloro, *Editors*

August 2020
Global Oral and Maxillofacial Surgery
Shahid Aziz, Steven Roser, and Jose M. Marchena, *Editors*

November 2020
Dentoalveolar Surgery
Somsak Sittitavornwong, *Editor*

RECENT ISSUES

November 2019
Advances in Oral and Maxillofacial Surgery
Jose M. Marchena, Jonathan W. Shum, and Jonathon S. Jundt, *Editors*

August 2019
Dental Implants, Part II: Computer Technology
Ole T. Jensen, *Editor*

May 2019
Dental Implants, Part I: Reconstruction
Ole T. Jensen, *Editor*

Preface

Orthodontics for the Oral and Maxillofacial Surgery Patient

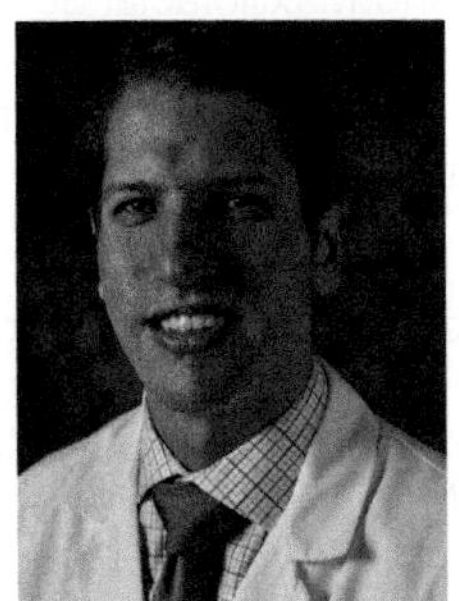

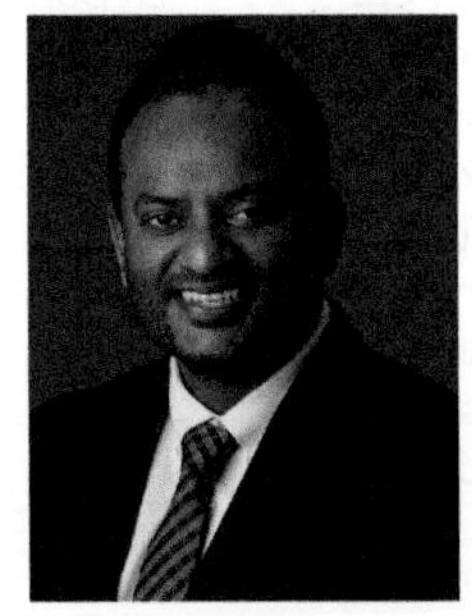

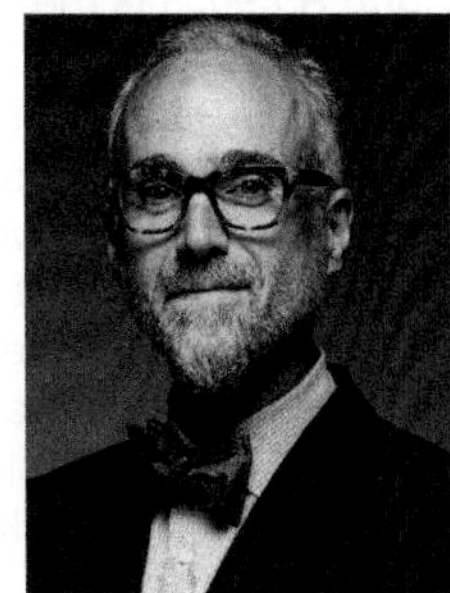

Michael R. Markiewicz, DDS, MPH, MD, FACS

Veerasathpurush Allareddy, BDS, PhD

Michael Miloro, DMD, MD, FACS

Editors

The specialties of Oral and Maxillofacial Surgery and Orthodontics are intimately related. In fact, it can be stated that, in many cases, "an Oral and Maxillofacial Surgeon (OMFS) is only as good as their Orthodontist." This relationship and collaboration between these 2 specialties are critical to the success of the orthodontist and surgeon, and, in turn, the success of their patient. This could not be more evident than in the field of orthognathic surgery, where the outcomes, and, in actuality, the frank ability of the surgeon to perform the procedure are dictated by the level of appropriate orthodontic preparation of that patient, based upon an the initial, and evolving, treatment plan determined by the surgeon, orthodontist, and patient.

However, the basic principles and clinical relevance of orthodontics to orthognathic surgery are often overlooked in an Oral and Maxillofacial Surgery residency training program. The rationale, planning, and execution of the orthodontic component of a combined orthodontic-oral and maxillofacial treatment are often lacking in the education of an OMFS surgeon and is often secondary to the attainment of surgical knowledge. The lack of appreciation for this crucial collaboration between specialties would be similar for dental implant surgery in which the OMFS trainee who does not understand or appreciate the prosthodontic components of those combined treatment approaches. Therefore, the development of this critical relationship may be delayed or inhibited from the outset and difficult to incorporate into the treatment paradigm at a later time. This relationship and knowledge of each other's specialties capabilities and limitations are essential, not only for orthognathic surgery and management of dentofacial deformities but also, for example, in the case of management of impacted teeth, the use of techniques for skeletal anchorage, the diagnosis and relevance of obstructive sleep apnea, and the need for adjunctive procedures, such as aesthetic facial surgery. In addition, a knowledge of dentofacial orthopedics and other common orthodontic maneuvers and techniques will allow the OMFS surgeon to

Oral Maxillofacial Surg Clin N Am 32 (2020) xiii–xiv
https://doi.org/10.1016/j.coms.2019.10.001
1042-3699/20/© 2019 Published by Elsevier Inc.

make more informed and appropriate decisions in the management of the "growing" patient. Therefore, we set out to produce a clinical reference for orthodontists and OMFSs in training and in clinical practice.

This issue of the *Oral and Maxillofacial Surgery Clinics of North America* is the first of a 2-part series. The second issue, "Orthodontics for the Craniofacial Surgery Patient," is intended to build upon the foundational framework of the information presented in this issue, however, with a further application of these principles to a more complex patient population—those patients with craniofacial anomalies, facial clefts, craniofacial dysostoses, and other congenital and acquired anomalies of the head and neck.

To accomplish our goal of providing current collaborative practice guidelines and engaging those individuals who we deemed to be authorities on the orthodontic and surgical aspects of the proposed topics, we utilized a unique approach in author recruitment. We solicited both an orthodontist and an OMFS, deemed to be an expert in each of their respective fields, to coauthor each article in a collaborative fashion. These individuals were chosen without concern of their institutional origin to avoid potential single-institutional bias in practice philosophies. This was an incredibly challenging endeavor since most clinicians are most experienced in publishing their literature with the team with whom they practice. Despite the potential risks of not identifying compatible authors, all of the authors graciously and enthusiastically accepted the invitation to be part of this project and looked forward to establishing a new relationship, and working with, another author with whom they may or may not have had the chance to interact with in the past. We believe that this unique approach to authorship for this issue highlights the importance of the collaboration between the orthodontist and OMFS and led to the production of this unique text produced herein. We thank all of those who have contributed as they are the value of this unique text.

Michael R. Markiewicz, DDS, MPH, MD, FACS
Department of Oral and Maxillofacial Surgery
School of Dental Medicine
University at Buffalo
3435 Main Street, 112 Squire Hall
Buffalo, NY 14214, USA

Department of Neurosurgery
Division of Pediatric Surgery
Department of Surgery
Jacobs School of Medicine and Biomedical Sciences

Craniofacial Center of Western New York
John R. Oishei Children's Hospital
Buffalo, NY, USA

Veerasathpurush Allareddy, BDS, PhD
Department of Orthodontics
College of Dentistry
University of Illinois at Chicago
801 South Paulina Street
138AD (MC841)
Chicago, IL 60612-7211, USA

Michael Miloro, DMD, MD, FACS
Department of Oral and Maxillofacial Surgery
College of Dentistry
University of Illinois at Chicago
801 South Paulina Street
M/C 835
Chicago, IL 60612-7211, USA

E-mail addresses:
mrm25@buffalo.edu (M.R. Markiewicz)
sath@uic.edu (V. Allareddy)
mmiloro@uic.edu (M. Miloro)

Digital Workflow for Combined Orthodontics and Orthognathic Surgery

Mohammed H. Elnagar, DDS, MS, PhD[a,*], Sharon Aronovich, DMD, FRCD(C)[b], Budi Kusnoto, DDS, MS[a]

KEYWORDS

- Computer-aided surgery • 3D orthognathic surgery simulation • Virtual model surgery
- Digital workflow

KEY POINTS

- 3D Data Acquisition and Processing for diagnostic and quantification of the dentofacial deformities.
- Developing 3D Virtual treatment planning and orthognathic surgery.
- Transfer the 3D Virtual treatment plan to Operating room.
- Future of Computer-assisted surgical planning.
- Teledentistry - Remote Monitoring and Follow up.

INTRODUCTION

Dentofacial deformities affect quality of life, self-image, social behavior, and public perception, leading to a perception that the individual is less attractive, less successful, and less socially acceptable based on societal norms. The treatment approach using combined orthodontics and orthognathic surgery is considered to be a very powerful tool to correct functional abnormalities, but also to alter soft tissues and facial form in order to improve overall facial esthetics.[1,2]

The establishment of a correct diagnosis and treatment plan is one of the most critical parts in the management of the orthognathic surgical patient. Computer technology has certainly enhanced the ability of the clinician to deliver a more precise treatment outcome, reduce risk, and achieve better outcomes.

Many software packages for computer-assisted surgery (CAS) are available, and some of them allow in-house CAS to be performed from the database (cone-beam computed tomography [CBCT], intraoral scans) and then transferred to the operating room with the generation of a surgical splint (eg, Dolphin 3D; Dolphin Imaging 11.9 Premium, Chatsworth, CA, USA). Furthermore, there are several commercially available systems, including Medical Modeling (3D Systems Healthcare, Littleton, CO, USA) and Maxilim (Medicim, Mechelen, Belgium) that can help to facilitate the process of virtual surgical planning (VSP). For a service fee, the commercial companies construct surface models from CBCT images and digital dental casts registered to the CBCT, perform the virtual surgery via Webinars with the surgeon and orthodontist, on occasion, and print the actual surgical splints. The various components of the digital workflow process are covered in this article.

Data Acquisition

In order to build an accurate model that can represent a realistic digital simulation, it must begin with proper data acquisition. Each of the end users, including the clinicians and

Disclosure Statement: The authors have nothing to disclose.

[a] Department of Orthodontics, College of Dentistry, University of Illinois at Chicago, 801 South Paulina Street, Room 131, Chicago, IL 60612-7211, USA; [b] Department of Oral and Maxillofacial Surgery, University of Michigan, 1500 E Medical Center Dr, Ann Arbor, MI 48109, USA
* Corresponding author.
E-mail address: melnagar@uic.edu

Oral Maxillofacial Surg Clin N Am 32 (2020) 1–14
https://doi.org/10.1016/j.coms.2019.08.004

technicians, should have the knowledge of how various methods of data acquisition might influence the outcomes of the treatment simulation. Data acquisition methods can be categorized into several methods, such as (a) surface scans, (b) volumetric scans, and (c) 4-dimensional (4D) video scans/movements. Each method of data acquisition must lead to 1 common goal, that is, to create precise replicas of the patient for the purpose of establishing a comprehensive diagnosis, treatment planning, treatment simulation, and design and delivery of orthodontic and surgical treatment. To be clear, accurate 3D virtual treatment planning for orthodontics and orthognathic surgery requires appropriate and accurate image acquisition to establish the proper database.

Image acquisition of the maxillofacial region (cone-beam computed tomography)

CBCT has become an increasingly important tool in treatment planning and diagnosis in implant dentistry, endodontics, orthodontics, and other dental and medical specialties. The benefits of CBCT in orthodontics include increased accuracy of image geometry and improved ability to record accurate measurements by eliminating image magnification, anatomic structure overlap, and image distortion commonly encountered with 2-dimensional (2D) radiographs (traditional cephalometry).[3] One of the concerns with the routine use of CBCT is the effects of increased exposure to ionizing radiation. The medical imaging industry has improved upon this technology over the past 2 decades of its increasingly widespread use in dentistry. With technologic advances, such as the use of flat panel detectors, the availability of different/limited fields of view, and the advances in computer science, improvements have been made toward the reduction of unnecessary radiation exposure by CBCT technology.[3,4]

For proper image acquisition of the maxillofacial region, the jaw relationship should be scanned with the mandible in "centric relation (CR)," and, ideally, in a "natural head position (NHP)." For a proper combined orthodontic and orthognathic surgery virtual planning, the patient's lips should be relaxed in repose with the teeth in a normal occlusal relationship (CR). With the advent of CBCT imaging, this has become feasible and reproducible. To ensure that the CBCT is acquired with the mandible in CR, the patient should be scanned while occluding into a bite registration material. A large field of view should be considered to include all anatomic structures required to plan the orthognathic surgery.[5,6] CBCT imaging is a 3D volume of Digital Imaging and Communications in Medicine (DICOM) data, consisting of a collection of "cubelike blocks" called "voxels."[7]

The CBCT DICOM data can be "rendered" to generate a 3D virtual image of the patient's head by (1) "surface rendering" or (2) "volume rendering." "Surface rendering" is a reconstruction of 3D structure surfaces by segmentation based on gray scales, and it allows digitization of 3D cephalometric landmarks, planning of 3D virtual osteotomies, definition of the 3D virtual occlusal relationship, maxillary and mandibular bony movements with additional soft tissue simulation, and 3D superimposition of datasets.[8] Moreover, it allows integration of 3D digital dental casts and 3D facial photographs into the CBCT scan.[9,10] "Volume rendering" is a direct reconstruction of 3D structures by rendering a volume of voxels. With regards to each voxel, color and opacity are assigned based on various shading algorithms. Volume rendering allows more detailed anatomy of the teeth and interdental spaces. However, it does not allow user actions and interactions, such as 3D virtual osteotomies, bone fragment movements, or additional soft tissue simulation or 3D integration of datasets. For optimal 3D virtual treatment planning of orthognathic surgery, both "surface rendering" and "volume rendering" are usually used in combination.[11]

Image acquisition of the dentition and occlusion

Images derived from a single CBCT scan cannot provide accurate detailed information regarding the dentition or interocclusal relationships, which are mandatory for proper orthodontic preparation and surgical treatment planning and appropriate generation of surgical splints.[10] Additional image acquisition of the patient's dentition in the form of 3D digital models is required in order to obtain accurate occlusal and intercuspation analysis. In addition, 3D digital models facilitate the measurement of tooth position in 3 dimensions, can be manipulated easily, may be segmentalized to analyze specific teeth, and allow 3D mapping of tooth movements in various treatment plans.[12]

These digital models may be obtained via an indirect method that requires digital scanning of previously obtained plaster casts or via impressions of the dentition. Various extraoral 3D scanners have been designed to capture 3D images for dental impressions or physical casts and then create 3D digital models. The scanning technology uses a nondestructive laser beam and several digital cameras to reproduce high-resolution 3D images of the target surfaces. Dental impressions, models, or bite registrations are positioned inside a chamber platform, which is automatically rotated and inclined during scanning, ensuring complete multiple angle coverage of the model's geometry. The laser light is projected onto the object, and the cameras acquire its mirror image from the surface. Upon completion of scanning, a rendered stereolithographic (STL) model is created.[13,14]

A direct method to capture the dentition could be obtained by using intraoral scanning systems to acquire digital intraoral impressions for the entire dental arch and can be used to replace orthodontic impression acquisition. The STL files of the scanners can be used to produce digital dental models.[15] Because intraoral scanning is a direct procedure, it may be more accurate than the indirect method, and inaccurate scanning could be corrected by rescanning a specific part of the scan. Intraoral scanners generate STL files as well as Polygon File Format (PLY) and OBJ format files, which contain all of the color information. The scanning process includes scanning each arch separately and then scanning the occlusion.[16] Accurate bite registration information should be established, and multiple bite registrations might be needed in cases involving a functional shift or dual bite situations with occlusal interferences.

Image acquisition of the texture of the face (facial three-dimensional scanning)

Facial 3D scanning uses the CBCT 3D facial soft tissue mask of the patient to assess the head texture and color. With the introduction of 3D photographs, a 3D camera is used to capture the soft tissue surfaces of the face with correct geometry and texture information, performed with nonionizing image acquisition.[13] It based on stereophotogrammetry, which is a method of obtaining an image by means of 1 or more stereo pairs of photographs being acquired simultaneously. The technique is based on the triangulation and fringe projection method. Image fusion (ie, registration of a 3D photograph on a CBCT) results in an accurate and photorealistic digital 3D data set of a patient's face.[2,17,18] Augmenting 3D facial soft tissue texture provides improved patient assessment and communication and the production of an individualized 3D virtual treatment plan.

Video/functional/dynamic database acquisition

The human face is highly dynamic and deformable and, recently, dynamic 4D image acquisition of the texture of the face has been introduced (eg, Temporal-3dMD Systems (4D), 3dMD, Atlanta, GA, USA).[19] The technology is very promising but still time consuming to implement in the clinical daily routine, and therefore, it has been used mainly for research purposes. Functional records (ie, jaw range of motion, jaw path of opening-closing, smile animation, speech, muscle tonicity, and soft tissue evaluation) should be documented well and synchronized to the rest of the database in order to establish a set of comprehensive visual treatment objectives.

Processing of Acquired Image Data/Records Synchronization

The accuracy of the computer simulation is very much influenced by the manner in which the records are obtained, standardized, and augmented. Clinicians often obtain records from different methods and sources to establish treatment objectives and comprehensive management of patients. Usually, clinicians assess each of these records individually. Unsynchronized records can also lead to a less than ideal treatment sequence and thus might produce compromised patient assessment and treatment outcomes.[20]

Creation of a three-dimensional virtual augmented model of the head

To create a "3D virtual augmented/composite model" of the patient's head, "rigid registration" is necessary. Many types of "rigid registration" exist, including point-based, surface-based, and voxel-based rigid registration.[21]

To integrate accurate occlusal and intercuspation data into the 3D patient model, "rigid registration," with or without markers, based on points, surfaces, voxels, or a combination, currently still must be performed.

The first step in the registration process locates/segments the major areas of the jaws that will be involved in the surgery using the patient's created surface representations of these areas; then, clean up the surface representations of the maxilla and mandible is usually needed to remove any extraneous information. If the patient had orthodontic braces when the scan was created, it is recommended to sculpt them out of the surface images (**Fig. 1**).

Integration of digital dental casts in cone beam computed tomography scans to augment the patient's dentition and occlusion By using a surface matching method, the digital dental models can be integrated into the CBCT scan (**Fig. 2**), especially by using small voxel size, and specific segmentation threshold selection. However, when the patient has orthodontic appliances, surface matching of a digital dental cast onto the dentition in the CBCT scan is difficult.[10] Using intraoral reference devices or bite jigs to locate fiducial markers outside the occlusal area improves the integration of digital dental casts into CBCT scans; however, this process can be time consuming.[22,23]

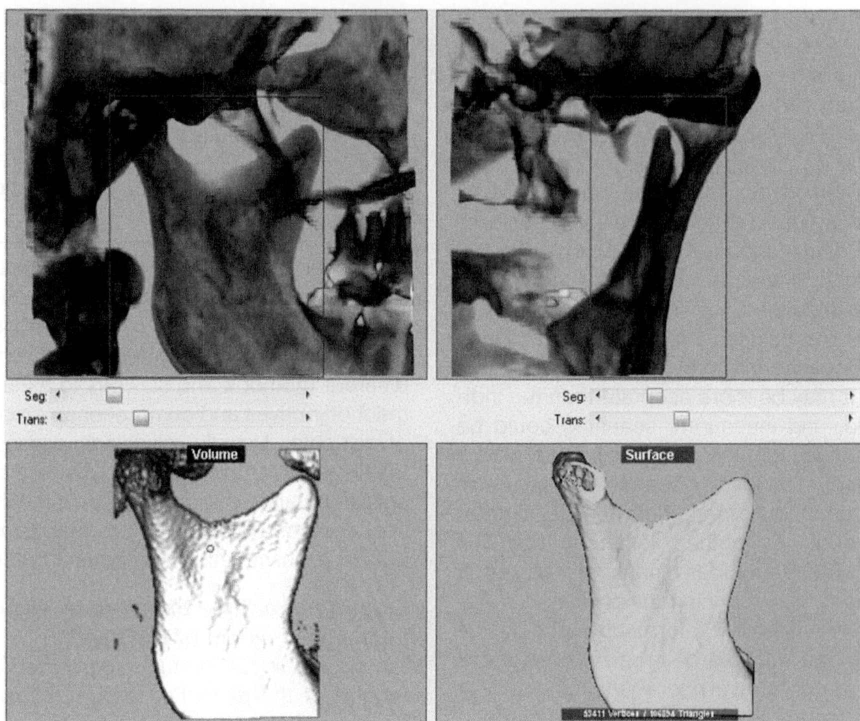

Fig. 1. Segmentation of the major areas that will be involved in the surgery. (*Courtesy of* Dolphin Imaging 11.9 Premium, Chatsworth, CA.)

Swennen and colleagues[24] used a triple scan method to integrate a high-resolution 3D image of the dentition into the CBCT scan. Their method is reliable and does not cause any soft tissue deformation. However, a disadvantage is that 2 CBCT scans are required for generation of the integration model. Rangel and colleagues[10] introduced a method whereby titanium markers were glued on to the gingiva, which were then used for the matching procedure.

Integration of three-dimensional photographs (head surface texture) Schendel and Lane[25] used surface-based automatic registration for the integration of 3D facial surface images into the CBCT data. Surface images can correct CBCT surface artifacts caused by several situations. Patient movement is more likely when the patient is upright rather than supine (ie, swallowing, breathing, head movement). The time interval to take the CBCT scans can vary among machines from 5 to 70 seconds, and a longer interval allows more potential for patient movement. CBCT device stabilization aids (eg. chin rest, forehead restraints) can distort the soft tissue surface anatomy recorded in the CBCT image. Also, surface images can supplement any missing anatomic data because a surface scan provides a more accurate representation of the soft tissues drape that reflects the patient's NHP.[9] Any errors in the integration of the 3D soft tissues and skull models could increase the cumulative errors of the prediction planning method and could transfer to errors in orthodontic or surgery planning or treatment.[26] 3D facial scanner technology, combined with a CBCT apparatus, has been introduced to evaluate the registration accuracy of CBCT and 3D facial surface scans that were obtained with the least possible time interval between scans. It has been reported that a CBCT followed immediately with a 3D facial surface scan, and then merged to correct any deficiencies in the facial surface rendering, can provide a superior version of the diagnostic

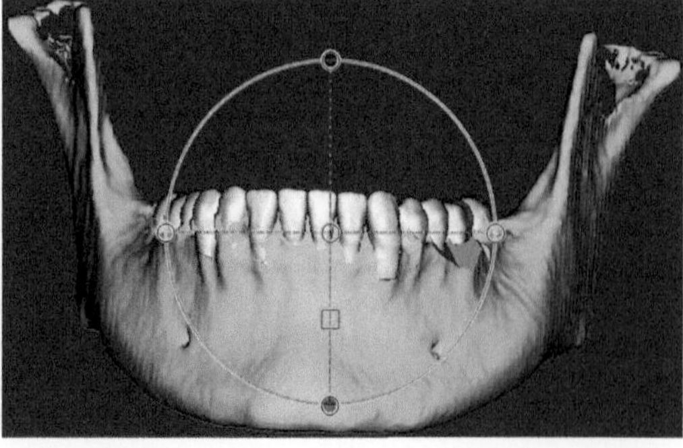

Fig. 2. Digital dental model can be integrated into the CBCT scan. (*Courtesy of* Dolphin Imaging 11.9 Premium, Chatsworth, CA.)

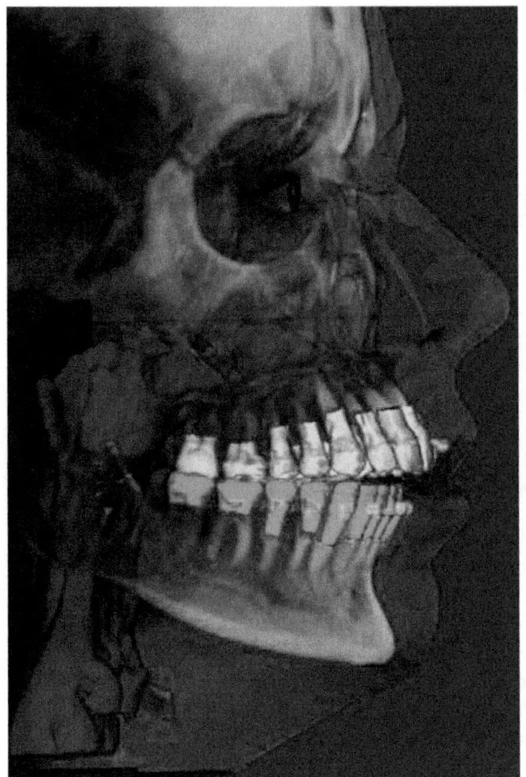

Fig. 3. Composite augmented head. (*Courtesy of* Dolphin Imaging 11.9 Premium, Chatsworth, CA.)

records and could provide better information for complex treatment planning that affects the esthetic facial appearance (**Fig. 3**).[9]

Orientation of three-dimensional virtual augmented/composite model of the patient's head to natural head position

Many patients with craniomaxillofacial deformities have significant skeletal asymmetries. The use of the NHP obviates internal landmarks and provides a reproducible reference framework.

Xia and colleagues[5] developed 2 techniques to orient the composite model to the NHP: the first one uses a 3D-calibrated laser surface scanner, and the second uses a digital orientation sensor. With the laser surface scanner method, the surface geometry of the facial soft tissues is captured while the patient's head is in the NHP, with the patient sitting on a calibrated chair at the center of the scanner. The scanner creates a correctly oriented 3D image of the face. The soft tissues of the composite model are then rendered, and the model is aligned to the NHP by matching its soft tissues to the scanned image. In the digital orientation sensor technique, a digital orientation is attached to the same face-bow. With the patient in the NHP, the pitch, roll, and yaw of the face are recorded, and these are then used to reorient the composite skull model. In the computer, a digital replica (computer-aided design [CAD] model) of the digital orientation sensor is registered to the composite skull model via the fiducial markers, and the 2 objects are merged with each other. Afterward, the recorded pitch, roll, and yaw are applied to the digital oriental sensor replica by reorienting the composite skull model to the NHP.[5]

Establishing a Proper Diagnosis and Quantification of the Deformity

3D inspection of the virtual composite model of the patient's head is a great diagnostic tool for a maxillofacial deformity. Both "volume rendering" and "surface rendering" offer a thorough in-depth 3D virtual inspection. Both viewing methods also incorporate CBCT slices, which allow 2D inspection of the patient's anatomy in the 3 standard planes (axial, sagittal, coronal) and multiplanar planes. A large amount of clinical information can be obtained (eg, condylar anatomy and location, maxillofacial bony and dental pathologic features, maxillary sinus pathologic features, nasal septum deviation, a restricted airway, dentoalveolar bone support to the teeth, and the pathway of the inferior alveolar nerve).[6]

A virtual approach was developed in which virtual lateral and frontal cephalograms were calculated from the CBCT data set of the patient and linked with the hard and soft tissue surface-rendered representations. This approach allowed the authors to bridge conventional cephalometry with 3D cephalometry of the facial soft tissue mask and underlying bone and teeth with a common 3D cephalometric reference frame.[27] Furthermore, a virtual dynamic diagnosis (4 dimensions) of the patient (eg, smile esthetics, habits) has recently been introduced and will likely be integrated into the future.[6] 3D cephalometric analysis is divided into 6 components: symmetry, transverse, vertical, pitch, Anteroposterior, and shape. These sections mimic the ideal order in which a diagnosis should be established and a 3D orthodontic and surgical treatment plan should be developed.

Developing Three-Dimensional Simulation

Osteotomy design

To develop a 3D simulation of surgery, the augmented/composite head model is initially prepared (precut) to simulate various osteotomies. Simulate various osteotomies, such as Le Fort I osteotomy, a sagittal split osteotomy, an intraoral vertical ramus osteotomy, an inverted "L"

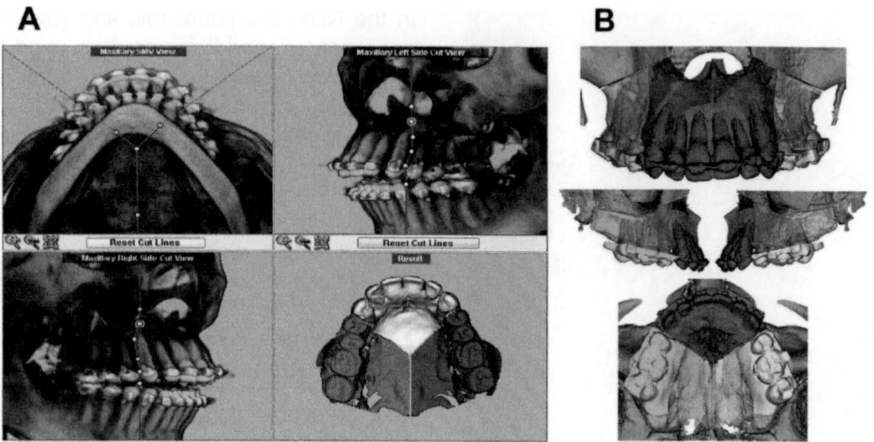

Fig. 4. (*A*) Defining the osteotomies. Three-piece (Le Fort I) surface and volume rendering used. (*B*) The final osteotomies to define the cuts. Three-piece (Le Fort I). (*Courtesy of* Dolphin Imaging 11.9 Premium, Chatsworth, CA.)

osteotomy, and/or a genioplasty. In this step, the clinician specifies the intended location and geometry of all osteotomies to be performed in the maxilla, proximal segments of the mandible, and anterior mandible (**Figs. 4** and **5**). Care should be taken during designing the cuts to avoid any injury to anatomic structures, such as tooth roots and the inferior alveolar canal. A combination between surface rendering and volume rendering should be used at this stage. In this step, the landmarks are digitized on the image so that the imaging software (eg, Dolphin Imaging) can track the movements of the osteotomy segments that will be specified in later steps of the 3D surgery planning process.

Treat and mobilizing bone segments

After the jaws are osteotomized, bony segments could be repositioned and rotated to the desired locations. In bimaxillary surgery, the maxilla is usually repositioned first, and the maxillary asymmetry is quantified by a triangular spline. The software reads the x, y, and z coordinates of the triangle vertices, calculates the discrepancy between the right and left sides, and then automatically

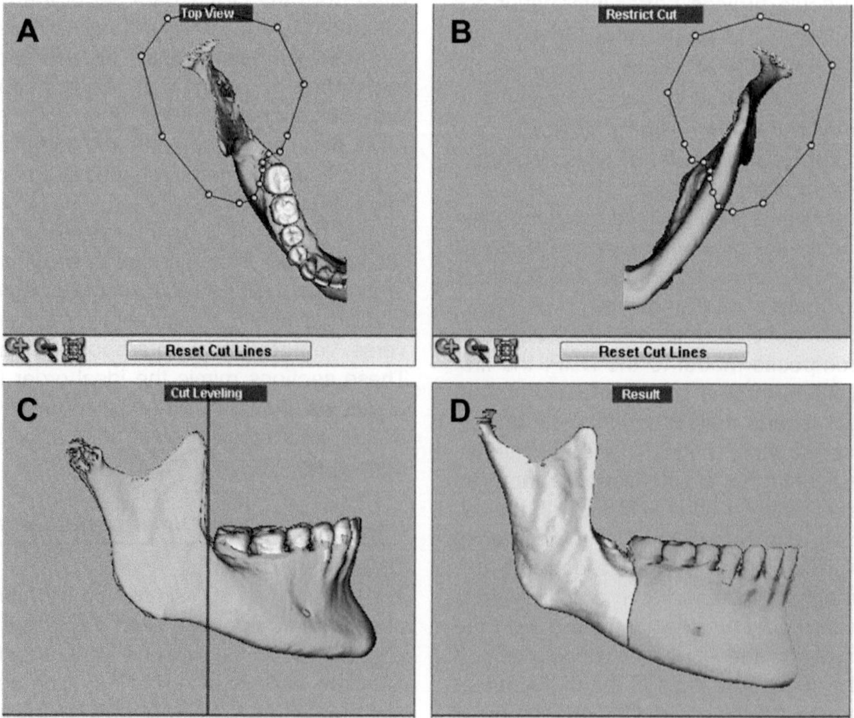

Fig. 5. Sagittal split osteotomy design. (*Courtesy of* Dolphin Imaging 11.9 Premium, Chatsworth, CA.)

moves/rotates the triangle to a position of symmetry (0° of roll and 0° of yaw). Then, the upper dental midline is corrected. After that, the maxillary pitch (occlusal plane inclination) is adjusted to the desired angle. If the dental arch is asymmetric, intervention is required to move/rotate the maxilla to the most balanced position. After the asymmetry of the maxilla has been corrected, the maxilla is moved anteroposteriorly and superoinferiorly to the desired position as determined by the cephalometric analysis and clinical measurements.

After the maxilla has been placed into its final position, the distal segment of the mandible is moved into maximal intercuspation, which may be difficult to establish on a computer. Once the distal segment is in position, the proximal segments of the mandible are aligned. If necessary, a genioplasty is also simulated, with avoidance of any collisions with the mandibular osteotomies or the inferior alveolar canal (**Fig. 6** and **7**).

In patients with facial asymmetries, the bones may not only be asymmetrically displaced but there also may be differences in size and shape from 1 side to the other. Using a mirror-image routine, one-half of the face is selected, copied, flipped (mirror image), and superimposed onto the contralateral side, so a decision can be made to add volume (grafting), remove volume (ostectomy), or adjust the position of the segments (camouflage).

The soft tissue changes associated with movements of bony segments can be simulated using the software algorithm. The latter may add value in the overall treatment plan and provides patients with an idea of the expected esthetic changes. However, currently a true prediction of the soft tissue changes in 3D planning remains challenging.

An alternative way of preparing for and executing a computerized surgical plan can involve the use of a laser level, with the patient in NHP, to guide placement of horizontal and vertical radiographic markers. A CBCT scan is obtained aligning the midsagittal and horizontal laser lines with the radiographic markers on the face, and with the patient in CR. 3D-printed dental models or casts are hand articulated into the desired final occlusion and set in a hinge-axis articulator. A medium-body polyvinyl siloxane material may be used to capture the final occlusal setup. Alternatively, an intraoral scanner may be used to capture the desired final occlusion. For segmental maxillary osteotomies, the maxillary model is segmented and glued into position based on the desired occlusal setup. The segmented CBCT data and dental scan are integrated and oriented in NHP based on the universal X-Y-Z coordinates.

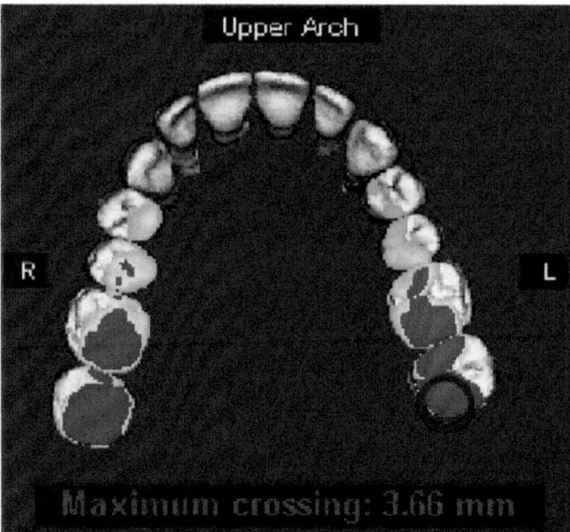

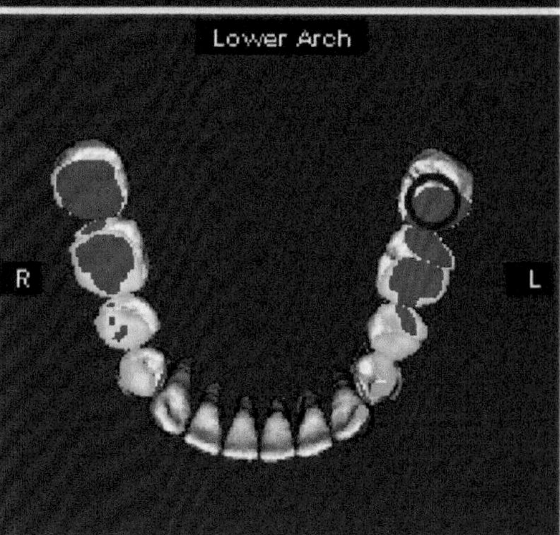

Fig. 6. Heat map showing occlusion collision. (*Courtesy of* Dolphin Imaging 11.9 Premium, Chatsworth, CA.)

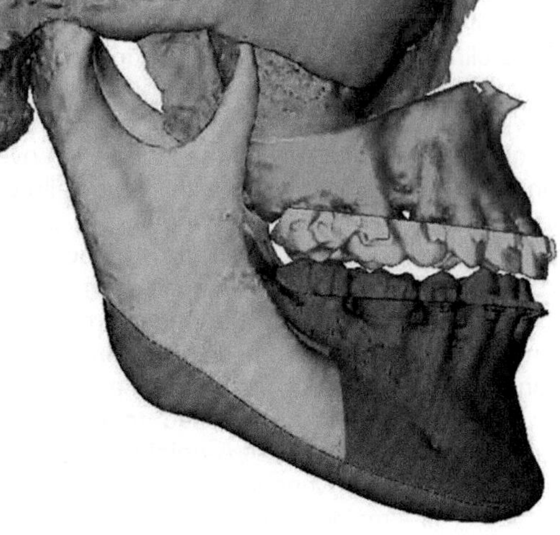

Fig. 7. 3D virtual simulation of surgical treatment. (*Courtesy of* Dolphin Imaging 11.9 Premium, Chatsworth, CA.)

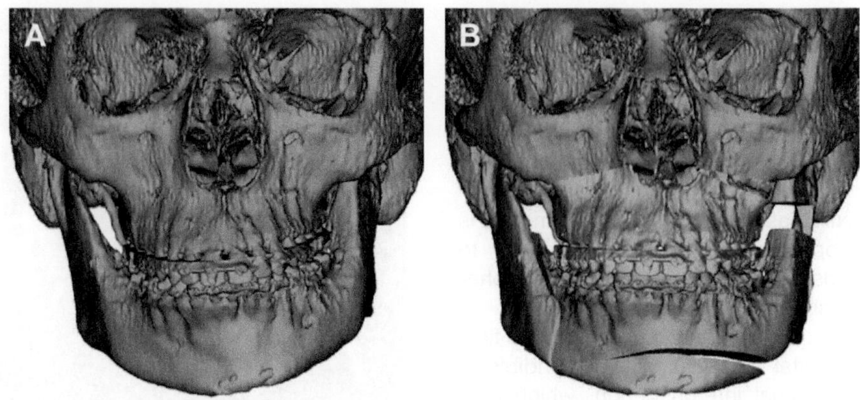

Fig. 8. (*A, B*) A patient with significant maxillary and mandibular canting secondary to left condylar fracture in childhood and shortened left ramus-condyle height. Occlusal and skeletal cant correction achieved with bimaxillary surgery, including sagittal ramus osteotomy on the right and inverted-L osteotomy on the left. An asymmetric genioplasty with interpositional bone graft designed to achieve skeletal symmetry in the lower facial third.

A workflow in the use of computer-assisted surgical simulation The condylar position is assessed in the glenoid fossa to ensure a proper CR. If necessary, the condyle may be seated more posteriorly and superiorly in the fossa before or after movement of the segmented anatomy. The mandible is related to the maxilla in the final occlusion. The maxillary dental midline is adjusted with transverse linear movements to coincide with the facial midline. Maxillary canting at the canine and mesiobuccal (MB) cusp tips of the first molars is assessed relative to the horizontal plane, which may or may not coincide with the infraorbital rims. Correction of the maxillary cant is accomplished with simultaneous attention to mandibular symmetry at the inferior border (**Fig. 8**).

Anterior-posterior and superior-inferior movements of the maxilla are then performed based on the clinical facial examination, taking into account the ideal maxillary incisor position, tooth show (incisor display), and the extent of soft tissue changes desired. Having the mandible move with the maxilla as a complex at this stage allows the surgeon to visualize the changes at B-point, pogonion, and the lower incisor tip. The occlusal and mandibular plane angles can be examined at this point, and changes to the pitch or occlusal plane may be performed based on desired facial changes. For instance, a clockwise rotation of the occlusal plane may be used to decrease chin projection and increase A-point and anterior nasal spine (ANS) advancement in a patient with a class III malocclusion. Occlusal plane rotation may also be considered to optimize the smile line and incisor angulation (**Figs. 9** and **10**).

A submental and bird's-eye view is then used to assess and correct the maxillomandibular yaw by using a midsagittal plane through nasion and foramen magnum. This plane provides a visual comparison of the discrepancy between the right and left maxillary canines and MB cusp of the maxillary first molars. In addition, the width discrepancy between the right and left gonial angles can be measured to the midsagittal plane and to the root of the zygomatic arches (**Figs. 11** and **12**).

The proximal segments of the mandible, as in a bilateral sagittal split osteotomy (BSSO), are

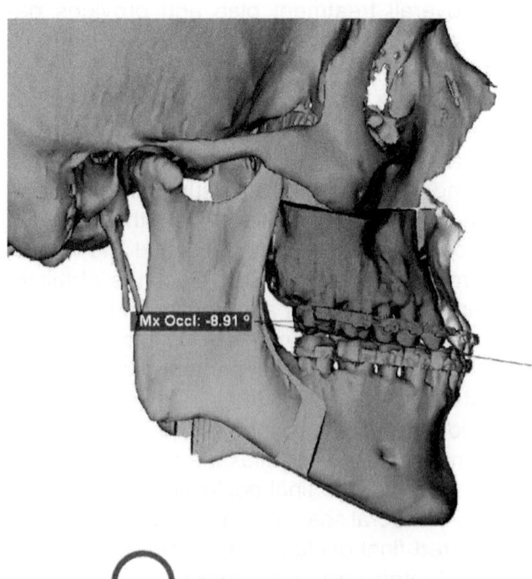

Fig. 9. A counterclockwise occlusal plane rotation in a patient with obstructive sleep apnea to achieve significant B-point advancement.

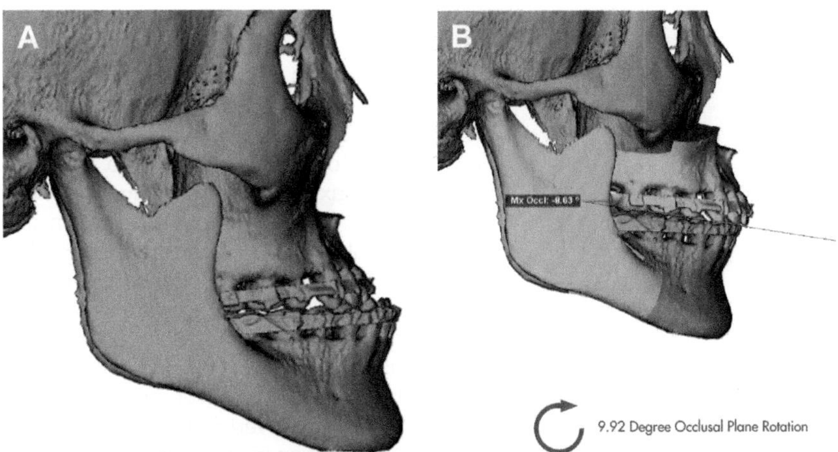

Fig. 10. (*A, B*) Clockwise rotation of the occlusal plane may be used to achieve ideal A- to B-point relationship while reducing chin projection and increasing midface advancement in a patient with a class III malocclusion and reverse occlusal plane angle.

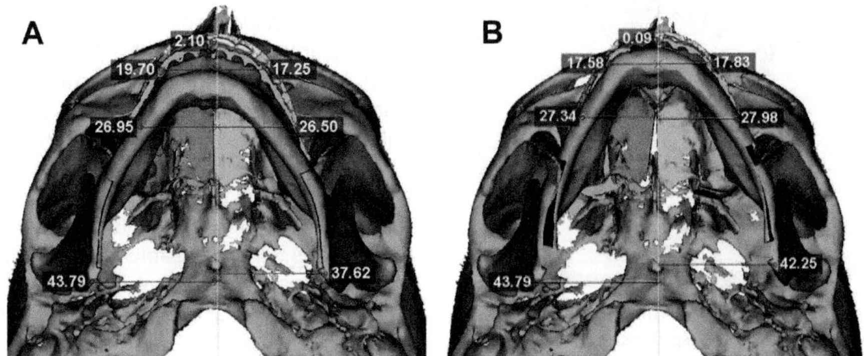

Fig. 11. (*A, B*) The submental view helps appreciate yaw and transverse changes achieved from baseline (*left*) to final simulated position (*right*). Note that position of the maxillary dental arch is improved based on maxillary canine and molar symmetry as well as gonial angle symmetry, using the midsagittal plane as a reference.

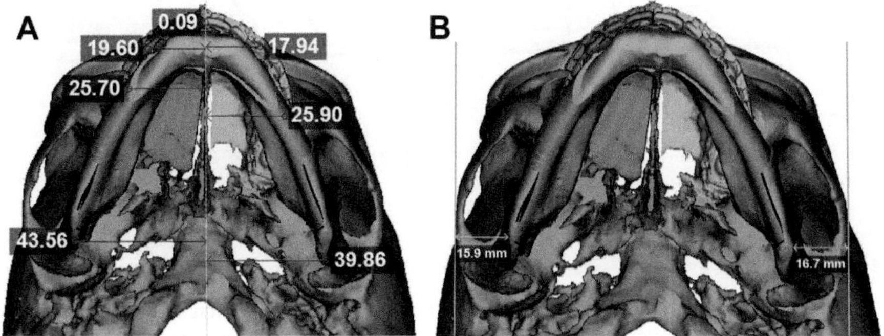

Fig. 12. (*A, B*) In cases of skull base asymmetry (*left*), the midsagittal plane may not provide an ideal landmark to gauge gonial angle symmetry. (*right*) Referencing the widest curvature of the zygomatic arch establishes balance between the widest portion of the midface (zygomatic arches) and lower face (gonial angles).

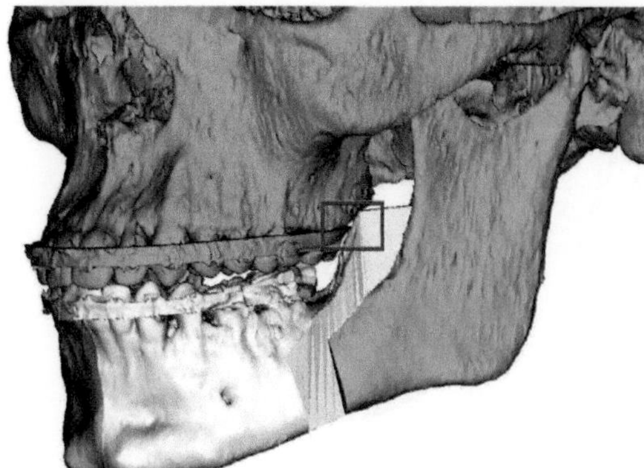

Fig. 13. Impingement of the anterior ramus onto the maxillary tuberosity identified and marked for reduction.

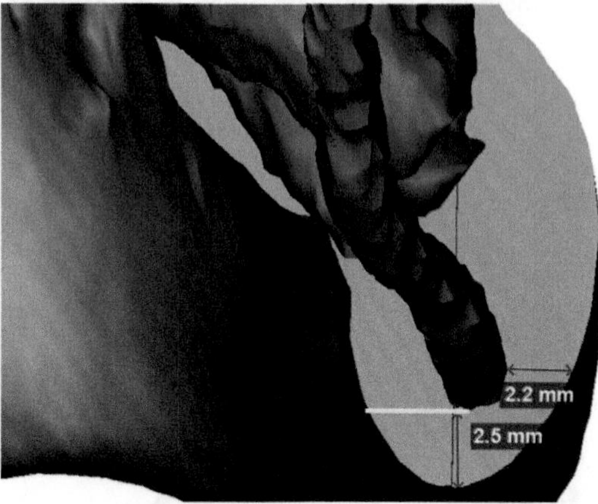

Fig. 14. Evaluation of nerve position at the anterior aspect of a simulated sagittal split osteotomy reveals a thin mandibular body, with an inferior alveolar nerve that is closely approximated with the lateral and inferior borders. In this case, a different osteotomy intraoral vertical ramus osteotomy was chosen to avoid damage to the Inferior Alveolar Nerve.

related to the distal segments to confirm transverse gonial symmetry and identify the location and extent of bony interferences to relieve during surgery. On occasion, large mandibular advancements with a clockwise mandibular rotation may lead to impingement of the anterior ramus onto the maxillary tuberosity (**Fig. 13**). The impingement can be identified on computer-assisted surgical simulation and reduced during surgery.

The caliber and location of the inferior alveolar nerve, as well as mandibular anatomy such as the thickness of the ramus and body, can be assessed during planning to identify anatomic variants that may favor an alternative osteotomy, such as an inverted-L osteotomy for advancement cases, or an intraoral vertical ramus osteotomy for mandibular setback cases (**Fig. 14**).

STL occlusal splints are designed and manufactured to reproduce the surgical plan in the operating room. For large advancement or cases where the condylar position is not ideal, a mandible first surgical simulation can be viewed with the intermediate occlusal splint aimed to reposition the mandibular before the maxilla (**Fig. 15**).

For segmental maxillary operations, the final splint may be altered to include a thicker palatal buildup or a palatal bar to aid in transverse retention. Holes are also incorporated to wire the splint to the maxillary dentition and further stabilize transverse changes. For segmental maxillary osteotomies, the available root divergence at interdental osteotomy sites is measured to ensure 3 mm of space is available in the apical half, and the trajectory of the interdental osteotomy is designed to minimize the risk of root trauma during surgery. CAD-computer-aided manufacturing (CAM) is used to design and fabricate marking guides that may index the dentition and locate

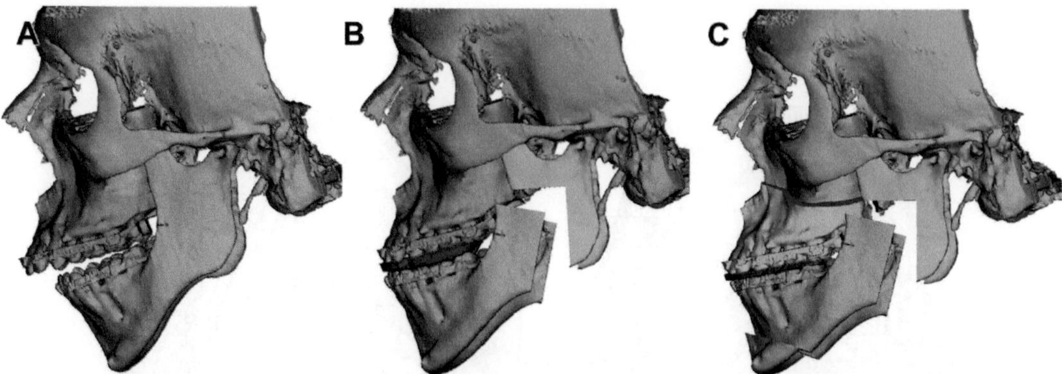

Fig. 15. (*A–C*) In this case, posterior condylar repositioning was performed as a first step in a patient with arrested condylar resorption secondary to juvenile idiopathic arthritis that was in remission. From baseline (*left*), a mandible first advancement is planned (*middle*) and a 3D printed model of the final mandibular position was used intraoperatively to prebend a reconstruction plate for fixation. Simulating the expected change in condylar/proximal segment position improves the fixation plate alignment and fit. Intermediate (*middle*) and final (*right*) STL splints allow transfer of the surgical plan to accurately reposition the maxillomandibular complex.

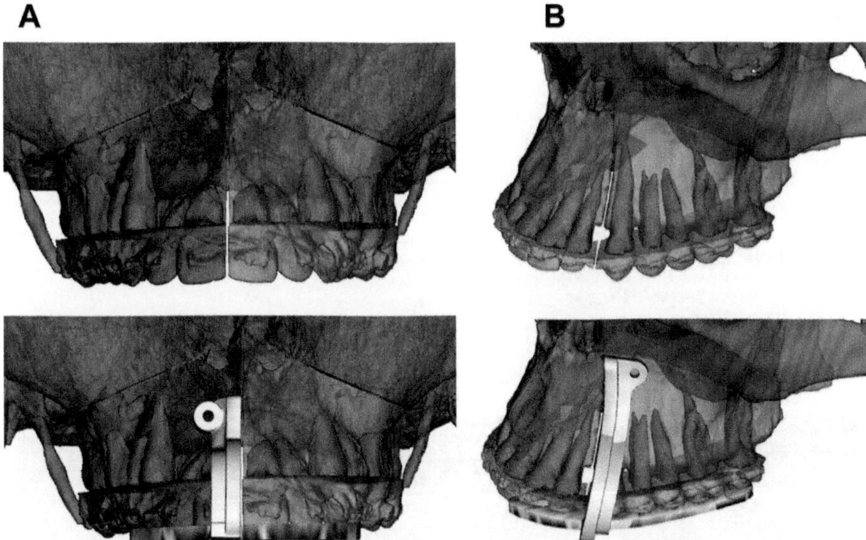

Fig. 16. (*A*, *B*) Midline and paramedial interdental osteotomies with less than optimal interradicular spacing. In cases where ideal root divergence cannot be obtained, CAD-CAM marking guides decrease the risk of damage to adjacent teeth.

the ideal location and trajectory for the saw during interdental osteotomy. The aim of the previously described producer is to increase the safety of surgery and help minimize dental or periodontal complications (**Fig. 16**).

Once the ideal maxillomandibular position is achieved, any residual skeletal bony asymmetries can be appreciated with linear measurements or mirror imaging. Corrective ostectomies can be performed with depth cuts for simple reductions, or with a CAD-CAM osteotomy guide.

When computer-assisted surgical simulations are based on the final occlusal position, the expected skeletal changes can be fully appreciated. This surgical simulation is also a useful tool to confirm plans for single jaw surgery by determining that the extent of bony advancement at known landmarks coincides with the desired facial change and allows assessment of yaw and symmetry as the operated jaw is related to the unoperated jaw.

Three-Dimensional Virtual Treatment Planning Presentation and Communication

3D virtual treatment planning has potential as a powerful communication tool. In the early stages of planning, the orthodontic and surgical treatment plan may be reviewed and presented to the patient, orthodontist, and the oral and maxillofacial surgeon. VSP provides various view options so that comparisons can be made between the preoperative state and the postoperative result. In addition, a movie simulation can be created to demonstrate the treatment plan. 3D virtual orthognathic surgery

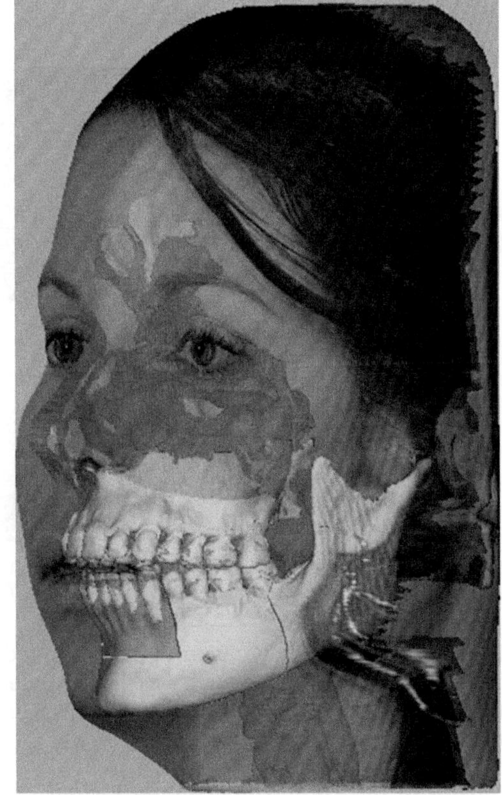

Fig. 17. Integrated treatment plan of the patient as a single virtual anatomic model, including the hard and soft tissues and teeth. (*Courtesy of* Dolphin Imaging 11.9 Premium, Chatsworth, CA.)

A

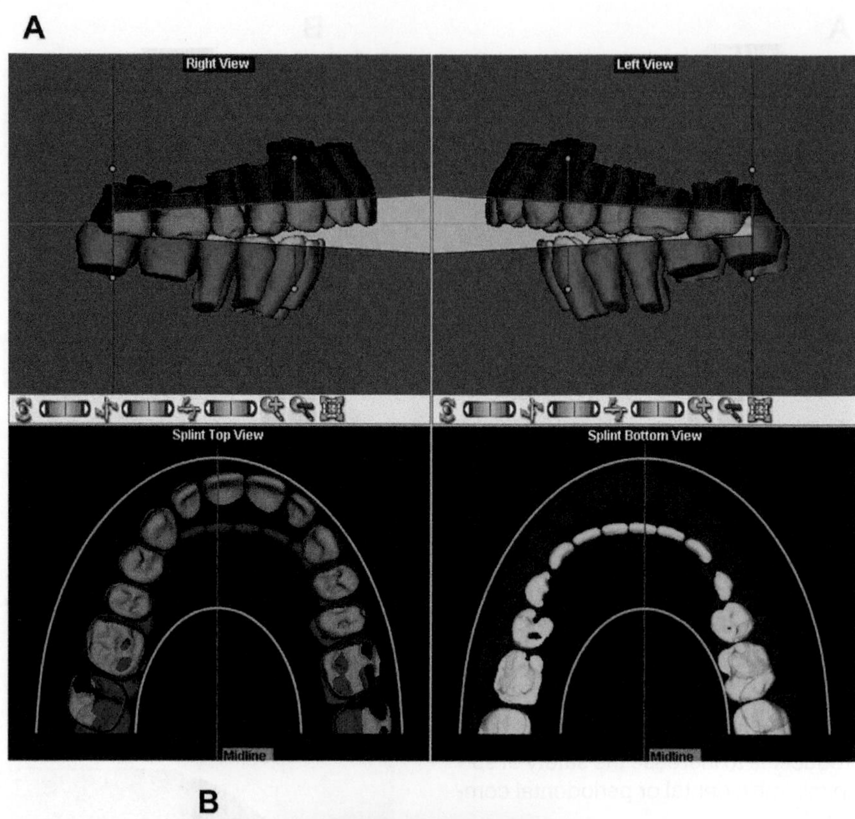

B

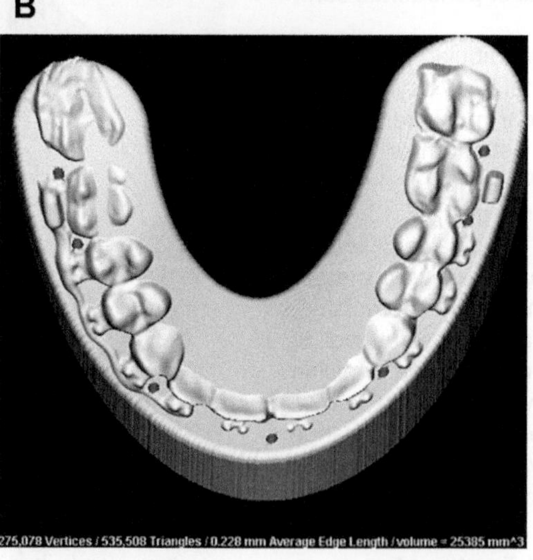

Fig. 18. (*A*) Inserting a digital wafer between the maxillary and mandibular dental arches. (*B*) 3D virtual surgical splint. (*Courtesy of* Dolphin Imaging 11.9 Premium, Chatsworth, CA.)

planning offers the visualization of an integrated treatment plan of the patient as a single virtual anatomic model, including the hard and soft tissues and teeth (**Fig. 17**).

Transfer of the Three-Dimensional Virtual Treatment Plan to Operating Room

After the creation of an integrated treatment plan, intermediate and final 3D virtual surgical splints can be generated using CAD/CAM techniques.[28] Surgical dental splints are created by a computational process after inserting a digital wafer between the maxillary and mandibular dental arches. In surgeries that do not involve the teeth (eg, genioplasty), digital surgical cutting and repositioning templates can be created. These guides are used during the actual surgery to help the surgeons achieve the desired results. The templates record the 3D surface geometry of the area of interest so that the template fits on the bone in a unique position. A guiding template for the osteotomy's surgical cuts can also be fabricated. Localizing bone fixation screws and prebending surgical miniplates also can be created to transfer the 3D virtual plan to the operation room.

The digital STL files are created for use in splint fabrication, and splints and templates are then sent to a rapid prototyping machine or 3D printing to fabricate physical splints and templates. These splints can then be sterilized and used at the time of the surgery (**Fig. 18**).[29]

Future of Computer-Assisted Surgical Planning

Although 3D virtual treatment planning of orthodontics and orthognathic surgery offers an unprecedented tool, the limitation of rendering and manipulation the 3D data on a 2D screen may still lead to some errors in planning. The implementation of virtual reality and haptic technology in the digital workflow could improve the accuracy and precision of the process and make it more user-friendly and may potentially decrease errors.

Teledentistry: Remote Monitoring and Follow-Up

The cycle of the digital dentistry workflow and 3D planning and treatment execution will not be complete without the ability to perform treatment progress (follow-up) precisely. In this era of digital dentistry, teledentistry is becoming a significant integral part of this interim follow-up process.

Dental Monitoring (DM) technology allows orthodontists and oral and maxillofacial surgeons to monitor their patients remotely. DM comprises 3 interconnected platforms: a smartphone application for patients; a patented tooth movement tracking algorithm; and an online Doctor Dashboard, where orthodontists and oral and maxillofacial surgeons can view patient treatment progress and pretreatment or posttreatment changes. It is a novel technology enabling orthodontists/oral and maxillofacial surgeons/dentists/dental professionals to follow orthodontic treatment progress (braces or clear aligners) remotely via a unique mobile app controlled using intelligence (AI) technology. This AI technology can also assess oral hygiene, development of periodontal disease, potential caries, and more than 50 other dental conditions that might arise during orthodontic treatment and certainly is in line with broadening access of oral health care, especially for patients who live far away, or cannot easily have access to regular dental visits, to be more closely monitored.[30]

REFERENCES

1. Naini FB, Moss JP, Gill DS. The enigma of facial beauty: esthetics, proportions, deformity, and controversy. Am J Orthod Dentofacial Orthop 2006; 130(3):277–82.
2. Elnagar MH, Elshourbagy E, Ghobashy S, et al. Three-dimensional assessment of soft tissue changes associated with bone-anchored maxillary protraction protocols. Am J Orthod Dentofacial Orthop 2017;152(3):336–47.
3. Kusnoto B, Kaur P, Salem A, et al. Implementation of ultra-low-dose CBCT for routine 2D orthodontic diagnostic radiographs: cephalometric landmark identification and image quality assessment. Semin Orthod 2015;21(4):233–47.
4. Lee HC, Song B, Kim JS, et al. An efficient iterative CBCT reconstruction approach using gradient projection sparse reconstruction algorithm. Oncotarget 2016;7(52):87342–50.
5. Xia JJ, Gateno J, Teichgraeber JF. New clinical protocol to evaluate craniomaxillofacial deformity and plan surgical correction. J Oral Maxillofac Surg 2009;67(10):2093–106.
6. Swennen GRJ, Mollemans W, Schutyser F. Three-dimensional treatment planning of orthognathic surgery in the era of virtual imaging. J Oral Maxillofac Surg 2009;67(10):2080–92.
7. Abramovitch K, Rice DD. Basic principles of cone beam computed tomography. Dent Clin North Am 2014;58(3):463–84.
8. Pauwels R, Araki K, Siewerdsen JH, et al. Technical aspects of dental CBCT: state of the art. Dentomaxillofac Radiol 2015. https://doi.org/10.1259/dmfr.20140224.
9. Nahm K-Y, Kim Y, Choi Y-S, et al. Accurate registration of cone-beam computed tomography scans to 3-dimensional facial photographs. Am J Orthod Dentofacial Orthop 2014;145:256–64.
10. Rangel FA, Maal TJJ, de Koning MJJ, et al. Integration of digital dental casts in cone beam computed tomography scans—a clinical validation study. Clin Oral Investig 2018;22(3):1215–22.
11. Swennen G, editor. 3D virtual treatment planning of orthognathic surgery. Berlin: Springer Berlin Heidelberg; 2017. https://doi.org/10.1007/978-3-662-47389-4.
12. Elnagar MH, Elshourbagy E, Ghobashy S, et al. Dentoalveolar and arch dimension changes in patients treated with miniplate-anchored maxillary protraction. Am J Orthod Dentofacial Orthop 2017;151(6): 1092–106.
13. Ghoneima A, Allam E, Kula K, et al. Three-dimensional imaging and software advances in orthodontics. Orthod - Basic Asp Clin Considerations.

IntechOpen; 2012. p. 9500. https://doi.org/10.5772/32037.

14. Correia GDC, Habib FAL, Vogel CJ. Tooth-size discrepancy: a comparison between manual and digital methods. Dental Press J Orthod 2014;19(4): 107–13. Available at: http://www.ncbi.nlm.nih.gov/pubmed/25279529. Accessed April 15, 2019.
15. Kravitz ND, Groth C, Jones PE, et al. Intraoral digital scanners. J Clin Orthod 2014;48(6):337–47. Available at: http://www.ncbi.nlm.nih.gov/pubmed/25083754. Accessed April 15, 2019.
16. Logozzo S, Zanetti EM, Franceschini G, et al. Recent advances in dental optics–part I: 3D intraoral scanners for restorative dentistry. Opt Lasers Eng 2014; 54:203–21.
17. Kapila SD, Nervina JM. CBCT in orthodontics: assessment of treatment outcomes and indications for its use. Dentomaxillofac Radiol 2015;44(1). https://doi.org/10.1259/dmfr.20140282.
18. Maal TJJ, Plooij JM, Rangel FA, et al. The accuracy of matching three-dimensional photographs with skin surfaces derived from cone-beam computed tomography. Int J Oral Maxillofac Surg 2008;37(7): 641–6.
19. Temporal-3dMD Systems (4D) | 3dMD. Available at: http://www.3dmd.com/static-3dmd_systems/dynamic-surface-motion-capture-4d/. Accessed April 17, 2019.
20. Kusnoto B. Two-dimensional cephalometry and computerized orthognathic surgical treatment planning. Clin Plast Surg 2007;34(3):417–26.
21. Almukhtar A, Ju X, Khambay B, et al. Comparison of the accuracy of voxel based registration and surface based registration for 3D assessment of surgical change following orthognathic surgery. PLoS One 2014;9(4):e93402.
22. Bobek S, Farrell B, Choi C, et al. Virtual surgical planning for orthognathic surgery using digital data transfer and an intraoral fiducial marker: the Charlotte method. J Oral Maxillofac Surg 2015; 73(6):1143–58.
23. Yang W-M, Ho C-T, Lo L-J. Automatic superimposition of palatal fiducial markers for accurate integration of digital dental model and cone beam computed tomography. J Oral Maxillofac Surg 2015;73(8):1616.e1-10.
24. Swennen GRJ, Mollemans W, De Clercq C, et al. A cone-beam computed tomography triple scan procedure to obtain a three-dimensional augmented virtual skull model appropriate for orthognathic surgery planning. J Craniofac Surg 2009;20(2): 297–307.
25. Schendel SA, Lane C, Harrell WE. 3D Orthognathic surgery simulation using image fusion. Semin in Orthod 2009;15:48–56.
26. Naudi KB, Benramadan R, Brocklebank L, et al. The virtual human face: superimposing the simultaneously captured 3D photorealistic skin surface of the face on the untextured skin image of the CBCT scan. Int J Oral Maxillofac Surg 2013;42(3):393–400.
27. Swennen GRJ, Schutyser F, Barth E-L, et al. A new method of 3-D cephalometry Part I: the anatomic Cartesian 3-D reference system. J Craniofac Surg 2006;17(2):314–25. Available at: http://www.ncbi.nlm.nih.gov/pubmed/16633181. Accessed April 18, 2019.
28. Xia JJ, Gateno J, Teichgraeber JF. Three-dimensional computer-aided surgical simulation for maxillofacial surgery. Atlas Oral Maxillofac Surg Clin North Am 2005;13(1):25–39.
29. Lin H-H, Lonic D, Lo L-J. 3D printing in orthognathic surgery—a literature review. J Formos Med Assoc 2018;117(7):547–58.
30. Hoye L, Morris R, Elnagar MH, et al. Accuracy of dental monitoring 3D digital dental models using photo and video modes. Am J Orthod Dentofacial Orthop 2019;156(3):420–8.

Orthodontic and Surgical Considerations for Treating Impacted Teeth

Veerasathpurush Allareddy, BDS, PhD[a,*], Jennifer Caplin, DMD, MS[b],
Michael R. Markiewicz, DDS, MPH, MD[c],
Daniel J. Meara, MS, MD, DMD, MHCDS[d,e]

KEYWORDS

- Tooth impactions • Orthodontist • Oral and maxillofacial surgeon • Cone beam CT
- Treatment planning • Closed versus open surgical exposure

KEY POINTS

- Tooth impactions are prevalent in clinical practice.
- Mandibular third molars are the most frequently impacted teeth, followed by maxillary third molars, maxillary canines, mandibular premolars, and maxillary incisors.
- Diagnosis is based on clinical examination coupled with imaging, especially cone beam CT (CBCT) scans.
- Good Orthodontic mechanics, surgical planning, and patient education is essential to success.
- Surgical considerations include local anatomic concerns, anesthesia method, flap design, bone removal/coronal exposure, surgical instrumentation, bonding material characteristics, tooth ankylosis, and minimization of surgical complications.

EPIDEMIOLOGY

Impacted teeth are often the most challenging condition that an orthodontist encounters. The prevalence of impacted teeth ranges from 1% to 3.5% in the general population,[1] but is as high as 23%.[2] The mandibular third molars are the most frequently impacted teeth, followed by maxillary third molars, maxillary canines, mandibular premolars, and maxillary incisors.[3–5] The prevalence of maxillary canine impactions has been reported to range from 0.8% to 2% in the general population. Most (85%) maxillary canines are impacted palatally.[6] Impacted teeth occur more often in females (70%) compared with males.[7,8] Racial and ethnic variations of impacted teeth have been reported with Asians and blacks having the least prevalence, whereas those in Greece and Turkey have the highest prevalence of impacted teeth.[9–11]

ETIOLOGY

A wide range of systemic and local factors have been shown to be associated with impacted teeth.[1,3,12] Some of the systemic factors that have been implicated include: endocrine deficiencies (hypothyroidism), cleidocranial dysplasia, and craniofacial dysostosis syndromes. Local factors include: severe teeth

[a] Department of Orthodontics, College of Dentistry, University of Illinois at Chicago, 801 South Paulina Street, 138AD (MC841), Chicago, IL 60612-7211, USA; [b] Department of Orthodontics, University of Illinois at Chicago College of Dentistry, 801 South Paulina Street, 138AD (MC841), Chicago, IL 60612-7211, USA; [c] Department of Oral and Maxillofacial Surgery, School of Dental Medicine, University at Buffalo, 112 Squire Hall, Buffalo, NY 14214, USA; [d] Department of Oral and Maxillofacial Surgery & Hospital Dentistry, Christiana Care Health System, 501 West 14th Street, Wilmington, DE 19801, USA; [e] Department of Physical Therapy, University of Delaware, Newark, DE 19713, USA
* Corresponding author.
E-mail address: sath@uic.edu

Oral Maxillofacial Surg Clin N Am 32 (2020) 15–26
https://doi.org/10.1016/j.coms.2019.08.005

size/arch length discrepancies, failure of root resorption of roots primary teeth, early loss of primary teeth and associated space loss, presence of supernumerary teeth, and trauma.[1,3,12] Two popular theories that attempt to establish a causal pathway include the genetic theory and the guidance theory.[13,14] Proponents of the genetic theory argue that a familial component (impacted teeth in siblings and parents) and presence of associated dental anomalies (eg, other concomitantly congenitally missing teeth, peg-shaped maxillary lateral incisors, enamel hypoplasia) indicated a strong polygenic multifactorial inheritance.[14,15] Proponents of the guidance theory postulate that local environmental factors, such as lack of appropriate contact between the erupting maxillary canine and lateral incisor root, lead to impaction of maxillary canines.[13] Currently, there is no conclusive evidence on either causal pathway for teeth impactions. It is likely that a combination of genetic and local environmental factors play a role in impacted teeth.

DIAGNOSIS

The earliest sign of an impacted maxillary canine is an absence of a canine bulge during routine orthodontic examinations at around 9 years of age when patients initially present for an orthodontic consultation. Panoramic and periapical radiographs have routinely been used to diagnose impacted teeth (**Fig. 1**). The case illustrated in **Fig. 1** is a panoramic radiograph that was exposed during an orthodontic consultation. The initial clinical examination of a 15-year-old patient showed a full complement of mandibular dentition (excluding the third molars), maxillary dentition (with exception of third molars and maxillary left permanent canine), and presence of a maxillary left primary canine. The panoramic radiograph evaluation showed an impacted maxillary left permanent canine and a supernumerary mandibular right premolar, which was also impacted.

The position (palatal or labial) of an impacted tooth is diagnosed with two-dimensional radiographs (frequently periapical or occlusal radiographs) using the vertical parallax and tube shift methods, also known as the SLOB (same side lingual, opposite side buccal) or BAMA (buccal always moves away) rules. The advent of 3-dimensional radiographs (cone beam computed tomography [CBCT]) has enabled practitioners to diagnose and accurately determine the position of impacted teeth (**Fig. 2**), judge the proximity of impacted teeth to roots of adjacent teeth (**Fig. 3**), and determine if there is resorption of roots of adjacent teeth (**Fig. 4**). Studies using three-dimensional images showed that close to two-thirds of patients had resorption of maxillary incisor roots adjacent to an impacted maxillary canine.[16,17] CBCT images are particularly useful when multiple impacted teeth and retained teeth are suspected (**Fig. 5**). The surgical exposures of impacted teeth and orthodontic traction mechanics is planned more accurately with CBCT images. A downside of CBCT images is radiation exposure involved. However, this is minimized by using "limited" field or "very limited" field images.

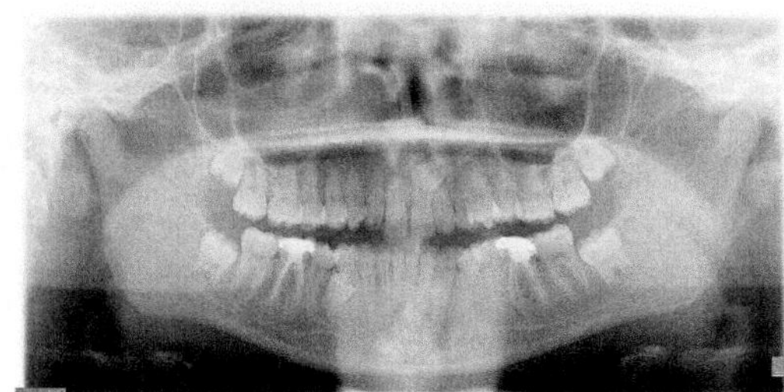

Fig. 1. Routine panoramic radiograph exposed during initial orthodontic consultation.

ORTHODONTIC PREPARATION AND SURGICAL EXPOSURE OF IMPACTED MAXILLARY CANINES

Aside from the third molars, the maxillary canines are the most frequently impacted teeth. In the following paragraphs, we provide an overview of orthodontic preparation and various surgical exposure techniques used for treating impacted maxillary canines. The surgical method used for exposures is largely dependent on individual preferences and is driven by the mesiobuccal location of impacted tooth (labial, palatal, or intra-alveolar), patient compliance with oral hygiene practices, and periodontal health.

CLOSED SURGICAL EXPOSURE

Before surgical exposure of impacted teeth, the orthodontist must prepare the maxillary arch (align, level, and create sufficient space for placing the impacted tooth in its correct position in the arch) and communicate with the oral and maxillofacial surgeon about the planned orthodontic traction mechanics so that the gold chain can be bonded by the oral and maxillofacial surgeon at the ideal location on an exposed tooth. Ideally, it is recommended that the orthodontist be present at the time of surgical exposure and

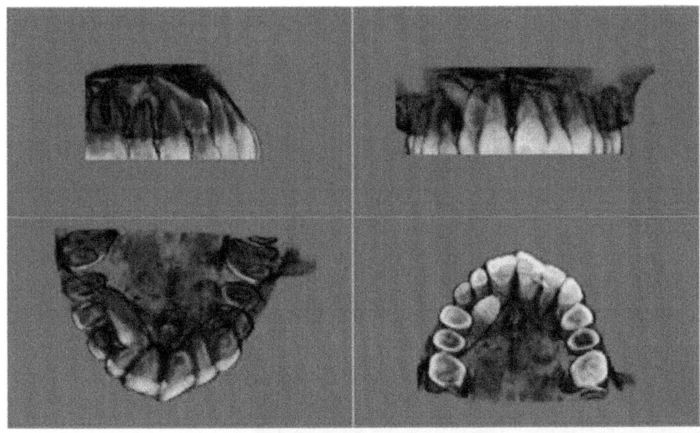

Fig. 2. CBCT images (limited field to reduce radiation exposure) to examine an impacted (palatally displaced) maxillary right canine.

bond the attachments to the exposed tooth. However, this is frequently not possible. Hence, communication between the two providers becomes a critical element of success because the flap is sutured back over the exposed tooth and the tooth is no longer visible clinically. In this technique, the surgeon creates a full-thickness flap to expose the impacted tooth and then proceeds with minimal bone removal.[18] The follicular tissue is removed to the extent that an attachment (usually a gold button attached to a gold chain) can be bonded to the exposed tooth. Utmost care should be taken at the time of acid etching and applying the bonding primer to the exposed tooth. Spillover of etchants to surrounding soft tissues should be prevented because they can cause localized reactions and necrosis of gingiva. Poor etching and priming frequently leads to bond failure and re-exposures (**Fig. 6**). Once the attachment is bonded, the flap is sutured back to its former position and covers the entire exposed area. The gold chain is drawn through the flap and attached to the orthodontic hardware with a nonresorbable suture (main arch wire, which is typically a stainless steel archwire, or an auxillary appliance) (**Fig. 7**). The gold chain should never be drawn through the gingival sulcus of another

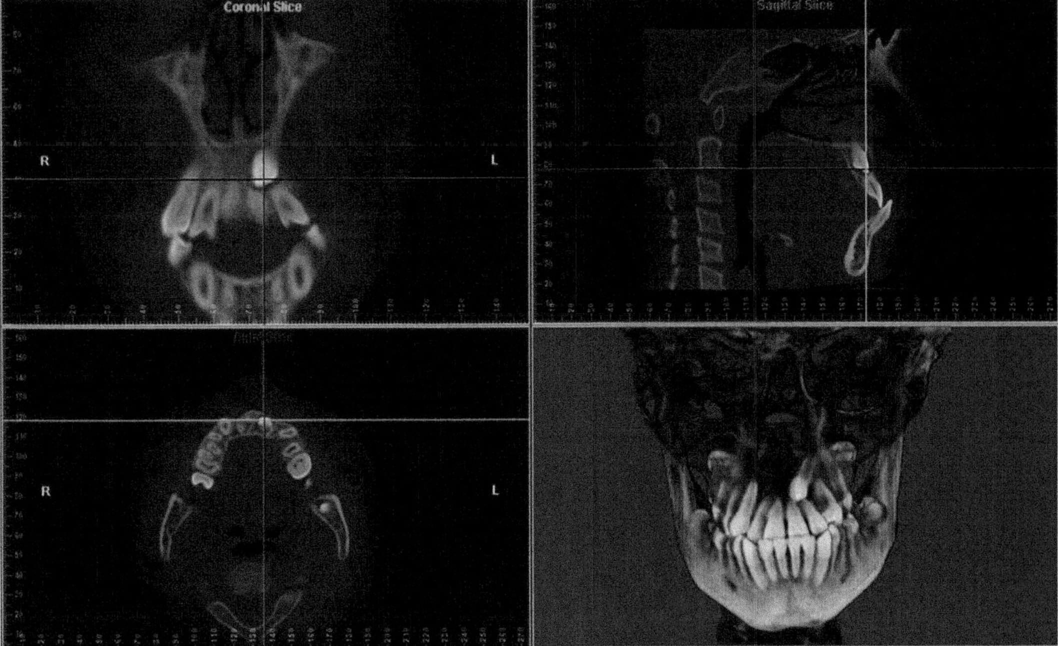

Fig. 3. Visualizing proximity of roots of teeth adjacent to impacted maxillary left canine.

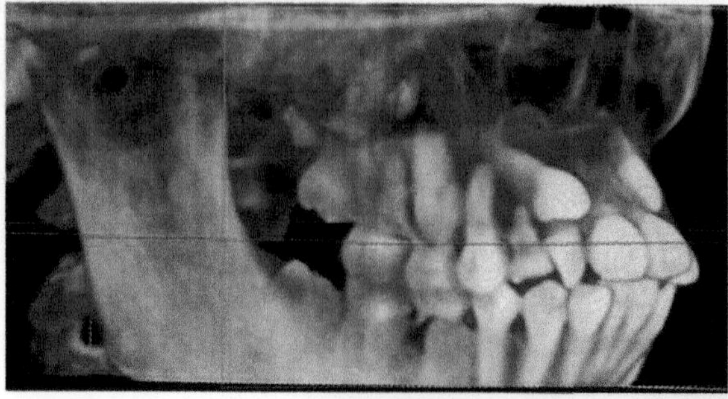

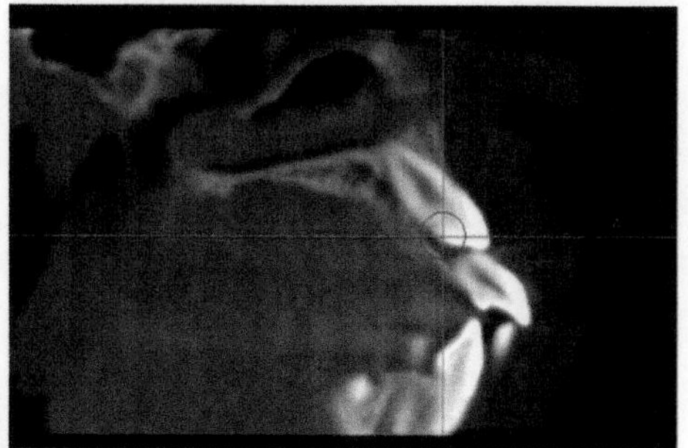

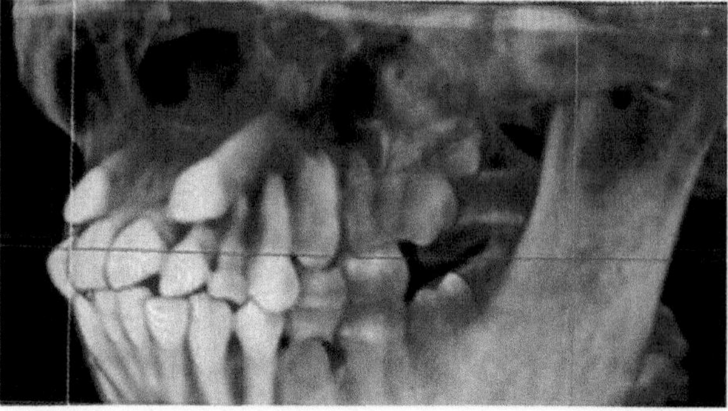

Fig. 4. Resorption of roots of maxillary right and left lateral incisors adjacent to impacted maxillary canines.

tooth because this may lead to significant periodontal defect. It can be drawn through an extraction socket if a primary canine or premolar was extracted at the same time, or a window for the gold chain should be cut in the flapped tissue adjacent to the impacted tooth.

The gold chain is activated immediately or as soon as is tolerated by the patient, postoperatively, to provide orthodontic traction on the impacted tooth. The chain is activated every 4 weeks and orthodontic mechanics are used to place the impacted tooth in its ideal position in the maxillary arch. Apart from gold chain tied to the main archwire, auxillary springs and cantilevers can also be used to move the impacted tooth into position (see **Fig. 7**; **Fig. 8**). The mechanics used for moving teeth is largely dependent on the preferences of the orthodontist.

OPEN SURGICAL EXPOSURE

In the open eruption technique, the bone is completely removed from the coronal aspect of the tooth.[19,20] A full-thickness flap is elevated from the first premolar to the midline. The bone encasing the impacted canine is gently removed until the crown of the tooth is exposed. The flap is sutured back while leaving a window for the exposed tooth to erupt. Typically, a periodontal

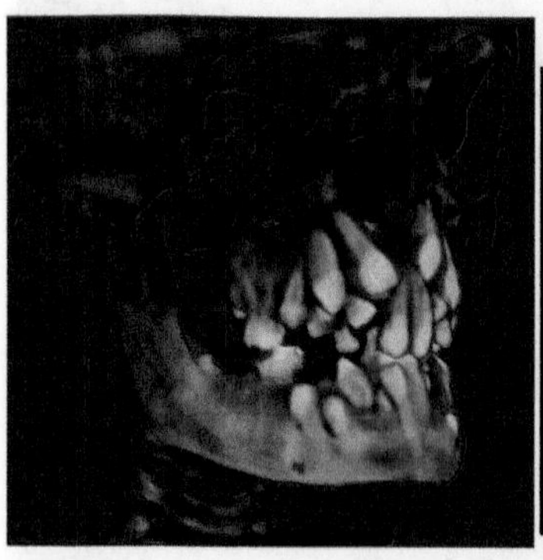

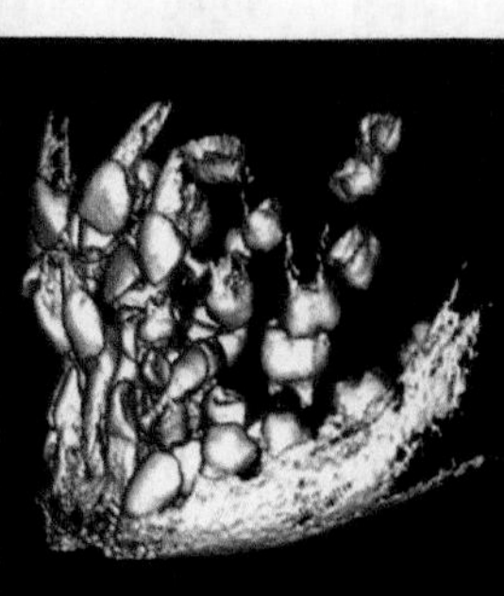

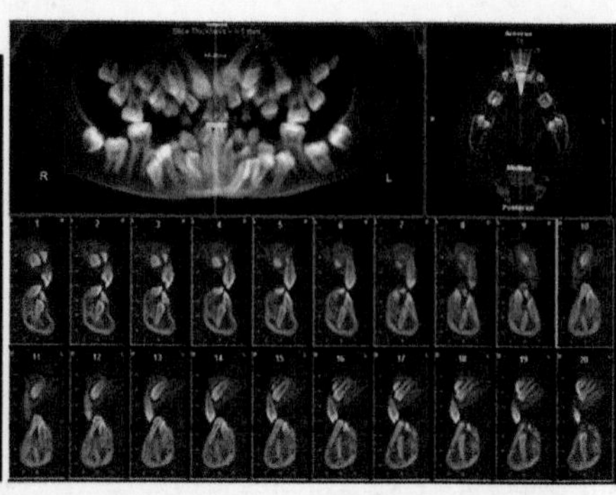

Fig. 5. CBCT images to examine multiple impacted teeth and supernumerary teeth in a patient with cleidocranial dysplasia.

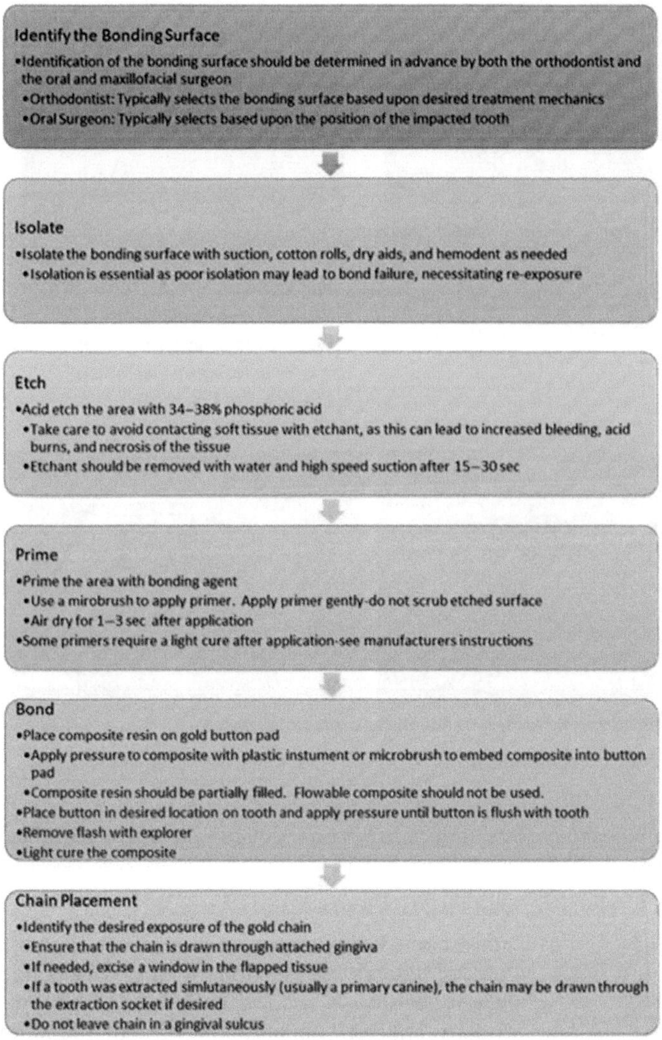

Identify the Bonding Surface
- Identification of the bonding surface should be determined in advance by both the orthodontist and the oral and maxillofacial surgeon
  - Orthodontist: Typically selects the bonding surface based upon desired treatment mechanics
  - Oral Surgeon: Typically selects based upon the position of the impacted tooth

Isolate
- Isolate the bonding surface with suction, cotton rolls, dry aids, and hemodent as needed
  - Isolation is essential as poor isolation may lead to bond failure, necessitating re-exposure

Etch
- Acid etch the area with 34–38% phosphoric acid
  - Take care to avoid contacting soft tissue with etchant, as this can lead to increased bleeding, acid burns, and necrosis of the tissue
  - Etchant should be removed with water and high speed suction after 15–30 sec

Prime
- Prime the area with bonding agent
  - Use a mirobrush to apply primer. Apply primer gently-do not scrub etched surface
  - Air dry for 1–3 sec after application
- Some primers require a light cure after application-see manufacturers instructions

Bond
- Place composite resin on gold button pad
  - Apply pressure to composite with plastic instument or microbrush to embed composite into button pad
  - Composite resin should be partially filled. Flowable composite should not be used.
- Place button in desired location on tooth and apply pressure until button is flush with tooth
- Remove flash with explorer
- Light cure the composite

Chain Placement
- Identify the desired exposure of the gold chain
  - Ensure that the chain is drawn through attached gingiva
  - If needed, excise a window in the flapped tissue
  - If a tooth was extracted simlutaneously (usually a primary canine), the chain may be drawn through the extraction socket if desired
  - Do not leave chain in a gingival sulcus

Fig. 6. Proper procedures for bonding gold chain to exposed impacted tooth.

dressing is placed over the surgical area and replaced periodically. Alternatively, the surgeon may just excise a window of mucosa overlying the impacted tooth, exposing the overlying bone and crown covering the tooth, and not reflect a flap. This is often indicated when the tooth is palpable. A gold chain may be attached at the time of surgery by the surgeon, or later by the orthodontist. Alternatively, the tooth is allowed to passively erupt into the arch up to the occlusal plane. It typically takes 6 to 9 months for this passive eruption.[20] Proponents of the open eruption technique recommend that the surgical exposure be performed during the mixed dentition stage and prefer to start the comprehensive phase of orthodontic treatment after the surgical exposure and eruption of impacted tooth to the level of occlusal plane to minimize the time in braces.[19,20] For canines that are close to the cementoenamel junction of the lateral or central incisors, a simple soft tissue punch may be performed.

There has been considerable controversy regarding the relative merits and demerits of the closed versus open surgical techniques, which is beyond the scope of this article, but Mathews and Kokich[20] and Becker and Chaushu[18] provide an excellent point/counterpoint discussion. A brief overview of the relative advantages and disadvantages of the closed surgical exposure and open eruption techniques is provided in **Table 1**.[18,20,21]

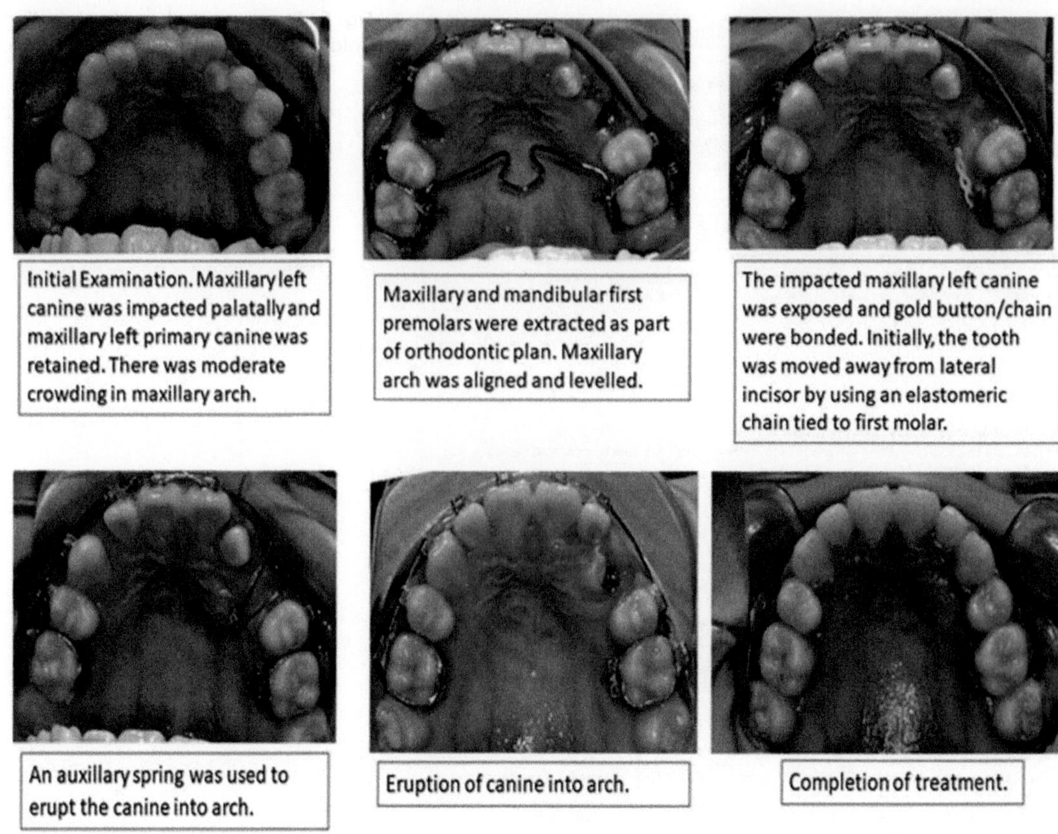

Initial Examination. Maxillary left canine was impacted palatally and maxillary left primary canine was retained. There was moderate crowding in maxillary arch.
Maxillary and mandibular first premolars were extracted as part of orthodontic plan. Maxillary arch was aligned and levelled.
The impacted maxillary left canine was exposed and gold button/chain were bonded. Initially, the tooth was moved away from lateral incisor by using an elastomeric chain tied to first molar.
An auxillary spring was used to erupt the canine into arch.
Eruption of canine into arch.
Completion of treatment.

Fig. 7. Exposure of impacted maxillary left canine using closed surgical exposure technique and use of gold chain and auxillary spring to move impacted tooth.

PROCEDURES FOR TREATING LABIALLY IMPACTED CANINES

Labially impacted maxillary canines can be uncovered by excisional uncovering (gingivectomy), apically positioned flaps, or by the closed eruption technique.[19] The most appropriate method for exposure of an impacted tooth is dependent on the labiolingual position of tooth, vertical position of the tooth relative to mucogingival junction, amount of gingiva in the area of the impacted tooth, and mesiodistal position of the canine in relation to the root of lateral incisor.[19] If a crown is coronal to mucogingival junction, any of the previously mentioned techniques can be used to uncover the tooth. If the crown of the impacted canine is apical to the mucogingival junction, an excisional technique is not recommended because there would not be any gingiva on the labial surface following eruption. An apically positioned flap is the preferred technique for periodontally compromised patients and is specifically indicated in those where there is a need for widening or preserving the zone of attached gingiva.[21] If the crown of the canine is positioned over the root of lateral incisor, the apically positioned flap procedure is recommended.[19,21] This procedure enables visualization of the impacted tooth and orthodontic traction can be applied immediately. The apically positioned flap procedure is technique sensitive and if performed poorly can lead to severe periodontal problems. Apically positioned flaps cannot be used for teeth that are deeply impacted or in the center of the alveolus. If there is sufficient gingiva to provide at least 2 to 3 mm of attached gingival over the crown of a tooth after it has erupted, then the excisional covering approach can be used. For canines that are positioned significantly apical to the mucogingival junction, the treatment of choice is the closed eruption technique.[19,21]

COMPLICATIONS OF TREATMENT

Keys to realizing excellent outcomes include: diagnosing and localizing the impacted tooth/teeth, establishing a treatment plan tailored to the patient, communication between the orthodontist

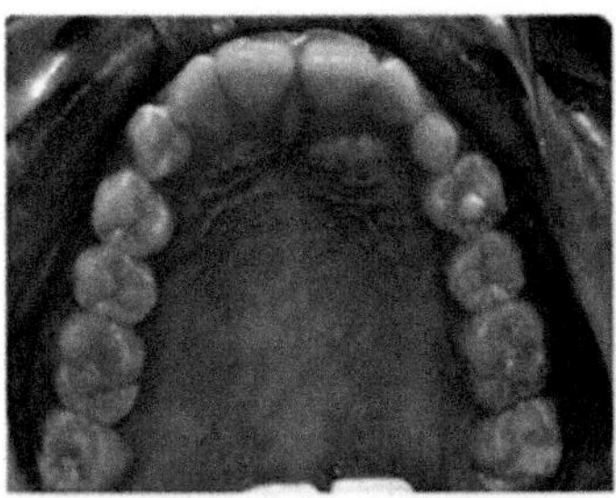

Initial Examination. Maxillary left canine was impacted palatally and maxillary left primary canine was retained.

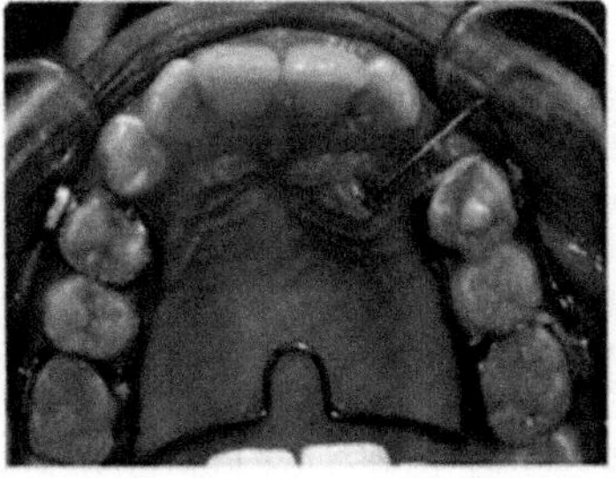

First premolars and molars were banded and transpatal arch was cemented. A cantilever was used to engage the exposed canine.

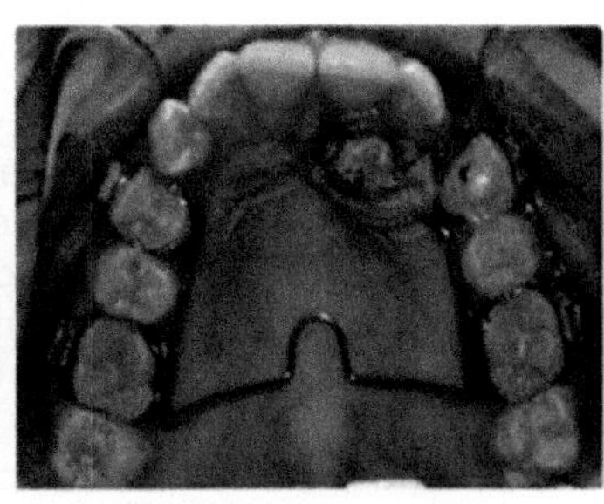

Cantilever was periodically activated and impacted canine was erupted into the arch.

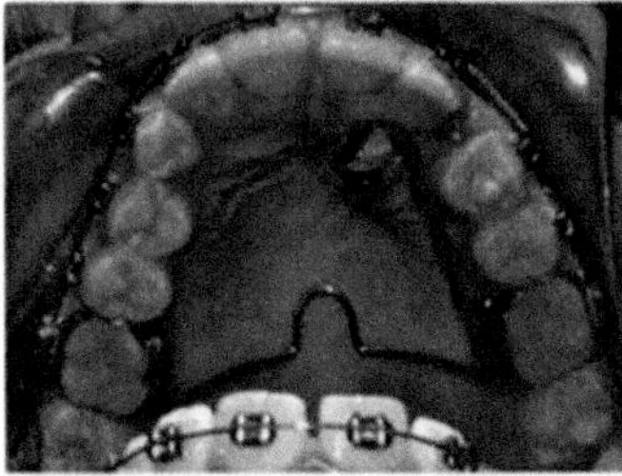

Maxillary arch was bonded and space was being created for placement of canine. An elastomeric chain was used to distalize the canine away from lateral incisor.

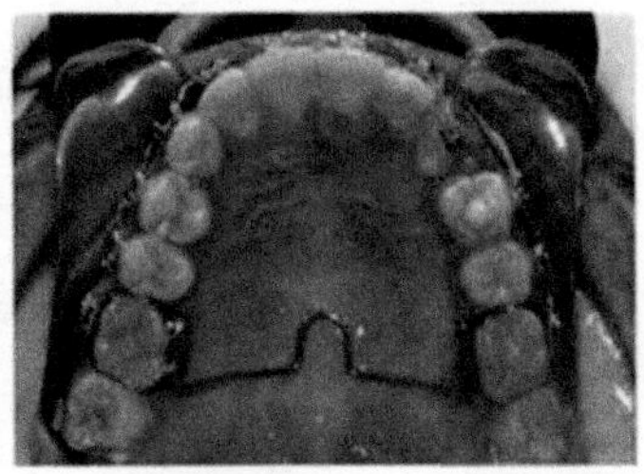

Maxillary left canine was placed into a good position in the arch.

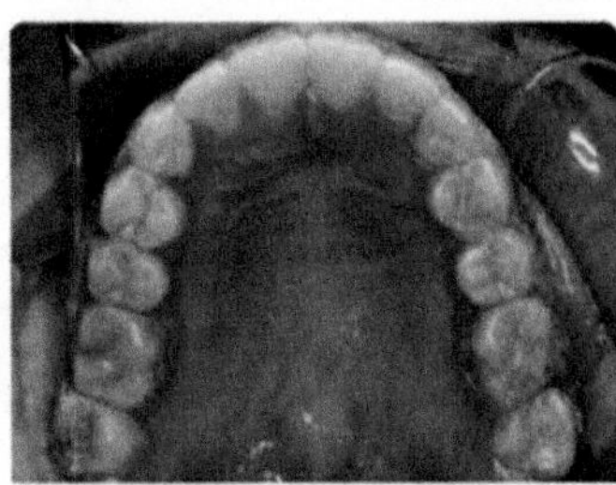

Completion of treatment

Fig. 8. Exposure of impacted maxillary left canine using closed surgical exposure technique and use of cantilever to move impacted tooth.

Table 1
Relative advantages and disadvantages of the closed surgical exposure and open eruption techniques

Feature	Closed Surgical Exposure	Open Eruption Technique
Orthodontic treatment	Orthodontic brackets are placed before the surgical exposure. Teeth are required to be aligned and leveled because orthodontic traction is placed immediately after exposure.	Impacted tooth is exposed and passively allowed to erupt. Braces are not placed until the tooth is close to the plane of occlusion. Consequently, treatment time with braces is minimized.
Visualization of exposed teeth	Not possible because a flap is placed over the exposure. Radiographs are necessary to visualize impacted tooth.	Tooth is clinically visible following exposure.
Bone removal	Less bone removal may be required.	Often a significant amount of bone removal is required.
Management	No periodontal packs need to be placed because there is no open wound.	Periodontal pack needs to be replaced periodically.
Need for re-exposures	Bond failures (buttons/brackets attached to impacted tooth) necessitate re-exposures.	There is no need for re-exposures unless there is tissue overgrowth over the exposed tooth.
Periodontal concerns	Minimal if gold chain is drawn through attached gingiva by the surgeon.	Higher risk of defects.

and oral and maxillofacial surgeon at the time of surgical exposure, and well planned orthodontic mechanics to move the impacted teeth. A breakdown in any of these can lead to poor outcomes. Some of the common pitfalls encountered in such situations are illustrated by the following cases.

One of the adverse outcomes associated with impacted teeth is ankylosis. This occurs more frequently in an impacted tooth with a closed apex. It is critical that an orthodontist identifies this as early as possible and plans for alternate treatment strategy should an impacted tooth undergo ankylosis. The following case illustrates a scenario where a labially impacted maxillary right canine in a 13-year-old patient was ankylosed and had to be extracted (**Fig. 9**). The long-term plan was to place an implant and implant-supported crown for the extracted maxillary right canine.

Failure to properly localize the position of an impacted tooth, in relation to adjacent root structures, and poorly planned orthodontic mechanics can often lead to catastrophic results as illustrated in the following case (**Fig. 10**).

Improper placement of the gold chain makes proper traction of the impacted tooth extremely difficult, and can lead to poor results (**Figs. 11** and **12**).

SURGICAL CONSIDERATIONS

- Planning
  - Maxilla versus mandible for site-specific anatomic structures
- Radiographs

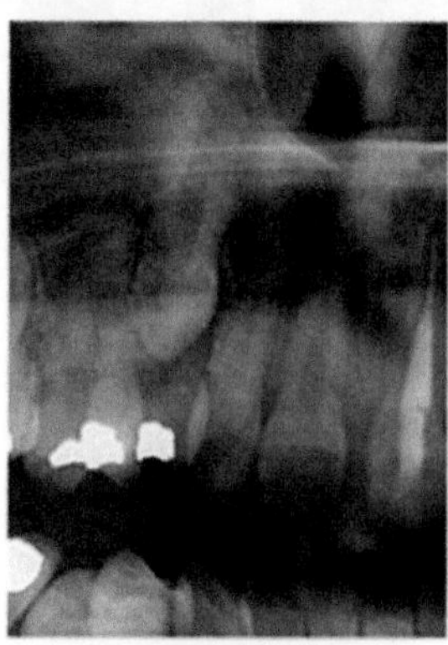

Periapical radiograph at initial Presentation at 13 years of age

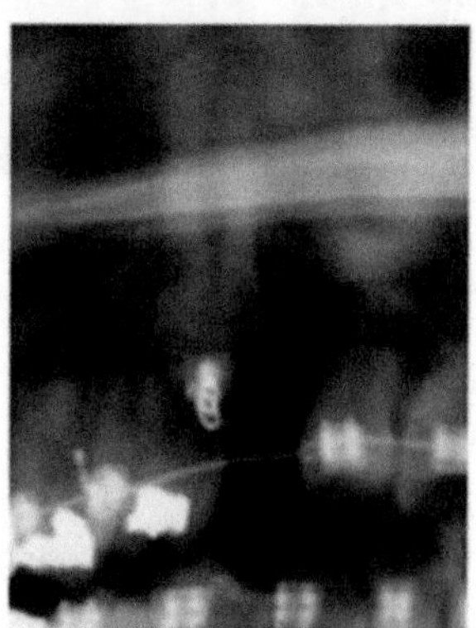

Periapical radiograph following orthodontic traction at 14 years of age

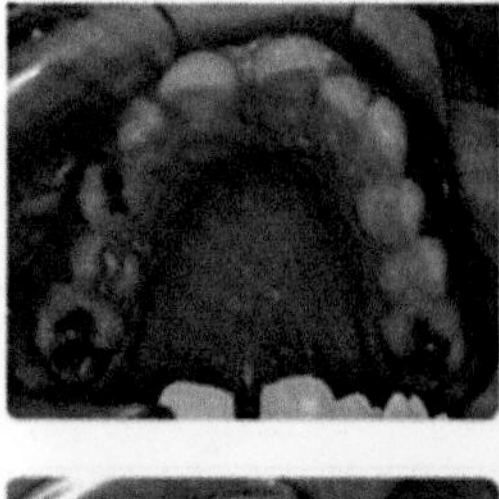

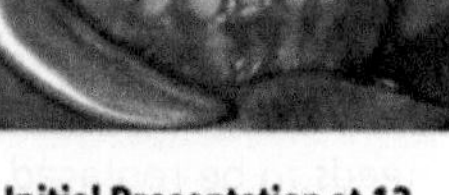

Initial Presentation at 13 years of age

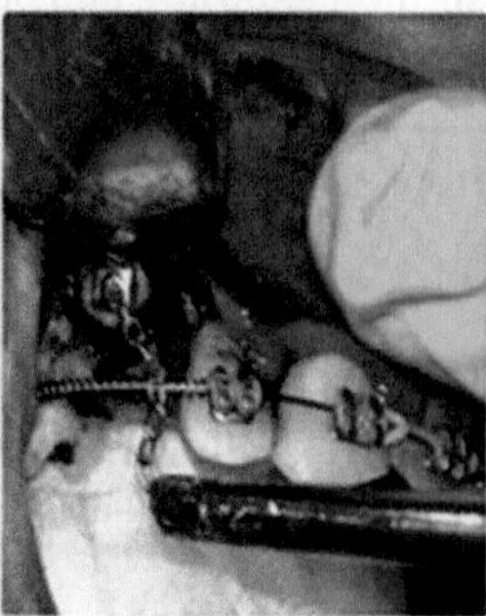

Surgical exposure of maxillary right canine

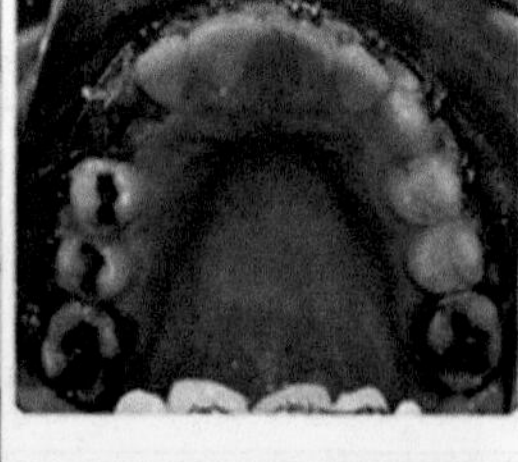

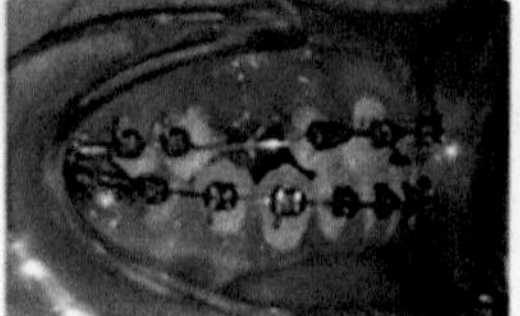

Start of Orthodontic traction

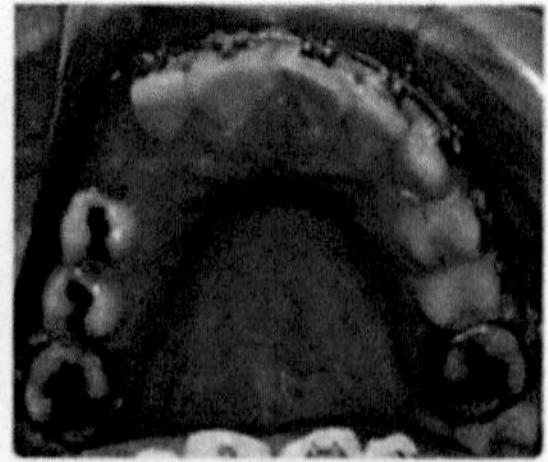

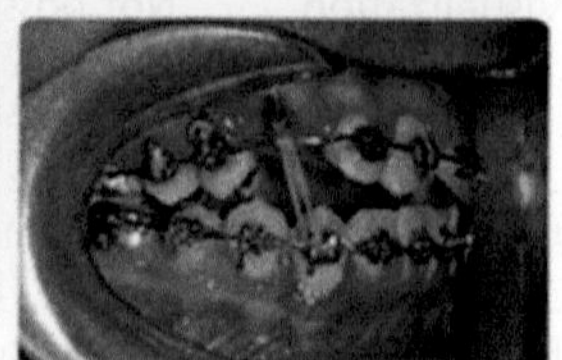

Ankylosed maxillary right canine leading to lateral/anterior open bite and intrusion of adjacent teeth

Fig. 9. Ankylosed Maxillary Right Permanent Canine.

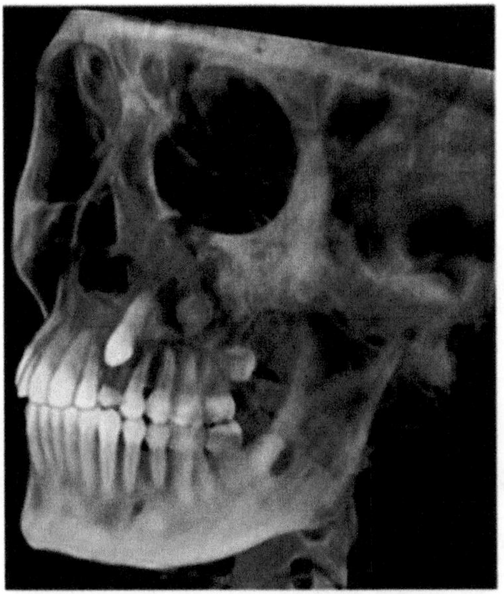

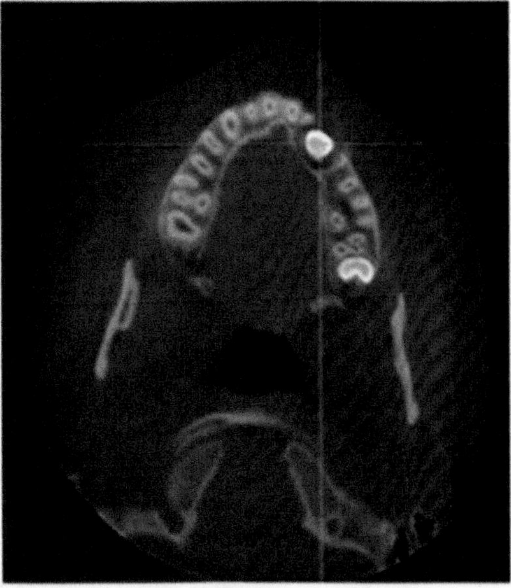

Initial Presentation – Note position of maxillary left canine in relation to maxillary left first premolar localized by CBCT

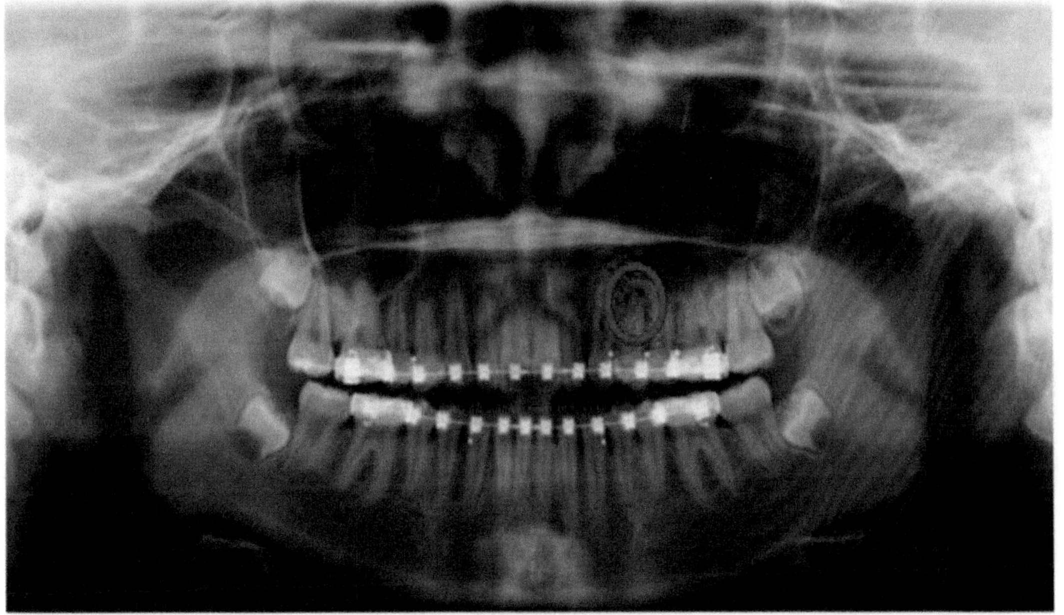

Progress – Resorption of root of maxillary left first premolar

Fig. 10. Poor orthodontic mechanics leading to root resorption of adjacent tooth.

- CBCT
  - Most definitive for determining position of impacted tooth and adjacent structures, such as neighboring teeth, nerves, and path of eruption

- Anesthesia
  - Operating room versus office
  - Local anesthesia versus intravenous sedation
- Flap design

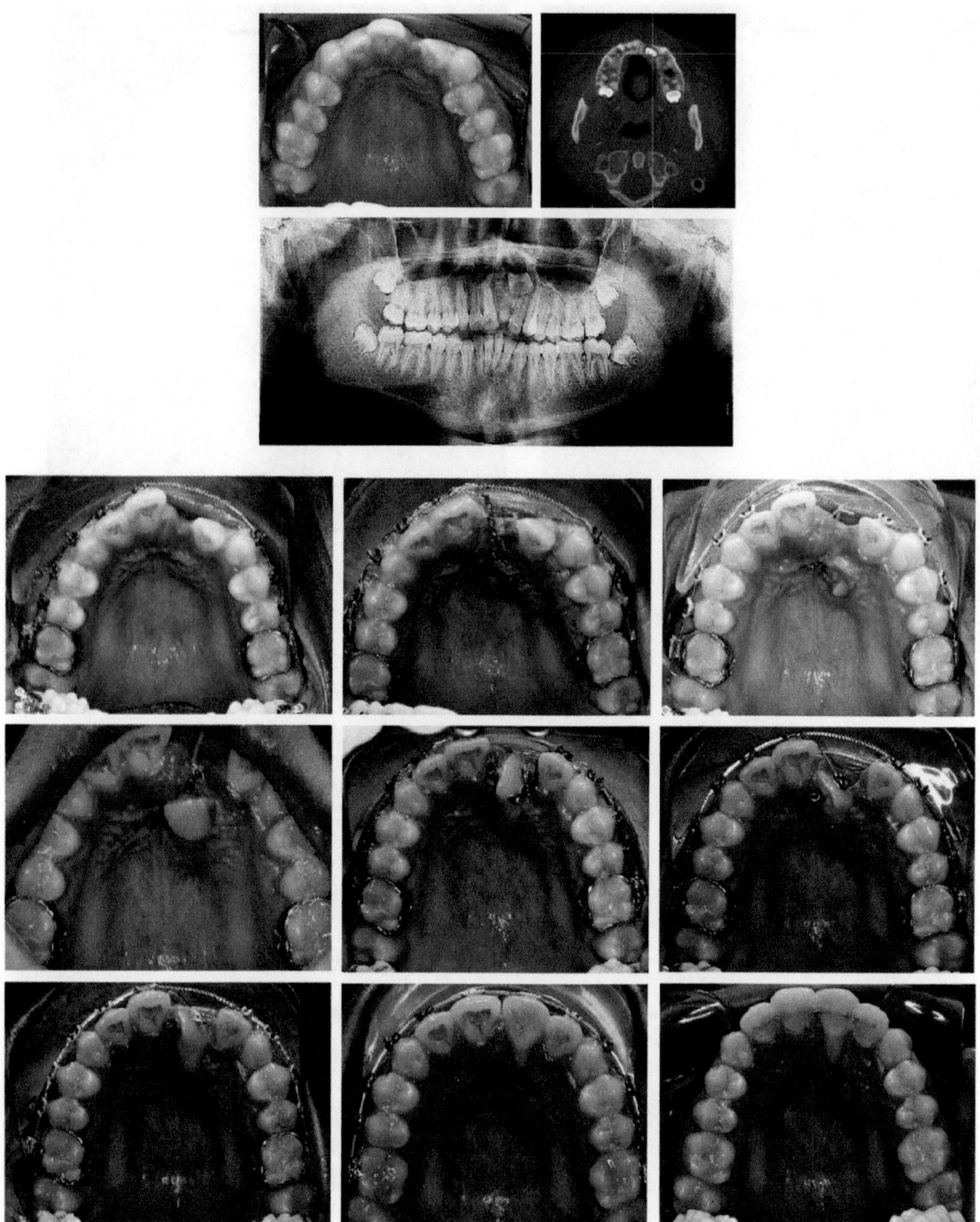

Fig. 11. Poorly planned bonding of impacted central incisor leads to bone loss. (*Top Two Rows*) Initial presentation. Note that the impacted central incisor is oriented properly and located in the alveolar bone. (*Bottom Three Rows*) Progress. Note how bonding the impacted central on the cingulum forced it to rotate 180° during traction. The tooth was also exposed at the level of the first premolars, despite its initial position in the alveolus. The following derotation and protraction resulted in loss of palatal bone.

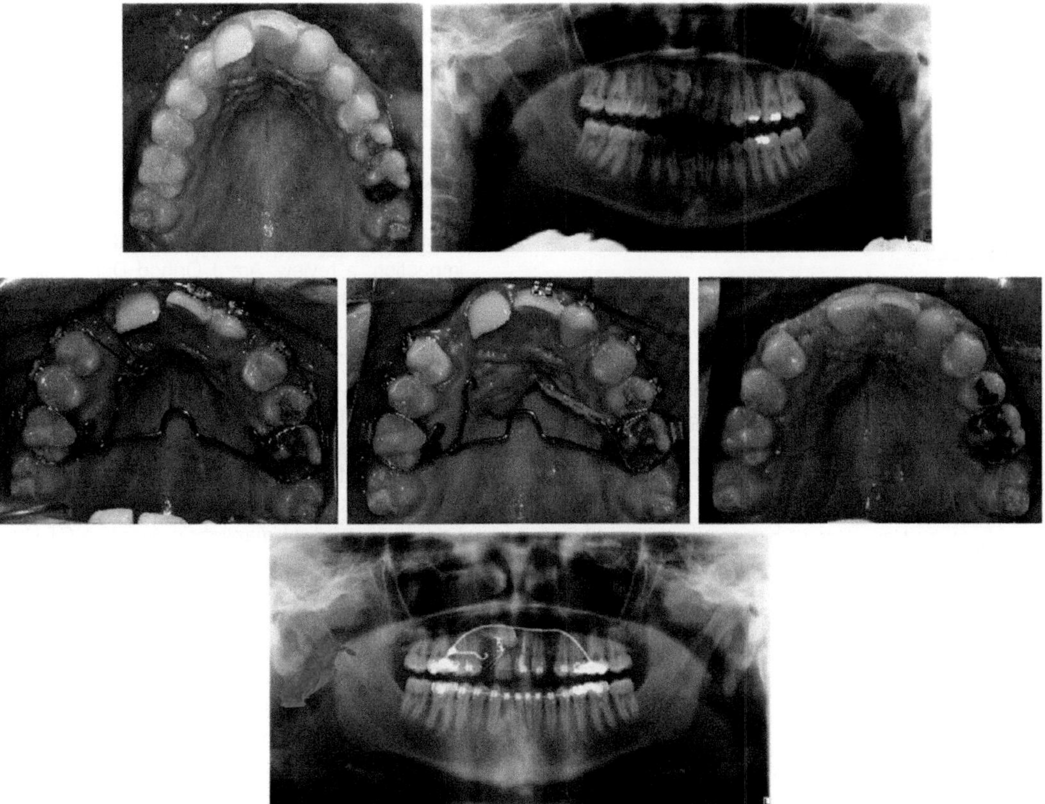

Fig. 12. Poorly planned bonding of impacted canine with short root leads to failure. (*Top Row*) Initial presentation. Note the short root on the impacted canine. (*Middle and Bottom Rows*) Progress. The impacted tooth was bonded on the cingulum, which was the center of resistance for this tooth because of the root length. The canine then erupted horizontally instead of vertically. This resulted in the impacted tooth erupting apex first, necessitating extraction.

  - Facial full-thickness mucoperiosteal flap with distal release versus envelope flap without release versus tissue punch
  - Flap size and exposure, especially on palatal aspect, to ensure adequate visualization and proper isolation of impacted tooth for gold chain bonding in dry environment
- Coronal tooth exposure
  - Rotary versus piezoelectric versus osteotome instrumentation for bone removal, tooth exposure, and prevention of iatrogenic injury to adjacent structures (teeth, nerves)
- Gold chain/button
  - Bonding materials and isolation require ments
  - Position of button; middle third versus other
- Ankylosis
  - Subapical osteotomy for small segment repositioning versus extraction
- Complications
  - Unnecessary surgical site because of misinterpretation of location of impaction
  - Damage to impacted tooth or adjacent teeth
  - Tearing of tissue flap
  - Early debonding of gold chain/button
  - Nerve injury
  - Anesthesia/patient management challenges

SUMMARY

Impacted teeth occur in a significant number of patients and require the coordinated efforts of orthodontists and oral and maxillofacial surgeons. Specifically, optimal results require a prompt orthodontic diagnosis and treatment plan with execution of either closed or open exposure of impacted teeth by the oral and maxillofacial surgeon. Failure to consider orthodontic mechanics and improper surgical technique can lead to suboptimal results. Thus, orthodontist/oral and maxillofacial surgeon communication is essential for success and patient education and shared decision-making is mandatory before initiating treatment.

DISCLOSURE

The authors have nothing to disclose.

REFERENCES

1. Becker A. Orthodontic treatment of impacted teeth. 3rd edition. New Jersey: Wiley-Blackwell; 2012.
2. Ferguson JW, Pitt SK. Management of unerupted maxillary canines where no orthodontic treatment is planned; a survey of UK consultant opinion. J Orthod 2004;31(1):28–33.
3. Chu FC, Li TK, Lui VK, et al. Prevalence of impacted teeth and associated pathologies: a radiographic study of the Hong Kong Chinese population. Hong Kong Med J 2003;9(3):158–63.
4. Dachi SF, Howell FV. A survey of 3874 routine full-mouth radiographs II. A study of impacted teeth. Oral Surg Oral Med Oral Pathol 1961;14:1165–9.
5. Rayne J. The unerupted maxillary canine. Dent Pract Dent Rec 1969;19:194–204.
6. Ericson S, Kurol J. Radiographic examination of ectopically erupting maxillary canines. Am J Orthod Dentofacial Orthop 1987;91(6):483–92.
7. Bishara SE. Impacted maxillary canines: a review. Am J Orthod Dentofacial Orthop 1992;101(2):159–71.
8. Roberts-Harry D, Sandy J. Orthodontics. Part 10: impacted teeth. Br Dent J 2004;196(6):319–27 [quiz: 362].
9. Aydin U, Yilmaz HH, Yildirim D. Incidence of canine impaction and transmigration in a patient population. Dentomaxillofac Radiol 2004;33(3):164–9.
10. Fardi A, Kondylidou-Sidira A, Bachour Z, et al. Incidence of impacted and supernumerary teeth: a radiographic study in a North Greek population. Med Oral Patol Oral Cir Bucal 2011;16(1):e56–61.
11. Kramer RM, Williams AC. The incidence of impacted teeth. A survey at Harlem hospital. Oral Surg Oral Med Oral Pathol 1970;29(2):237–41.
12. Kaczor-Urbanowicz K, Zadurska M, Czochrowska E. Impacted teeth: an interdisciplinary perspective. Adv Clin Exp Med 2016;25(3):575–85.
13. Becker A, Chaushu S. Etiology of maxillary canine impaction: a review. Am J Orthod Dentofacial Orthop 2015;148(4):557–67.
14. Peck S, Peck L, Kataja M. The palatally displaced canine as a dental anomaly of genetic origin. Angle Orthod 1994;64(4):249–56.
15. Leonardi R, Peck S, Caltabiano M, et al. Palatally displaced canine anomaly in monozygotic twins. Angle Orthod 2003;73(4):466–70.
16. Ericson S, Kurol PJ. Resorption of incisors after ectopic eruption of maxillary canines: a CT study. Angle Orthod 2000;70(6):415–23.
17. Walker L, Enciso R, Mah J. Three-dimensional localization of maxillary canines with cone-beam computed tomography. Am J Orthod Dentofacial Orthop 2005;128(4):418–23.
18. Becker A, Chaushu S. Palatally impacted canines: the case for closed surgical exposure and immediate orthodontic traction. Am J Orthod Dentofacial Orthop 2013;143(4):451–9.
19. Kokich VG. Surgical and orthodontic management of impacted maxillary canines. Am J Orthod Dentofacial Orthop 2004;126(3):278–83.
20. Mathews DP, Kokich VG. Palatally impacted canines: the case for preorthodontic uncovering and autonomous eruption. Am J Orthod Dentofacial Orthop 2013;143(4):450–8.
21. Sherwood K. Evidence-based surgical-orthodontic management of impacted teeth. Atlas Oral Maxillofac Surg Clin North Am 2013;21(2):199–210.

Temporary Skeletal Anchorage Techniques

Jason P. Jones, DDS, MD[a], Mohammed H. Elnagar, DDS, MSc[b,*], Daniel E. Perez, DDS[a,*]

KEYWORDS

• TADs • Skeletal anchorage • Miniscrews • Miniplates • BAMP • MARPE

KEY POINTS

- Basics of biomechanics of temporary skeletal anchorage.
- Types of temporary skeletal anchorage devices.
- Indications and surgical application of miniplates and miniscrews.
- Skeletal anchorage for orthopedic growth modification.

THE INTRODUCTION OF TEMPORARY SKELETAL ANCHORAGE DEVICES

The term orthodontic anchorage was first introduced by Edward Angle and can be explained as resistance to unwanted movement. The goal is to maximize desired tooth movements and minimize the unwanted ones.[1] As orthodontic treatment advanced in complexity and in frequency, more recent techniques, using temporary skeletal anchorage, were developed to help correct more severe discrepancies. These techniques allowed the orthodontist to move teeth against a rigid fixation, allowing for more focused movements of teeth. This type of rigid fixation allowed for greater interaction between the orthodontist and the oral and maxillofacial surgeon and vastly enhanced the treatment planning for the orthodontist.[2]

Although only recently used in mainstream orthodontic treatment planning, the idea of temporary skeletal anchorage dates back to 1945, when Gainsforth and Higley[3] unsuccessfully used vitalium screws and stainless steel wires in dogs as appliances for traction. Thereafter, in 1970, Linkow[4] used blade implants for class II elastic forces and throughout the 1970s and into the 1990s, many investigators used dental implants[5,6] as skeletal anchorage. In 1995, Block and Hoffman[7] used an implant in the palate as an orthodontic anchor device. In 1998, Costa and associates[8] used titanium miniscrews for oral and maxillofacial surgery plating fixation systems as skeletal anchorage. Then, in 1999, a rigid fixation plate traditionally used for fixation of fractures was modified by Umemori and coworkers.[9] This began a quick trajectory of the development of many more temporary skeletal anchorage techniques that allow the orthodontist to create movements in all 3 spatial planes[10] with absolute anchorage. In 2010, only 5.9% of published articles in 6 major orthodontic journals were associated with skeletal anchorage, and in 2015 and 2016, the number of articles nearly doubled at 10.4% and 10.5% of all published articles, respectively.[11]

BIOMECHANICS OF TEMPORARY SKELETAL ANCHORAGE DEVICES

Being skeletally anchored and not bearing force on existing dentition, the orthodontic force is applied in a much more continuous manner and creates less undesired movement of the adjacent dentition. The forces from the skeletal anchorage can

Disclosure Statement: The authors have nothing to disclose.

[a] Department of Oral and Maxillofacial Surgery, UT Health San Antonio, 8210 Floyd Curl Drive, MC 8124, San Antonio, TX 78229, USA; [b] Department of Orthodontics, College of Dentistry, University of Illinois at Chicago, 801 South Paulina Street, Room 131, M/C 841, Chicago, IL 60612-7211, USA
* Corresponding authors.
E-mail addresses: melnagar@uic.edu (M.H.E.); perezd5@uthscsa.edu (D.E.P.)

Oral Maxillofacial Surg Clin N Am 32 (2020) 27–37
https://doi.org/10.1016/j.coms.2019.08.003
1042-3699/20/Published by Elsevier Inc.

be applied either directly or indirectly. Direct forces are applied from the anchorage to the tooth or teeth segment that is to be moved, such as used when trying to intrude teeth. Indirect forces incorporate the skeletal anchorage into the design of teeth with the desired movement, using more traditional orthodontic mechanics as a result, such as used when trying to distalize an entire segment of teeth. This is advantageous in that it helps to make moves that would have already been treatment planned by the orthodontist much more efficiently, but does not change any of the traditional vectors or appliance designs. When to use what type of forces is case dependent and, in most scenarios, either type of force may be chosen to reach the desired and individualized treatment goal. These forces, have created a new segment of the population that can be treated with orthodontics alone and have allowed orthodontists to better reach a population that would have otherwise been much more difficult to treat using traditional orthodontic mechanics.

TYPES OF TEMPORARY SKELETAL ANCHORAGE DEVICES

Fig. 1 provides a classification of the types of temporary skeletal anchorage devices.

Miniscrews: Mechanics and Design

As a derivative of the original adaptation of miniplate bone screws used by Costa and associates,[8] various types of bone screws have been used for temporary orthodontic anchorage, are now commercially available for use, and have been described by several different authors.[2,6] Now, there are both self-tapping and self-drilling screws as well as a variety of screw lengths available for different indications to be further discussed, although screws less than 8 mm in length and 1.2 mm in diameter should generally be avoided.[12]

As with other combined orthodontic and oral and maxillofacial surgery procedures, the placement of miniscrews is dictated by the overall orthodontic treatment goal. Proper preoperative surgical planning in the determination of the appropriateness of a person to undergo a surgical procedure is a necessity and includes a clinical examination, any necessary radiographic imaging, any laboratory examinations deemed necessary, and a clear treatment plan determined by the oral and maxillofacial surgeon and the orthodontist.

The surgical procedure is one that is much less invasive than the placement of miniplates, but a thorough clinical evaluation of the treatment planned placement sites of miniscrews must be performed as to what type of miniscrew must be used and whether or not the surrounding tissue is favorable. For example, the maxilla is a much more favorable site for a self-drilling screw because the outer cortex of the maxilla is much more penetrable than that of the mandible, often necessitating a self-tapping screw in the mandible. Further, in areas where there is excess tissue, tissue may need a small incision for access or may be altogether avoided owing to concern of tissue growth over the skeletal anchorage device of choice.

Miniscrews: Indications

Miniscrews have many indications for use as temporary skeletal anchorage and were the first of the devices to be used in a variety of ways including:

1. Distalization of teeth[13,14]
2. Palatal expansion[15,16]
3. Extrusion of teeth[17,18]
4. Insufficient tooth-only anchorage[19]

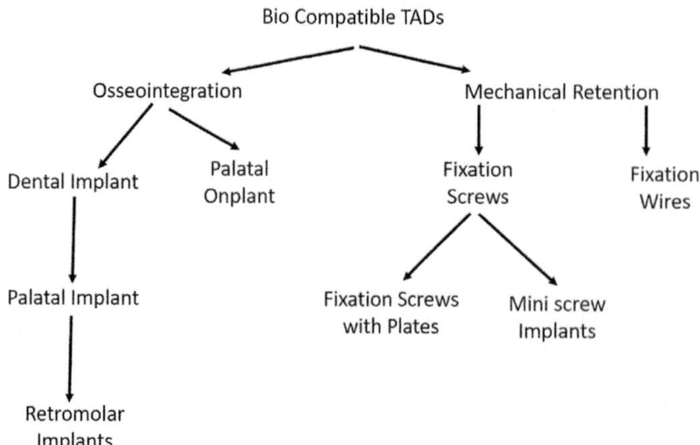

Fig. 1. Classification of skeletal anchorage devices. TADs. (*Adapted from* Cope JB. Temporary anchorage devices in orthodontics: a paradigm shift. Semin Orthod. 2005;11(1):6; with permission.)

5. Intrusion of teeth (often single teeth)[20,21]
6. Lingual orthodontics[22,23]
7. Orthopedic growth modification[24,25]
8. Protraction of teeth[26,27]
9. Retraction of anterior teeth[28,29]
10. Uprighting molars[6,30]

Miniscrews: Surgery

The surgical procedure is begun by placing local anesthetic in the treatment planned sites for placement of miniscrews via simple infiltration.[31] If a self-tapping screw is being used, as is often the case in the mandible, a pilot hole is created using a surgical handpiece and then the self-tapping anchorage screw is placed in the same fashion as the placement of other bone screws. If a self-drilling screw is used, as is often the case in the maxilla, the screw can be placed without any type of creation of a pilot hole.

Miniscrews and Palatal Expansion

Maxillary transverse deficiency is a common dentofacial deformity; rapid maxillary expansion (RME) is indicated in growing patients to widen the maxillary transverse dimension. Tooth-borne RME treatment in growing children results in separation of midpalatal and several circum-maxillary sutures contributing to an increase in transverse dimension.[32–34] In addition to skeletal changes, RME also produces both dental and alveolar tipping.[35] Younger children demonstrate greater skeletal expansion, whereas older children show greater dental tipping.[36] As people age, midpalatal and circum-maxillary sutures show greater resistance to expansion and RME produces mainly dentoalveolar effects that may cause undesired periodontal effects.[37,38]

Miniscrew assisted RPE can offer an alternative approach for maxillary expansion without extensive surgical intervention in young adults. This appliance is tooth borne and bone borne and has a rigid element that connects to 4 miniscrews that are inserted into the paramidsagittal area, to provide an orthopedic expansion force directly to the basal bone (**Figs. 2** and **3**).[38] Preliminary reports show that miniscrew assisted RPE efficiently provides midfacial expansion of the maxilla and zygomatic arches.[39]

Miniplates: Mechanics and Design

As a derivative of the original adaptation of a bone fixation plate used by Umemori and coworkers,[9] more specific plating systems were derived and have been used for temporary orthodontic anchorage and are also available for commercial use, being used and described by several different authors.[2,40–42] Plates have the advantage over most of the screw designs in that they allow for immediate loading with no need for osseointegration. Contrarily, they offer the disadvantage of needing incision and dissection for both placement and removal.

As with the miniscrews, the placement of miniplates is dictated by the overall orthodontic treatment goal and necessitates proper preoperative surgical planning. The specific type of miniplate can be prefabricated or custom fabricated by the surgeon and/or orthodontist to achieve the patient's treatment plan. Regardless of the type of plate used, there is typically 1 component that is screwed into the bone with traditional bone screws and a transmucosal arm or tail that extends into the area determined to be the skeletal anchorage point. The arm or tail should exit around

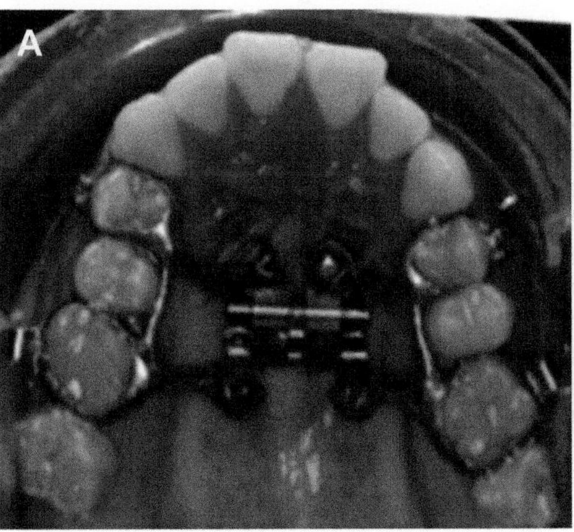

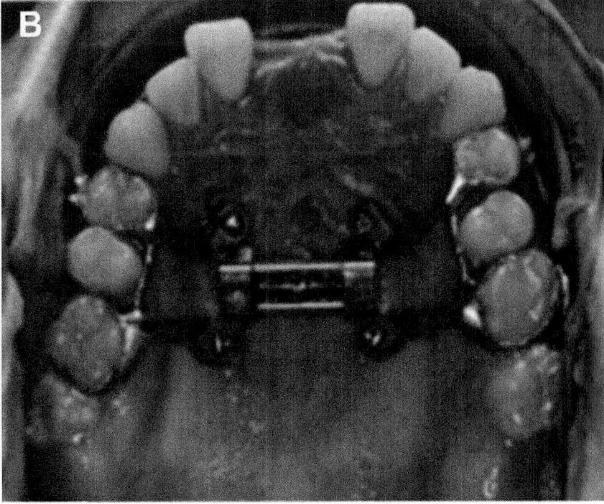

Fig. 2. Miniscrew assisted rapid maxillary expansion intraoral occlusal view (*A*) before and (*B*) after expansion. (*Courtesy of* Mohammed H. Elnagar, DDS, MSc, Chicago, IL.)

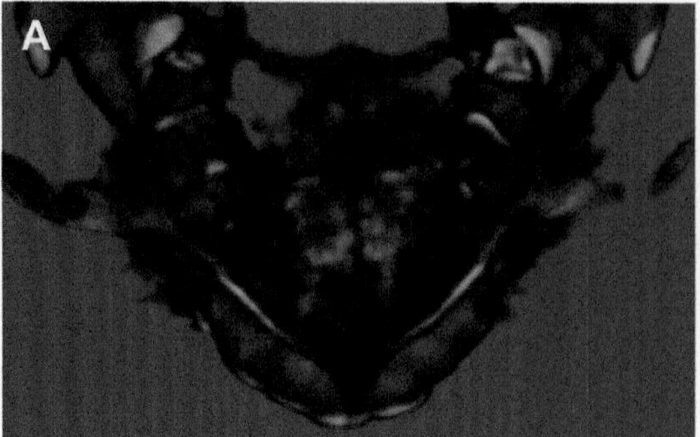

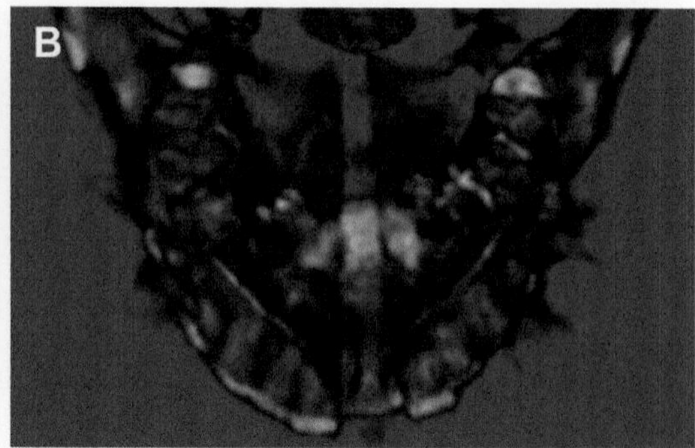

Fig. 3. Cone beam computed tomography scan showing the opening of the mid-palatal suture after miniscrew assisted rapid maxillary expansion in young adult. (*A*) Before expansion. (*B*) After expansion. (*Courtesy of* Mohammed H. Elnagar, DDS, MSc, Chicago, IL.)

the mucogingival line being careful to avoid nonattached, nonkeratinized tissues. There should also be extra care given to avoid tooth roots at the time of surgery, as well as ensuring that the placement of a screw does not impede planned future tooth movements. A minimum of 2 screws should be used to secure the plate, although better results are achieved when 3 screws are used for stability.

Care must be taken to avoid key anatomic structures, just as in orthognathic surgery, located in both the maxilla and mandible, such as the infraorbital neurovascular bundle if placing maxillary miniplates and the mental nerve and mandibular canal if placing mandibular miniplates as well as the roots of any adjacent teeth in both the maxilla and mandible.

Miniplates: Indications

Miniplates, although currently having fewer indications than miniscrews, show much promise in the future of orthodontic anchorage and are the preference of many surgeons and orthodontists at this time. The indications currently described are as follows:

1. Distalization of teeth[14,43,44]
2. Insufficient tooth-only anchorage[45]
3. Intrusion of teeth[9,46]
4. Orthopedic growth modification[2,47]
5. Retraction of anterior teeth[48,49]
6. Protraction of anterior teeth[50]
7. Closure of anterior open bite[9]

Miniplates: Surgery

The surgical procedure is begun by the administration of sedation if preferred by the patient and local anesthesia via infiltration[31] in the area where the skeletal anchorage plates are to be placed. An incision is then made from the mucogingival junctional toward the depth of the vestibule in a vertical fashion with a horizontal releasing incision along the inferior aspect of the vertical incision, either anterior or posterior to provide release and adequate visualization. A full-thickness mucoperiosteal flap is raised along the incision with adequate retraction of the flap to provide visualization. The designed miniplate is then inserted and ensured to have no space between the plate and bone to which it will be applied and secured using self-drilling or self-tapping monocortical screws. Copious irrigation and closure of the created flap is performed with a resorbable suture for the conclusion of the surgical procedure.

Miniplates and Orthopedic Growth Modification

The use of skeletal anchorage in orthopedics can minimize the dentoalveolar changes and maximize the skeletal changes.

Class III malocclusion growth modification

A facemask is the most commonly used therapy for treatment of class III patients with maxillary deficiency; however, the indirect application of the orthopedic forces by stretching elastics between intraoral tooth-borne appliances and the facemask limits the orthopedic effects and makes many undesirable changes.[51,52] Many skeletal anchorage protocols have been introduced to apply the orthopedic force directly to the maxillofacial skeleton. One protocol is to anchor the facemask with miniplates fixed in the zygomatic buttress with curvilinear miniplates fixed with at least 3 or 4 screws with placement of heavy elastics between the miniplates and the facemask (**Figs. 4** and **5**).[53] Another protocol consists of straight miniplates fixed at the infrazygomatic crest and symphyseal miniplates in the mandible connected by class III elastics (**Figs. 6** and **7**).

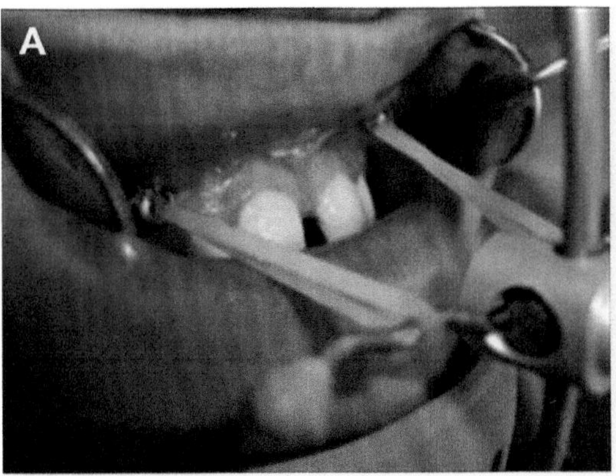

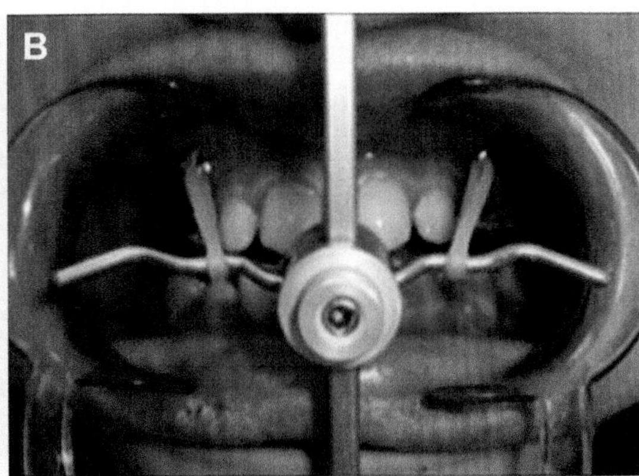

Fig. 4. Application of facemask to miniplates. (*A*) Lateral view. (*B*) Frontal view. (*From* Elnagar MH, Elshourbagy E, Ghobashy S, et al. Comparative evaluation of 2 skeletally anchored maxillary protraction protocols. Am J Orthod Dentofac Orthop. 2016;150(5):753; with permission.)

These 2 protocols apply orthopedic force directly to the maxilla without dissipation of forces through the teeth and both resulted in maxillary advancement and elimination of treatment-induced tooth movement.[53,54] Bone-anchored maxillary protraction protocols showed significant advancement of the soft tissues of the upper lip and the middle of the face, in addition to redirection of the sagittal soft tissue growth in the lower lip and mandible areas, which led to the improvement of the class III concave soft tissue profile.[55] However, class III elastics to miniplates can provide greater vertical closing of the mandibular plane than facemasks anchored with miniplates.[53]

Class II malocclusion growth modification

Fixed, functional appliances used for treatment of growing class II malocclusion patients with mandibular deficiency can be used to stimulate the mandibular growth and have the advantage over removable appliances of not requiring patient compliance.[56] Fixed functional intermaxillary devices are

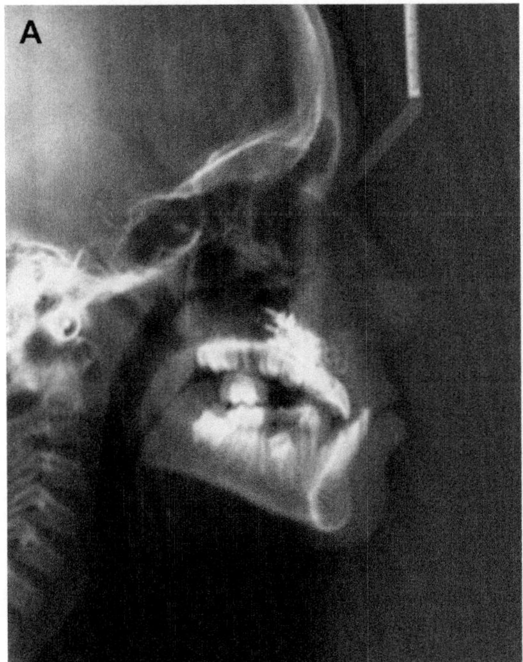

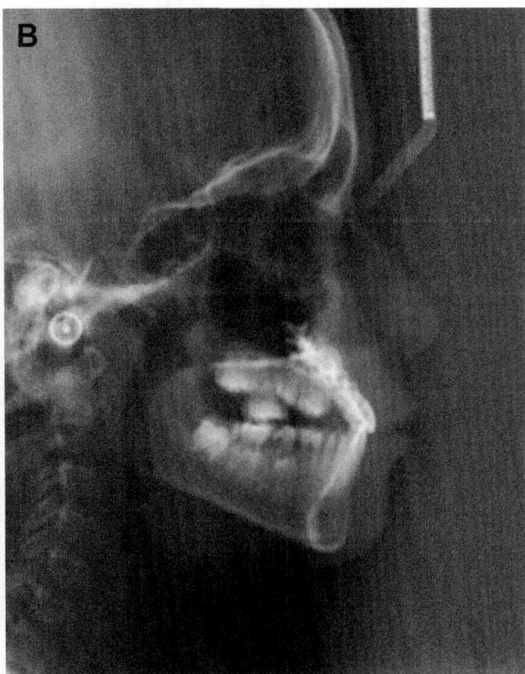

Fig. 5. Cephalograms (*A*) before and (*B*) after maxillary protraction by a skeletally anchored facemask with miniplates. (*From* Elnagar MH, Elshourbagy E, Ghobashy S, et al. Comparative evaluation of 2 skeletally anchored maxillary protraction protocols. Am J Orthod Dentofac Orthop. 2016;150(5):759; with permission.)

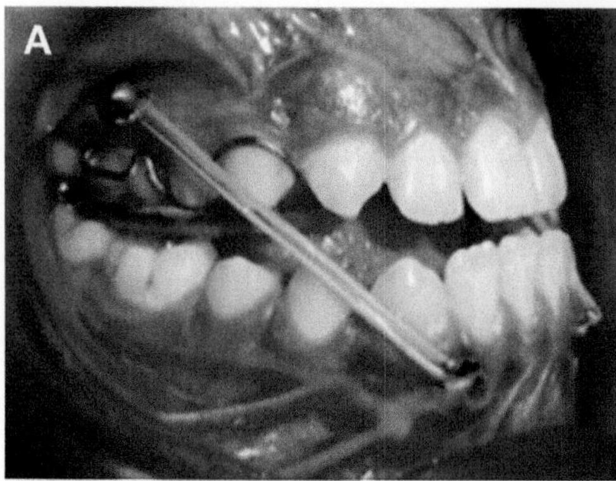

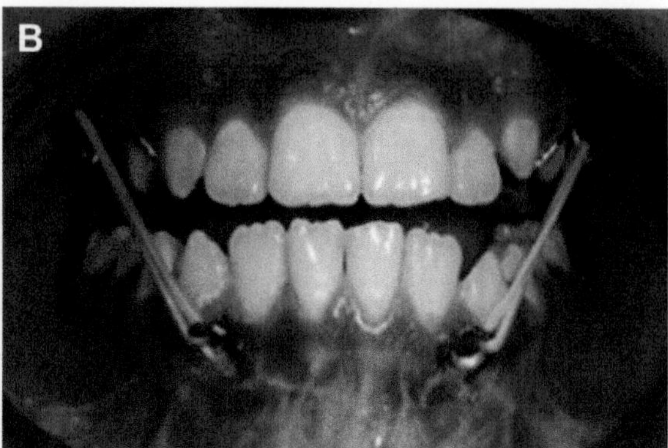

Fig. 6. Application of class III elastics extending from the infrazygomatic miniplates in the maxilla to the symphyseal miniplates in the mandible. (*A*) Lateral view. (*B*) Frontal view. (*From* Elnagar MH, Elshourbagy E, Ghobashy S, et al. Comparative evaluation of 2 skeletally anchored maxillary protraction protocols. Am J Orthod Dentofac Orthop. 2016;150(5):754; with permission.)

categorized as rigid (Herbst, MARA, DynaFlex, St. Ann, MO), flexible (Jasper Jumper) or as Hybrid (The Eureka Spring, The Forsus Fatigue Resistant Device).[57] These appliances provide mandibular advancement in a more forward position and maxillary molar distalization or retrusion of the maxillary dentition, but they also create unwanted intrusion and protrusion or proclination of the mandibular anterior teeth.[57] Fixed functional appliances have been combined with skeletal anchorage to reduce the mandibular incisor proclination by use of miniscrews or miniplates.[58,59]

In 1 protocol, mandibular miniplates placed in the posterior buccal area inferior to and between the mandibular first and second molar above the external oblique ridge, maxillary miniplates were placed in the anterior labial area with the arm centered slightly distal to the lateral incisor and orthopedic force applied using class II intermaxillary elastics (**Fig. 8**).[60]

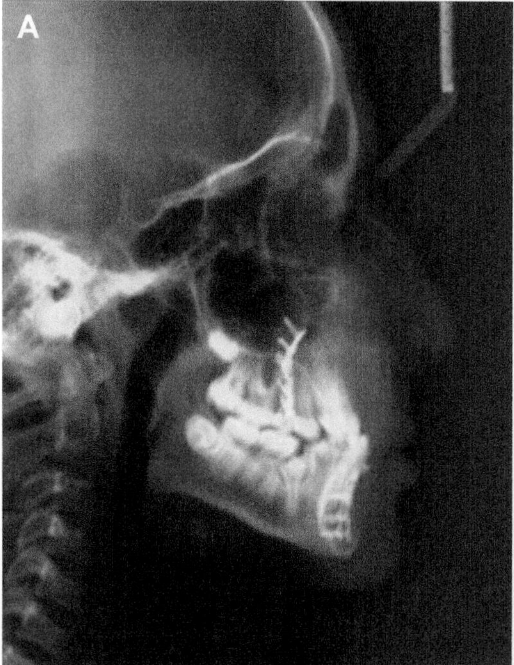

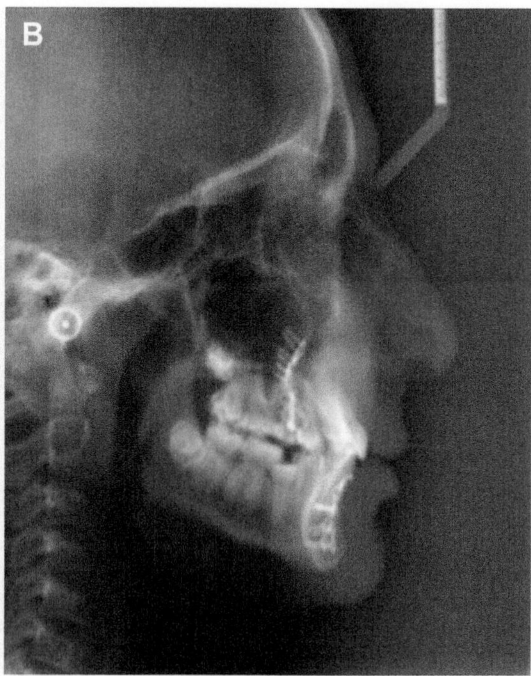

Fig. 7. Cephalograms (*A*) before and (*B*) after maxillary protraction by class III elastics extending from infrazygomatic miniplates to symphyseal miniplates. (*From* Elnagar MH, Elshourbagy E, Ghobashy S, et al. Comparative evaluation of 2 skeletally anchored maxillary protraction protocols. Am J Orthod Dentofac Orthop. 2016;150(5):760; with permission.)

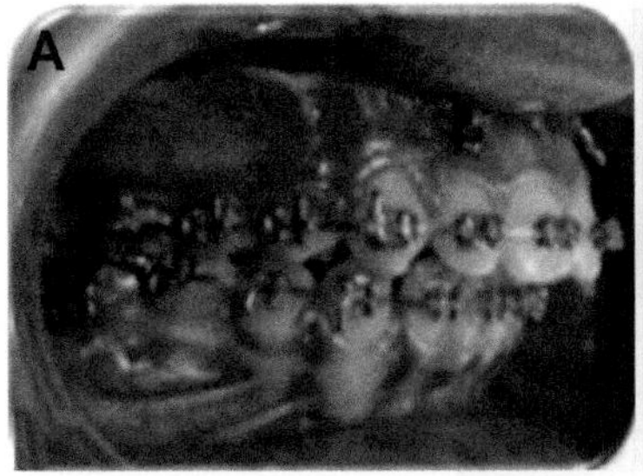

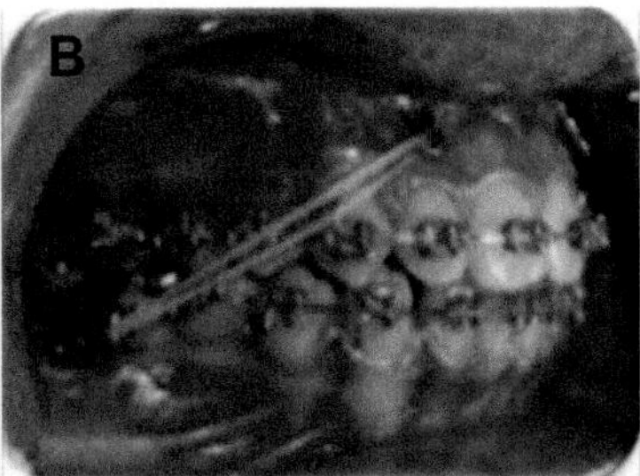

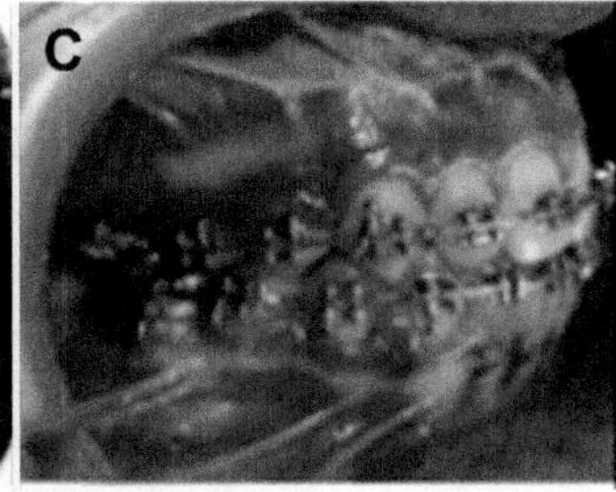

Fig. 8. The miniplates after the healing period. (*A*) Preexisting malocclusion. (*B*) Application of the intermaxillary elastic. (*C*) Finishing to class I molar and canine relationships. (*From* Al-Dumaini AA, Halboub E, Alhammadi MS, et al. A novel approach for treatment of skeletal Class II malocclusion: miniplates-based skeletal anchorage. Am J Orthod Dentofac Orthop. 2018;153(2):241; with permission.)

CASE: USING MINIPLATES TO CORRECT ANTERIOR OPEN BITE

An example of using miniplates to correct anterior open bite in provided in **Fig. 9**.

POSTOPERATIVE CARE AND COMPLICATIONS

In the immediate postoperative interval, the authors advise the use of postoperative radiography in the form of a panoramic radiograph or cone-beam computed tomography to ensure the desired placement of skeletal anchorage and relation to surrounding anatomic structures of concern. Depending on the overall treatment plan, the orthodontist may load or activate the designed skeletal anchorage immediately.

In the ensuing postoperative interval, the patient must adhere to proper and frequent oral hygiene taking care to not allow food or debris to pool around the miniplate or miniscrew. Chlorhexidine mouth rinses also aid with topical debridement and reduce soft tissue inflammation and risk of infection. It is also recommended to give antibiotic coverage for 5 to 7 days as the surgical sites heal because miniscrews and miniplates are transmucosal and represent an area for oral bacteria to communicate with the underlying soft tissues and bone. Pain associated with the surgical procedures should not be significant, but the specific analgesic protocol is up to the surgeon. Although there are many different postoperative complications that can occur, it must be noted that long-term follow-up data is still needed to monitor the complication rates of these procedures.[61] Overall, the 2 means by which the majority of complications can occur are those that are surgeon and/or orthodontist dependent and those that are patient dependent.

Those complications that are surgeon and/or orthodontist dependent can primarily depend on surgical technique and/or experience of the surgeon, poor treatment or surgical design, or excessive loading. Stripping of the interface between the bone and screw can occur during placement and can lead to mechanical failure of the screw during loading. This can also lead to complete loss of the screw head ultimately leaving the threaded portion of the screw embedded in bone (**Fig. 10**). Poor primary stability of the screw may occur in places with poor bone quality owing to patient-dependent factors or in areas known to have less quality bone such as those overlying the maxillary sinus. Individuals with less surgical experience may be more prone to complications such as wound dehiscence, hardware infection, or improper initial placement of miniscrews creating a hindrance in the initial orthodontic treatment plan. Root repair following contact by a miniscrew has also been studied and the quality of repair is associated with the damage caused by the miniscrew.[62] Orthodontist-dependent complications are those of improper loading putting too much stress on a miniscrew without proper distribution of forces or improper initial treatment planning creating undesirable force vectors leading to improper tooth or arch movements not initially intended.

Complications that occur owing to the patient are typically those of compliance or those with presurgical risk factors for complications such as poor wound healing associated with a medical history of diabetes, a history of radiation therapy, or bisphosphonate use. If patients fail to complete their initial antibiotic course or fail to continue proper oral hygiene with brushing and through the use of chlorhexidine rinses, there is an increased risk for infection of the surgical sites. Further, patients who smoke are also prone to mucosal breakdown, infection, and failure of the devices themselves.[2]

Despite these complications, the overall success rate for all orthodontic skeletal anchorage appliances was greater than 80%.[11] The success

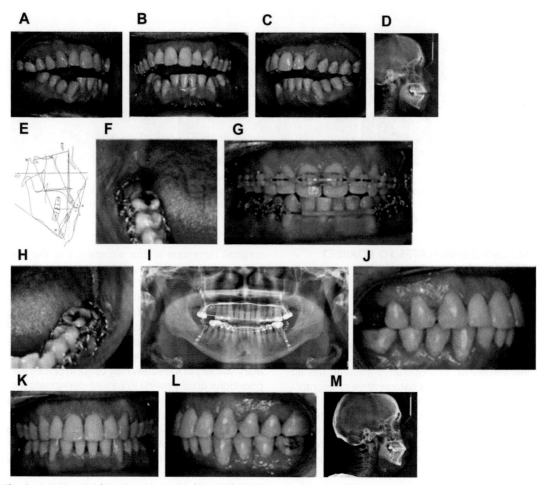

Fig. 9. A patient with an anterior open bite that developed with an unknown etiology who desired to not have orthognathic surgery. Posterior skeletal anchorage placed in the maxilla and mandible with miniplates. The open bite was then corrected by intrusion of posterior maxillary and mandibular dentition and eventually, and in much quicker time than traditional orthodontics, the anterior open bite is corrected with a total treatment time of 25 months. (*A–C*) Preoperative intraoral photographs. (*D, E*) Preoperative cephalometric radiograph and tracing demonstrating an anterior open bite. (*F–H*) Photographs of the skeletal anchorage in place after several weeks. (*I*) Panoramic radiograph demonstrating placement of skeletal anchorage. (*J–L*) Postorthodontic treatment intraoral photographs at the time of debanding. (*M*) Postorthodontic treatment cephalometric radiograph at the time of debanding. (*Courtesy of* Edward Ellis III, DDS, MS, San Antonio, TX.)

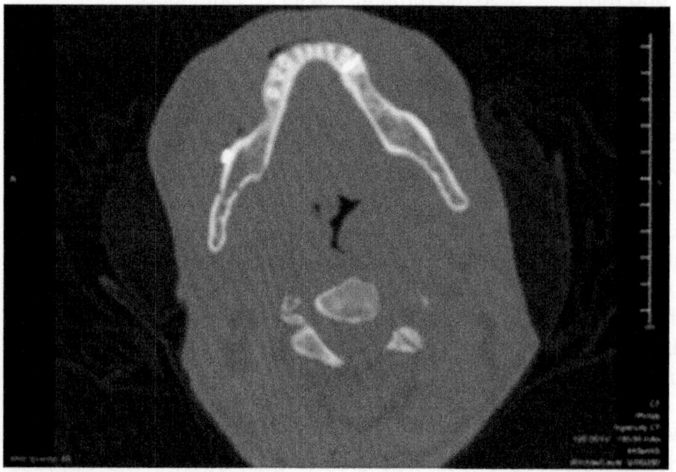

Fig. 10. Miniscrew with head stripped and broken during placement leaving the threaded portion of the screw embedded in bone between the left mandibular canine and first premolar.

rate is higher in the maxilla than in the mandible.[63,64] Palatal miniscrews have high success rates that are greater than 95%.[65,66] As discussed elsewhere in this article, longer miniscrews are more successful than shorter screws and proper location of placement is important for success.

FUTURE OF TEMPORARY SKELETAL ANCHORAGE DEVICES

Recently, virtual surgical planning has been described as a method for making surgical guides for the insertion of anchorage devices.[67] This strategy parallels the recent uptrend in using virtual surgical planning in orthognathic surgery and has the same surgical and planning advantages in the application of temporary skeletal anchorage.

SUMMARY

Skeletal anchorage allows the oral and maxillofacial surgeon and orthodontist to predictably make changes that were resorted to orthognathic surgery alone previously. Careful planning is to be discussed between the orthodontist and surgeon because this is not a technique that replaces orthognathic surgery and moderate to severe cases still require surgical correction. Ultimately, informed consent needs to be obtained explaining to the patient or their parents or surrogates that surgery may still be necessary if these techniques fail to obtain the desired outcomes. Although it is still a relatively new concept, it provides promise to the future of orthodontic treatment with relatively good literature to support its use in current practice today. The authors project that skeletal anchorage to be a growing field that allows for interdisciplinary collaboration in expanding the patient's and provider's repertoire of treatment options to allow a satisfactory end point of treatment as determined by the patient.

REFERENCES

1. Proffit WR, Fields HW, Larson BE, et al. Contemporary orthodontics.
2. Costello BJ, Ruiz RL, Petrone J, et al. Temporary skeletal anchorage devices for orthodontics. Oral Maxillofac Surg Clin North Am 2010;22(1):91–105.
3. Gainsforth BL, Higley LB. A study of orthodontic anchorage possibilities in basal bone. Am J Orthod Oral Surg 1945. https://doi.org/10.1016/0096-6347(45)90025-1.
4. Linkow LI. Endosseous blade-vent implants: A two-year report. J Prosthet Dent 1970. https://doi.org/10.1016/0022-3913(70)90011-9.
5. Smith JR. Bone dynamics associated with the controlled loading of bioglass-coated aluminum oxide endosteal implants. Am J Orthod 1979. https://doi.org/10.1016/0002-9416(79)90208-2.
6. Shapiro PA, Kokich VG. Uses of implants in orthodontics. Dent Clin North Am 1988;32(3):539–50.
7. Block MS, Hoffman DR. A new device for absolute anchorage for orthodontics. Am J Orthod Dentofacial Orthop 1995. https://doi.org/10.1016/S0889-5406(95)70140-0.
8. Costa A, Raffaini M, Melsen B. Miniscrews as orthodontic anchorage: a preliminary report. Int J Adult Orthodon Orthognath Surg 1998;13(3):201–9.
9. Umemori M, Sugawara J, Mitani H, et al. Skeletal anchorage system for open-bite correction. Am J Orthod Dentofacial Orthop 1999. https://doi.org/10.1016/S0889-5406(99)70345-8.
10. Leung MTC, Lee TCK, Rabie ABM, et al. Use of miniscrews and miniplates in orthodontics. J Oral Maxillofac Surg 2008;66(7):1461–6.
11. Kyung HM, Ly NTK, Hong M. Orthodontic skeletal anchorage: up-to-date review. Orthod Waves 2017;76(3):123–32.
12. Crismani AG, Bertl MH, Čelar AG, et al. Miniscrews in orthodontic treatment: review and analysis of published clinical trials. Am J Orthod Dentofacial Orthop 2010. https://doi.org/10.1016/j.ajodo.2008.01.027.
13. Ozkan S, Bayram M. Comparison of direct and indirect skeletal anchorage systems combined with 2 canine retraction techniques. Am J Orthod Dentofacial Orthop 2016. https://doi.org/10.1016/j.ajodo.2016.04.023.
14. Da Costa Grec RH, Janson G, Branco NC, et al. Intraoral distalizer effects with conventional and skeletal anchorage: a meta-analysis. Am J Orthod Dentofacial Orthop 2013. https://doi.org/10.1016/j.ajodo.2012.11.024.
15. Harzer W, Schneider M, Gedrange T. Rapid maxillary expansion with palatal anchorage of the hyrax expansion screw–pilot study with case presentation. J Orofac Orthop 2004. https://doi.org/10.1007/s00056-004-0346-7.
16. Garib Gamba D, Navarro De Lima R, Francischone CE, et al. Rapid maxillary expansion using palatal implants. J Clin Orthod 2008;42(11):665–71.
17. Roth A, Yildirim M, Diedrich P. Forced eruption with microscrew anchorage for preprosthetic leveling of the gingival margin. Case report. J Orofac Orthop 2004. https://doi.org/10.1007/s00056-004-0430-z.
18. Da Costa Filho LC, Soria ML, De Lima EM, et al. Orthodontic extrusion anchored in osseointegrated implants: a case report. Gen Dent 2004;52(5):416–8.
19. Ödman J, Lekholm U, Jemt T, et al. Osseointegrated implants as orthodontic anchorage in the treatment of partially edentulous adult patients. Eur J Orthod 1994. https://doi.org/10.1093/ejo/16.3.187.

20. Creekmore TD, Eklund MK. The possibility of skeletal anchorage. J Clin Orthod 1983;17(4):266–9. Available at: https://www.unboundmedicine.com/medline/citation/6574142/The_possibility_of_skeletal_anchorage.
21. Xun CL, Zhao H, Zeng XL, et al. Intrusion of overerupted maxillary molars with miniscrew implant anchorage: a radiographic evaluation. J Huazhong Univ Sci Technolog Med Sci 2013. https://doi.org/10.1007/s11596-013-1197-5.
22. Kyung H-M, Park H-S, Bae S-M, et al. The lingual plain-wire system with micro-implant anchorage. J Clin Orthod 2004;38(7):388–95.
23. Hong RK, Heo JM, Ha YK. Lever-arm and mini-implant system for anterior torque control during retraction in lingual orthodontic treatment. Angle Orthod 2005. https://doi.org/10.1043/0003-3219(2005)075<0129:LAMSFA>2.0.CO;2.
24. Henry PJ, Singer S. Implant anchorage for the occlusal management of developmental defects in children: a preliminary report. Pract Periodontics Aesthet Dent 1999;11(6):699–706 [quiz: 708].
25. Enacar A, Giray B, Pehlivanoglu M, et al. Facemask therapy with rigid anchorage in a patient with maxillary hypoplasia and severe oligodontia. Am J Orthod Dentofacial Orthop 2003. https://doi.org/10.1016/S0889-5406(03)00052-0.
26. Kyung S-H, Choi J-H, Park Y-C. Miniscrew anchorage used to protract lower second molars into first molar extraction sites. J Clin Orthod 2003;37(10):575–9. Available at: https://www.unboundmedicine.com/medline/citation/14617846/Miniscrew_anchorage_used_to_protract_lower_second_molars_into_first_molar_extraction_sites.
27. Mimura H. Protraction of mandibular second and third molars assisted by partial corticision and miniscrew anchorage. Am J Orthod Dentofacial Orthop 2013. https://doi.org/10.1016/j.ajodo.2012.08.030.
28. Park H-S, Kwon O-W, Sung J-H. Microscrew implant anchorage sliding mechanics. World J Orthod 2005; 6(3):265–74.
29. Wahabuddin S, Mascarenhas R, Iqbal M, et al. Clinical Application of Micro-Implant Anchorage in Initial Orthodontic Retraction. J Oral Implantol 2015. https://doi.org/10.1563/AAID-JOI-D-12-00227.
30. Allgayer S, Platcheck D, Vargas IA, et al. Mini-implants: mechanical resource for molars uprighting. Dental Press J Orthod 2013. https://doi.org/10.1590/S2176-94512013000100025.
31. Lehnen S, McDonald F, Bourauel C, et al. Patient expectations, acceptance and preferences in treatment with orthodontic mini-implants: a randomly controlled study on insertion techniques. J Orofac Orthop 2011. https://doi.org/10.1007/s00056-011-0013-8 [in English, German].
32. Kapila SD, Nervina JM. CBCT in orthodontics: assessment of treatment outcomes and indications for its use. Dentomaxillofac Radiol 2015;44(1). https://doi.org/10.1259/dmfr.20140282.
33. Habeeb M, Boucher N, Chung C-H. Effects of rapid palatal expansion on the sagittal and vertical dimensions of the maxilla: a study on cephalograms derived from cone-beam computed tomography. Am J Orthod Dentofacial Orthop 2013;144(3): 398–403.
34. Woller JL, Kim KB, Behrents RG, et al. An assessment of the maxilla after rapid maxillary expansion using cone beam computed tomography in growing children. Dental Press J Orthod 2014; 19(1):26–35.
35. Kraus CD, Campbell PM, Spears R, et al. Bony adaptation after expansion with light-to-moderate continuous forces. Am J Orthod Dentofacial Orthop 2014;145(5):655–66.
36. Kanomi R, Deguchi T, Kakuno E, et al. CBCT of skeletal changes following rapid maxillary expansion to increase arch-length with a development-dependent bonded or banded appliance. Angle Orthod 2013. https://doi.org/10.2319/082012-669.1.
37. Wertz RA. Skeletal and dental changes accompanying rapid midpalatal suture opening. Am J Orthod 1970;58(1):41–66.
38. Lim HM, Park YC, Lee KJ, et al. Stability of dental, alveolar, and skeletal changes after miniscrew-assisted rapid palatal expansion. Korean J Orthod 2017;47(5):313–22.
39. Cantarella D, Dominguez-Mompell R, Moschik C, et al. Midfacial changes in the coronal plane induced by microimplant-supported skeletal expander, studied with cone-beam computed tomography images. Am J Orthod Dentofacial Orthop 2018. https://doi.org/10.1016/j.ajodo.2017.11.033.
40. Sherwood KH, Burch JG, Thompson WJ. Closing anterior open bites by intruding molars with titanium miniplate anchorage. Am J Orthod Dentofacial Orthop 2002. https://doi.org/10.1067/mod.2002.128641.
41. Sherwood KH, Burch J, Thompson W. Intrusion of supererupted molars with titanium miniplate anchorage. Angle Orthod 2003. https://doi.org/10.1043/0003-3219(2003)073<0597:IOSMWT>2.0.CO;2.
42. Cornelis MA, Scheffler NR, De Clerck HJ, et al. Systematic review of the experimental use of temporary skeletal anchorage devices in orthodontics. Am J Orthod Dentofacial Orthop 2007;131(4 SUPPL): 52–8.
43. Jenner JD, Fitzpatrick BN. Skeletal anchorage utilising bone plates. Aust Orthod J 1985;9(2):231–3. Available at: https://www.unboundmedicine.com/medline/citation/3870084/Skeletal_anchorage_utilising_bone_plates.
44. Sugawara J, Kanzaki R, Takahashi I, et al. Distal movement of maxillary molars in nongrowing patients with the skeletal anchorage system. Am J

Orthod Dentofacial Orthop 2006. https://doi.org/10.1016/j.ajodo.2005.08.036.
45. Fukunaga T, Kuroda S, Kurosaka H, et al. Skeletal anchorage for orthodontic correction of maxillary protrusion with adult periodontitis. Angle Orthod 2006. https://doi.org/10.1043/0003-3219(2006)076[0148:SAFOCO]2.0.CO;2.
46. Sherwood KH, Burch JG. Skeletally based miniplate supported orthodontic anchorage. J Oral Maxillofac Surg 2005;63(2):279–84.
47. Kircelli BH, Pektaş ZO, Uçkan S. Orthopedic protraction with skeletal anchorage in a patient with maxillary hypoplasia and hypodontia. Angle Orthod 2006. https://doi.org/10.1043/0003-3219(2006)076[0156:OPWSAI]2.0.CO;2.
48. De Clerck H, Geerinckx V, Siciliano S. The zygoma anchorage system. J Clin Orthod 2002;36(8):455–9. Available at: http://www.ncbi.nlm.nih.gov/pubmed/12271935.
49. Bengi AO, Karacay S, Akin E, et al. Use of zygomatic anchors during rapid canine distalization: a preliminary case report. Angle Orthod 2006. https://doi.org/10.1043/0003-3219(2006)076[0137:UOZADR]2.0.CO;2.
50. Cha BK, Choi DS, Ngan P, et al. Maxillary protraction with miniplates providing skeletal anchorage in a growing Class III patient. Am J Orthod Dentofacial Orthop 2011. https://doi.org/10.1016/j.ajodo.2009.06.025.
51. Altug Z, Arslan AD. Skeletal and Dental Effects of a Mini Maxillary Protraction Appliance 2006;76:360–8.
52. Kircelli BH, Pektas ZÖ. Midfacial protraction with skeletally anchored face mask therapy: a novel approach and preliminary results. Am J Orthod Dentofacial Orthop 2008;133(3):440–9.
53. Elnagar MH, Elshourbagy E, Ghobashy S, et al. Comparative evaluation of 2 skeletally anchored maxillary protraction protocols. Am J Orthod Dentofacial Orthop 2016;150(5):751–62.
54. Elnagar MH, Elshourbagy E, Ghobashy S, et al. Dentoalveolar and arch dimension changes in patients treated with miniplate-anchored maxillary protraction. Am J Orthod Dentofacial Orthop 2017;151(6):1092–106.
55. Elnagar MH, Mohammed H, Khedr M, et al. Three-dimensional assessment of soft tissue changes associated with bone-anchored maxillary protraction protocols. Am J Orthod Dentofacial Orthop 2017;152(3):336–47.
56. O'Brien K, Wright J, Conboy F, et al. Effectiveness of treatment for class II malocclusion with the Herbst or twin-block appliances: a randomized, controlled trial. Am J Orthod Dentofacial Orthop 2003;124(2):128–37.
57. Papadopoulos MA. In: Papadopoulos MA, editor. Skeletal anchorage in orthodontic treatment of class II malocclusion. Elsevier; 2015. https://doi.org/10.1016/C2009-0-63214-1.
58. Manni A, Mutinelli S, Pasini M, et al. Herbst appliance anchored to miniscrews with 2 types of ligation: effectiveness in skeletal class II treatment. Am J Orthod Dentofacial Orthop 2016;149(6):871–80.
59. Aslan BI, Kucukkaraca E, Turkoz C, et al. Treatment effects of the Forsus Fatigue Resistant Device used with miniscrew anchorage. Angle Orthod 2014;84(1):76–87.
60. Al-Dumaini AA, Halboub E, Alhammadi MS, et al. A novel approach for treatment of skeletal Class II malocclusion: miniplates-based skeletal anchorage. Am J Orthod Dentofacial Orthop 2018;153(2):239–47.
61. Lai EHH, Yao CCJ, Chang JZC, et al. Three-dimensional dental model analysis of treatment outcomes for protrusive maxillary dentition: comparison of headgear, miniscrew, and miniplate skeletal anchorage. Am J Orthod Dentofacial Orthop 2008. https://doi.org/10.1016/j.ajodo.2007.05.017.
62. Alves M, Baratieri C, Mattos CT, et al. Root repair after contact with mini-implants: systematic review of the literature. Eur J Orthod 2013. https://doi.org/10.1093/ejo/cjs025.
63. Samrit V, Kharbanda OP, Duggal R, et al. Bone density and miniscrew stability in orthodontic patients. Aust Orthod J 2012;28(2):204–12.
64. Suzuki M, Deguchi T, Watanabe H, et al. Evaluation of optimal length and insertion torque for miniscrews. Am J Orthod Dentofacial Orthop 2013. https://doi.org/10.1016/j.ajodo.2013.03.021.
65. Karagkiolidou A, Ludwig B, Pazera P, et al. Survival of palatal miniscrews used for orthodontic appliance anchorage: a retrospective cohort study. Am J Orthod Dentofacial Orthop 2013. https://doi.org/10.1016/j.ajodo.2013.01.018.
66. Lee J, Miyazawa K, Tabuchi M, et al. Midpalatal miniscrews and high-pull headgear for anteroposterior and vertical anchorage control: cephalometric comparisons of treatment changes. Am J Orthod Dentofacial Orthop 2013. https://doi.org/10.1016/j.ajodo.2013.03.020.
67. Antunes KT, d'Ornellas MC, Noedel DD, et al. Three dimensional virtual planning through cone beam computed tomography for surgical guidance production. Stud Health Technol Inform 2017. https://doi.org/10.3233/978-1-61499-830-3-1250.

Interceptive Dentofacial Orthopedics (Growth Modification)

Jennifer Caplin, DMD, MS[a,*], Michael D. Han, DDS[b],
Michael Miloro, DMD, MD[b], Veerasathpurush Allareddy, BDS, PhD[a],
Michael R. Markiewicz, DDS, MPH, MD[c]

KEYWORDS

- Dentofacial deformity • Skeletal malocclusion • Growth modification • Growth assessment
- Dentofacial orthopedics • Orthognathic surgery

KEY POINTS

- Considering growth when managing dentofacial deformities is key, especially when determining the timing and type of treatment.
- The clinician must be familiar with growth evaluation and interceptive orthopedic options for the management of dentofacial deformities.
- Understanding the options available for growth modification and the ideal timing for correction of various dentofacial deformities allows the clinician to provide the most appropriate care for patients.

INTRODUCTION

Facial growth is a key consideration in the management of dentofacial deformities and skeletal malocclusions. Some deformities may be intercepted and managed during growth, whereas others can only be definitively managed after cessation of growth. The clinician must be cognizant of the significance of growth, and not view the dentofacial deformity as a snapshot. This article focuses on clinical considerations of growth in managing dentofacial deformities, and discusses methods to evaluate the status of growth, and management considerations for different types of dentofacial deformities in the context of growth modification.

GROWTH EVALUATION

Evaluation of growth is critical in determining the timing and type of treatment of dentofacial deformities. In the growing patient growth modification can be considered, which may minimize surgical movements, or even obviate surgery altogether. In the nongrowing patient, verifying cessation of growth is essential in minimizing relapse of Class III correction from latent mandibular growth.[1]

This section discusses evaluation of growth as it pertains to clinical management: anteroposterior growth of the mandible and anteroposterior and transverse growth of the maxilla (**Table 1**).

Disclosure Statement: The authors have nothing to disclose.

[a] Department of Orthodontics, University of Illinois at Chicago, 801 South Paulina Street, M/C 841, Chicago, IL 60612, USA; [b] Department of Oral and Maxillofacial Surgery, University of Illinois at Chicago, 801 South Paulina Street, M/C 835, Chicago, IL 60612, USA; [c] Department of Oral and Maxillofacial Surgery, School of Dental Medicine, University at Buffalo, 112 Squire Hall, Buffalo, NY 14214, USA
* Corresponding author.
E-mail address: jcapli3@uic.edu

Oral Maxillofacial Surg Clin N Am 32 (2020) 39–51
https://doi.org/10.1016/j.coms.2019.08.006
1042-3699/20/

Table 1
Comparison of growth prediction methods

	Advantages	Disadvantages
Maxilla		
Clinical examination	Noninvasive Minimal use of resources	Difficult to quantify and analyze
Chronologic age	Easy, noninvasive No resources required	Lacks ability to account for individual variations
Cephalometric analysis	Easy access Easy interpretation	Ionizing radiation if not using existing routine cephalometric radiograph
Cone beam computed tomography	Quantifiable 3-dimensional analysis possible Improved ability to account for individual variations, especially in transverse growth	Ionizing radiation Varying levels of access and cost
Mandible		
Hand-wrist radiographs	Good correlation with mandibular growth Easy access and straightforward interpretation	Ionizing radiation
Third finger middle phalanx maturation	Satisfactory correlation with mandibular growth Easy access and interpretation Minimizes ionizing radiation	Variable sensitivity
Cervical vertebrae	Use of existing routine cephalometric imaging	Questionable reproducibility
Dental development	Use of existing routine imaging (eg, panoramic radiograph) Straightforward interpretation	Unreliable
Biomarkers	Quantifiable Relatively noninvasive	Unclear accuracy with limited evidence Cost and availability
Special imaging (eg, scintigraphy)	Useful adjunct for abnormal growth (eg, hemimandibular hyperplasia)	Ionizing radiation Cost and availability

Mandibular Growth

When discussing mandibular growth in the context of dentofacial deformity management, a distinction must be made between timing of growth and growth cessation. Timing of growth, such as peak growth during puberty, is significant because it can guide the clinician in determining the timing and type of growth modification treatment of skeletal Class II or Class III deformities. However, verifying cessation of growth is required when managing a skeletal Class III deformity with mandibular prognathism to minimize the risk of relapse from latent mandibular growth after surgical correction.

Various methods have been developed to assess mandibular growth. With the exception of superimposition of serial lateral cephalometric radiographs, all of these methods are indirect assessments of mandibular growth. Commonly used methods involve the hand and wrist, cervical vertebrae, dental development, statural height, and secondary sex characteristics. Other methods using biomarkers and special imaging have also been described. Some of these methods are used without serial comparisons, although serial comparisons yield greater accuracy.

Hand-wrist radiographs

The most commonly used technique is the hand-wrist maturation method (HWM) (**Fig. 1**). Originally described by Todd in 1937, various modifications have been proposed. Studies that have attempted to correlate variations of the HWM

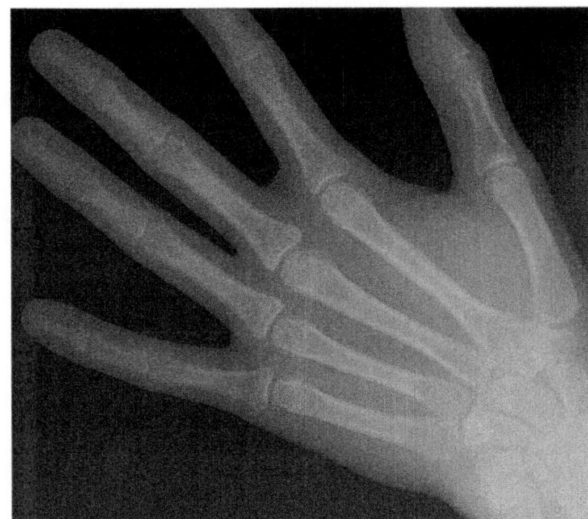

Fig. 1. Hand-wrist radiograph.

with peak mandibular growth have shown reasonable correlation.[2,3]

The third finger middle phalanx maturation method has been described as an alternative to HWM.[4–6] Longitudinal correlations with peak mandibular growth have shown satisfactory correlation, but with some variability in sensitivity, as is the case in other evaluation methods. The advantages of this method include easy access and execution, straightforward interpretation, and decreased radiation compared with the HWM, because it is obtained using standard periapical films.

Cervical vertebrae

The cervical vertebral maturation method (CVM) was originally introduced by Lamparski (**Fig. 2**). Several variations followed. This method is attractive in that no additional radiographs need to be taken because the analysis is performed on lateral cephalometric images. Despite this advantage, longitudinal studies have shown weaker correlation with mandibular growth when compared with hand radiograph-based methods. Also, some studies have shown poor intrarater reliability, further questioning the utility of this method.[7,8] Although this method should be used with caution, it may be appropriate to use as an adjunct to other analyses, because the CVM can be done without need for additional imaging.

Dental development

Timing of primary tooth exfoliation and permanent tooth eruption and dental maturation, such as calcification and root development, have been described as means to assess mandibular growth.[9–12] However, various studies have shown unsatisfactory correlations with mandibular growth.[13]

Statural height and secondary sex characteristics

Statural height and secondary sex characteristics, such as menarche for females and voice changes for males, have been studied in relation to mandibular growth.[3,14] No strong evidence exists that these are suitable methods to assess mandibular growth, leaving these methods only as adjunctive screening tools.

Biomarkers

Some biomarkers have been studied as potential indicators for mandibular growth. These include serum IGF-1, IGFBP-3, and gingival crevicular fluid biomarkers.[15,16] Only one study attempted to correlate a biomarker (IGF-1) with mandibular growth, where mild to moderate correlation was shown.[17] Other studies involving IGF-1, IGFBP-3,[18] and gingival crevicular fluid alkaline phosphatase[16] have shown statistically significant correlations with CVM stages, but not with mandibular growth. Although there is potential for biomarkers to be used in growth assessment, current evidence does not seem to justify the resources and cost.

Special imaging

Bone scintigraphy has been described as a method of assessing mandibular growth by analyzing the blood flow and metabolic activity in different parts of the mandible.[19] However, occasional use of this method is largely limited to special circumstances, such as hemimandibular hyperplasia or mandibular condylar hyperplasia, where the status of abnormal growth is critical in determining the optimal timing and method of surgical correction.[20–22]

Maxillary Growth

Unlike the mandible, methods to monitor sagittal growth of the maxilla are limited, and are largely restricted to clinical examination and routine cephalometric analyses. Instead, the focus of growth evaluation of the maxilla is typically on the axial plane for transverse discrepancies. The most common methods used for this purpose are chronologic age and imaging.

Chronologic age

Use of chronologic age is based on classical studies on cadaveric specimens, in which cessation of palatal sutural growth and subsequent

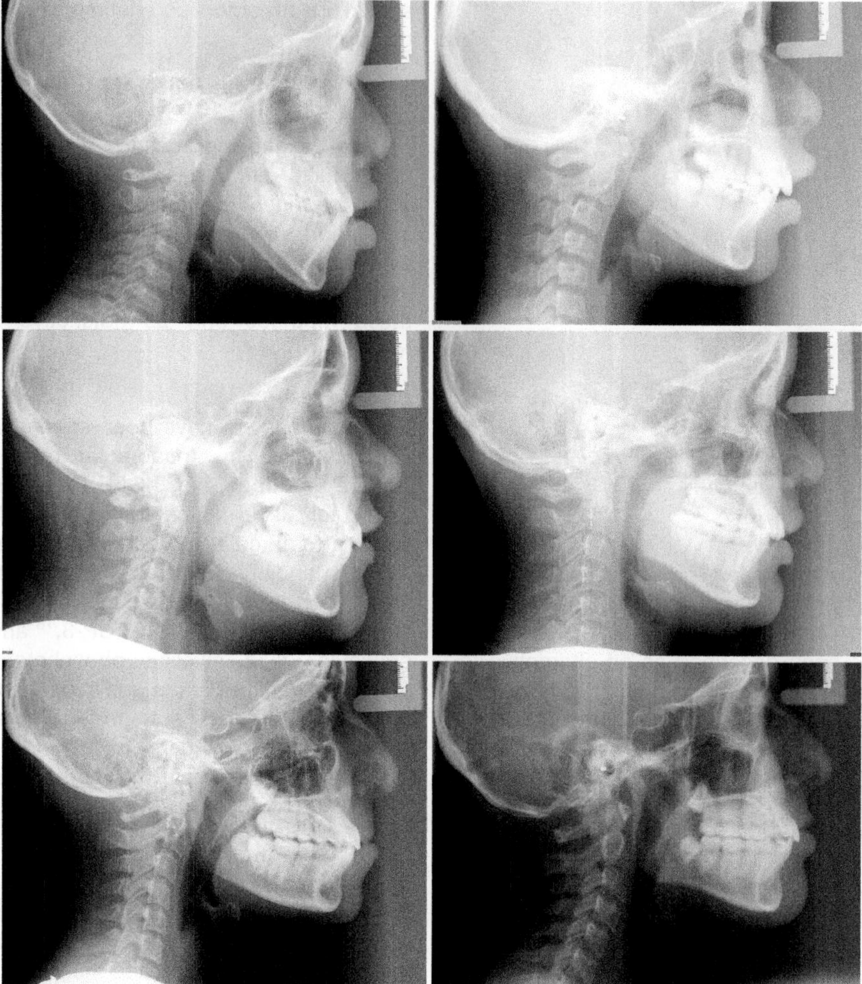

Fig. 2. Examples of cervical vertebra evaluation from stage 1 to 6.

apposition were noted to occur at predictable age groups for each sex.[23,24] Chronologic age is perhaps the most widely used evaluation strategy for maxillary transverse management. Although this is a reasonable and accepted method, some clinical studies involving different nonsurgical expansion techniques challenge this traditional view.[25–27]

Imaging

Some authors have suggested use of cone beam computed tomography as a means to assess midpalatal suture maturity in a more accurate and patient-specific manner.[28–30] Because of ease of access and its increasing routine use in nonsurgical orthodontics and dentofacial orthopedics, cone beam computed tomography–based evaluation methods show promise as adjunctive tools.

PALATAL EXPANSION

Palatal expansion has many uses in orthodontics. It is used to correct posterior crossbites, increase arch circumference to aid in crowding resolution, and increase arch width to improve smile esthetics, among others.

Rapid Expansion Versus Slow Expansion

There are two main types of expansion: slow and rapid. Rapid expansion involves the use of a fixed expander that is typically activated by an expansion screw that is turned one to two times per day by the patient or parents. Rapid expansion splits the maxillary sutures, allowing for true skeletal expansion of the maxilla (**Fig. 3**).[31] Slow expansion is typically achieved via arch development, applying gentle buccal pressure to teeth to encourage development of alveolar bone. Slow

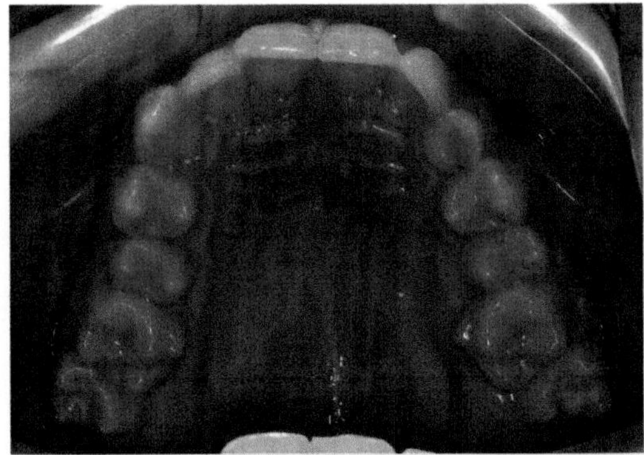
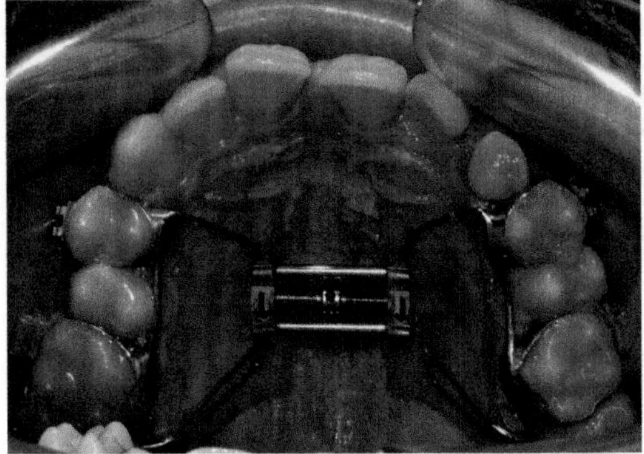

Fig. 3. Patient treated with rapid palatal expansion. Note the diastema between the upper central incisors, which indicates a separation of the midpalatal suture.

expansion does not orthopedically expand the maxilla. Instead, it results in increased width of the dental arch. Both rapid and slow expansion are effective and stable.[32–34]

Treatment Timing

The best time to rapidly expand the palate is during the growth period.[35–38] There is some evidence, however, that sutural expansion is achieved in adults.[25] Surgically assisted expansion has historically been recommended for many patients who require expansion as adults. Although this remains an excellent option, the use of bone anchored expanders offers a less invasive option (see skeletal anchorage in Jason P. Jones and colleagues' article, "Temporary Skeletal Anchorage Techniques," in this issue).

CLASS II

Class II malocclusions are the most common type of skeletal malocclusion.[39] Because of their prevalence, orthodontists must be proficient at diagnosing and treatment planning the myriad presentations of Class IIs, in growing and nongrowing patients. When approached correctly, with proper diagnosis and mechanics, most Class II malocclusions can be treated orthodontically.

Treatment Timing

The best time to correct a Class II is during the pubertal growth phase. Growth modification coupled with dentoalveolar change is effective, efficient, predictable, and stable if performed during the pubertal growth spurt and can be achieved with a single phase of orthodontic treatment.[40–46]

Class II correction is achieved during the mixed dentition phase using headgear, functional appliances, or other Class II correctors. However, this correction has not been shown to be stable. After Class II correction in the mixed dentition the patient continues to grow in a Class II skeletal pattern, resulting in relapse and the need for a second phase of orthodontic treatment.[41,42] The primary benefit to early Class II correction is a decrease in the rate of trauma to the upper incisors.[47,48]

After growth cessation, growth modification is no longer available as a treatment option. The only modes of Class II correction include dentoalveolar movements with or without extraction of teeth, or orthognathic surgery.[49]

Growth modification

Headgear Headgear applies a backward force to the maxilla, restricting forward growth and thereby allowing the mandible to grow into a Class I relationship.[50] The headgear can also be used to distalize maxillary molars in growing and nongrowing patients.[51] This is the appliance of choice for patients with a protrusive maxilla and well-positioned mandible. Additionally, because it does not apply force to the mandible or mandibular teeth, side effects that are common with many other Class II correctors, such as proclination of the lower incisors, does not occur.

Functional appliances A functional appliance is an appliance that postures the mandible forward. These appliances are either fixed or removable, and selection is based on the age of the patient, the severity of the Class II, patient compliance, and operator preference. By posturing the mandible forward into a Class I occlusion, any remaining growth potential in the mandible is encouraged to occur in a horizontal direction (**Fig. 4**). There is also some evidence that this posturing of the mandible encourages remodeling of the condyle and the glenoid fossa to displace the body of the

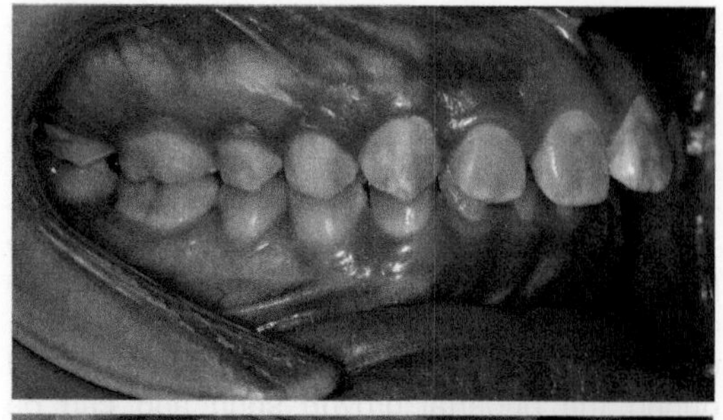

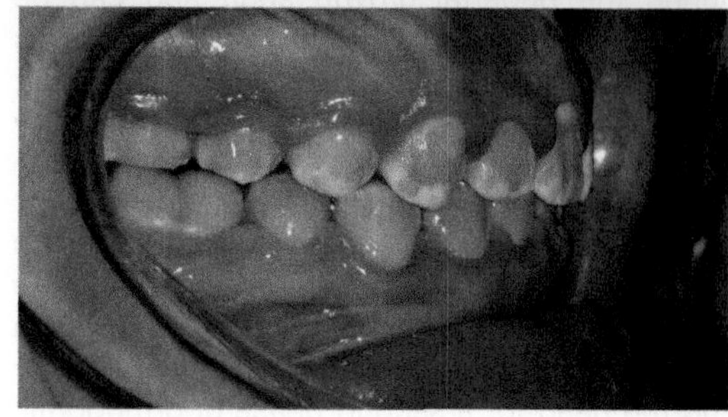

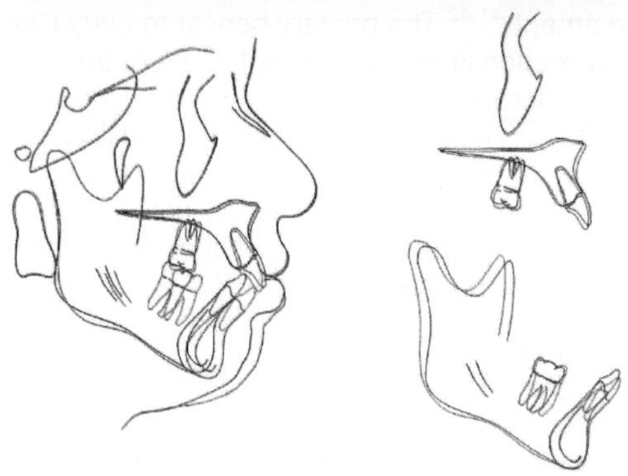

Fig. 4. Class II patient with significant growth potential treated with a functional appliance.

mandible into a more anterior position, but this is controversial.[52–54] Functional appliances can also exert a "headgear effect" on the maxilla. By applying a backward force to the maxilla as a counterforce to the protrusion of the mandible, maxillary growth restriction is observed.[49] Although skeletal change is the most desired effect of functional appliances, the quantity and stability of these effects are debated in the literature.[55]

An important role of functional appliances is their ability to induce dentoalveolar change. Functional appliances apply a distalizing force to maxillary teeth, resulting in distalization of molars and retroclination of upper incisors. The mesial force on mandibular teeth mesializes mandibular molars and proclines and protrudes lower incisors.[56] These changes effectively correct a Class II, and this correction is stable. Class II elastics are the simplest functional appliance. They induce a similar dentoalveolar effect and are effective at correcting Class II malocclusions (**Fig. 5**).[57]

Nongrowth modification

For patients who have ceased growing, the options for correcting a Class II decrease. Extraction of maxillary first premolars is a common solution to eliminate excess overjet. Maxillary canines are retracted into a Class I position while the Class II molar is maintained (**Fig. 6**). Extraction of upper first premolars and lower second premolars can also be used to aid in Class II correction and crowding resolution. Another option is distalization of maxillary teeth into a Class I occlusion. These changes are entirely dentoalveolar and are used in growing patients and nongrowing patients depending on the patient's need. If skeletal change or significant profile

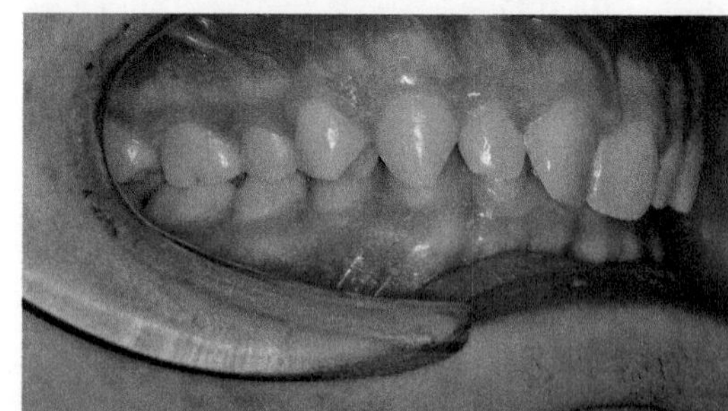

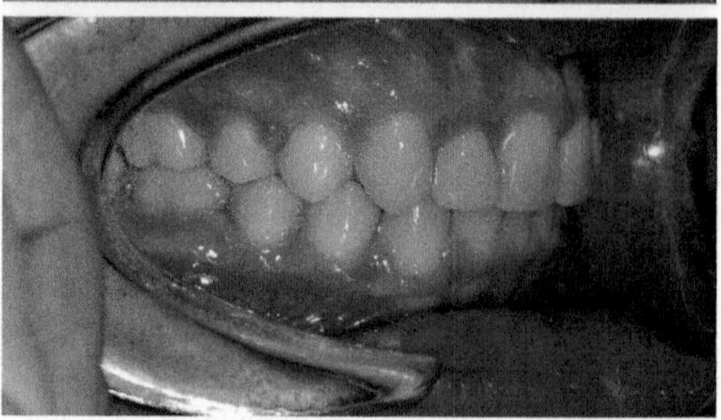

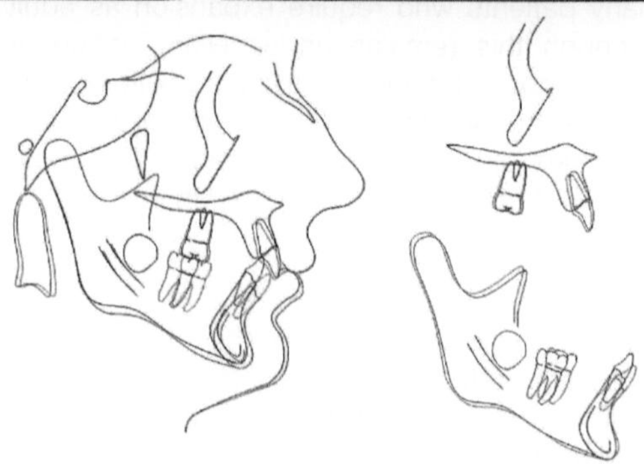

Fig. 5. Class II patient with limited growth potential treated with a functional appliance.

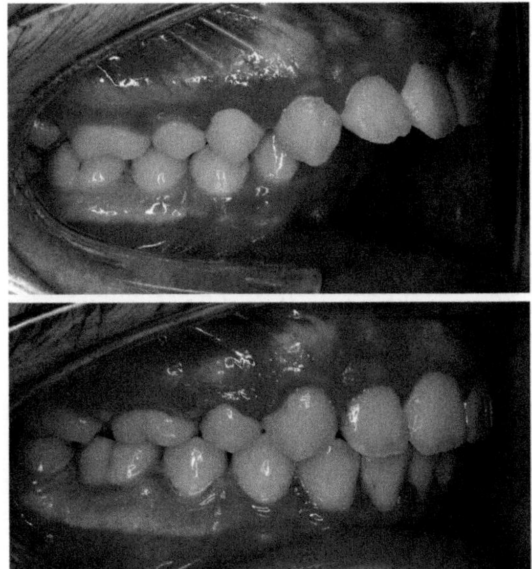

Fig. 6. Nongrowing Class II patient treated with upper first premolar extractions.

change is desired in nongrowers, orthognathic surgery is recommended.[58]

CLASS III

Class III patients present a special challenge for orthodontists. The mandible is one of the last bones to cease growing, and controlling this growth is highly complex. Predicting the magnitude of mandibular growth, and thereby predicting the eventual severity of a skeletal Class III in a growing patient, is poorly understood and unreliable. Many Class III patients must either remain in active orthodontic treatment for many years while the orthodontist attempts to control growth, or the patient must live through the formative years of high school with a visible Class III while waiting for growth cessation and orthognathic surgery. In many severe Class III cases, orthodontics alone is insufficient and orthognathic surgery is required to properly correct a skeletal Class III.

Reverse Pull Headgear

The maxilla is a much more plastic bone than the mandible because of the abundance of maxillary sutures. The reverse pull headgear, or facemask, is an extraoral orthopedic device that encourages downward and forward growth of the maxilla to mimic the natural growth pattern of the human face (**Fig. 7**). The reverse pull headgear is a highly effective appliance for decreasing the severity of a skeletal Class III,

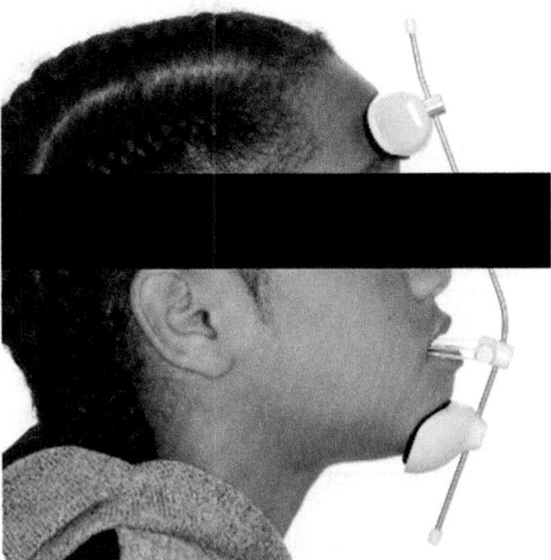

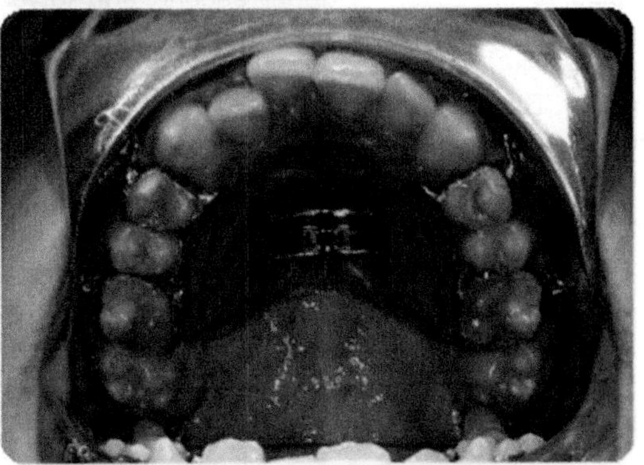

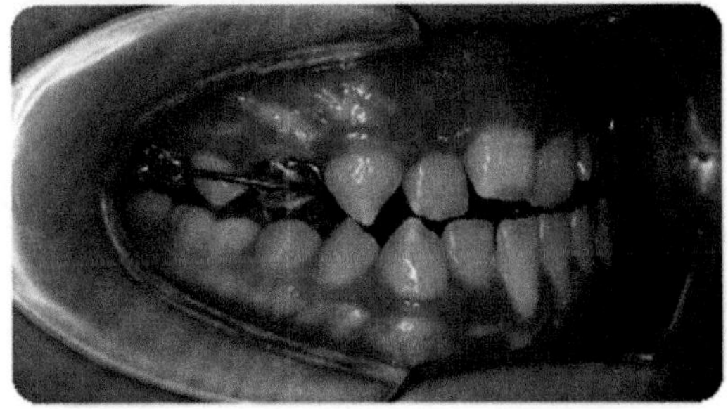

Fig. 7. Class III patient wearing a reverse pull headgear. Elastics are worn from an intraoral anchorage unit to the reverse pull headgear. Note the downward and forward elastic vector to mimic a normal growth pattern.

especially if used during the mixed dentition.[59–64] The earlier the reverse pull headgear is used, the more effective it is at encouraging orthopedic growth of the maxilla.[59] Achieving Class III correction during pubertal growth is more effective with skeletal anchorage (see skeletal anchorage in Jason P. Jones and colleagues' article, "Temporary Skeletal Anchorage

Techniques," in this issue.) Early correction with a reverse pull headgear is stable and decreases the likelihood that the patient will require orthognathic surgery in the future (**Fig. 8**).[60,65–68] The correction achieved is just as stable as correction with Le Fort I advancement.[69] Use of the reverse pull headgear also results in positive long-term profile changes.[70]

Dental Camouflage

In patients with mild Class III malocclusions, dental camouflage is used in place of orthognathic surgery. Proclination of upper incisors and retroclination of lower incisors can mask a Class III skeletal pattern (**Fig. 9**). Care must be taken to avoid dehiscence of incisor roots and to obtain a functional and esthetic result. Various extraction patterns can also be used to aid in dental camouflage, including extraction of upper second and lower first premolars, extraction of lower first premolars exclusively (**Fig. 10**), or extraction of a lower incisor. Dental camouflage is only recommended for patients who are past their peak growth period, because premature camouflage can lead to worsening problems if the Class III growth pattern continues.

Decompensation Before Orthognathic Surgery

Despite the effectiveness of early Class III correction, some patients still require orthognathic surgery to correct their severe Class III malocclusion.[68] These patients typically present with similar dental patterns. The upper incisors are often proclined and the lower incisors are retroclined as a natural compensation to the existing negative overjet.

Before orthognathic surgery, the orthodontist attempts to correct the natural compensation of the incisors and obtain ideal incisor angulation. This process is called "decompensation" (**Fig. 11**). Decompensation involves orthodontically increasing negative overjet before orthognathic surgery by moving the incisors into the final desired angulation. This allows for increased skeletal movement during the surgical procedure,

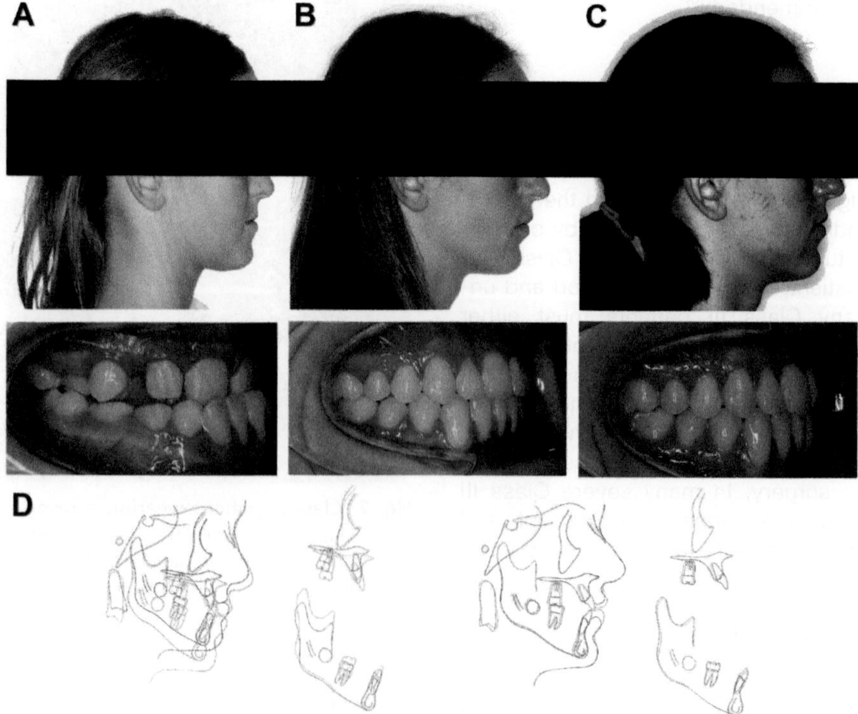

Fig. 8. Long-term follow-up of a Class III patient treated with a reverse pull headgear. (*A*) Initial (T1): the patient was 9 years, 4 months old when treatment began. (*B*) Final (T2): the patient wore a reverse pull headgear for 22 months. The total treatment time, including reverse pull headgear and comprehensive orthodontic treatment, was 38 months. (*C*) Retention (T3): the patient was brought back for a retention visit 26 months after debonding. The results are stable with no maxillary growth and minimal mandibular growth. The patient was 14 years, 9 months old at this retention visit and is unlikely to exhibit significant future growth. (*D*) Superimpositions for T1-T2 and T2-T3.

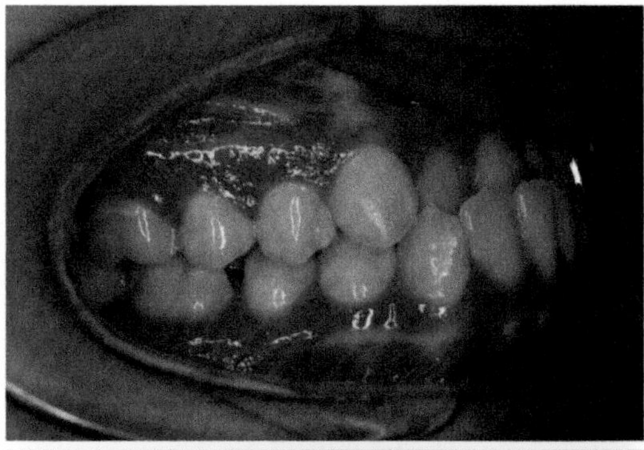

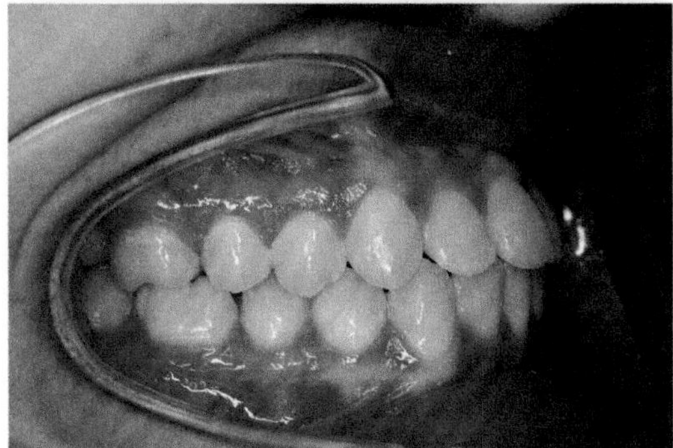

Fig. 9. Patient with a mild Class III malocclusion treated with dental camouflage.

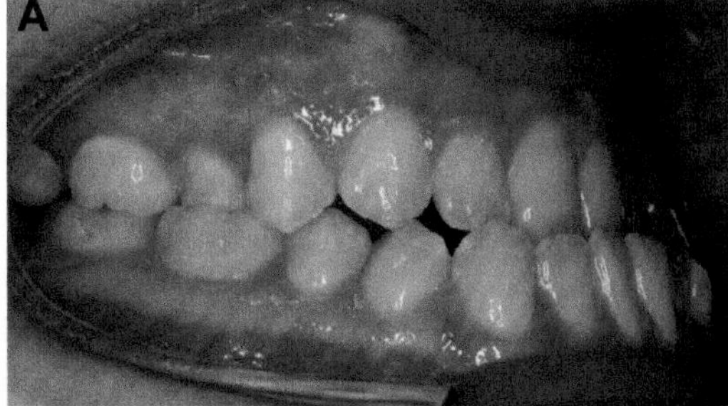

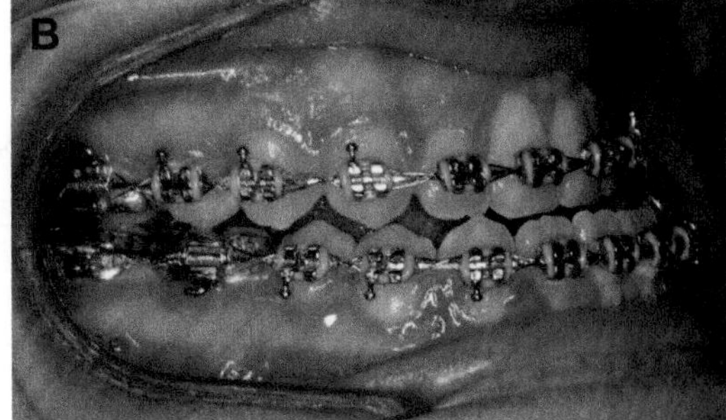

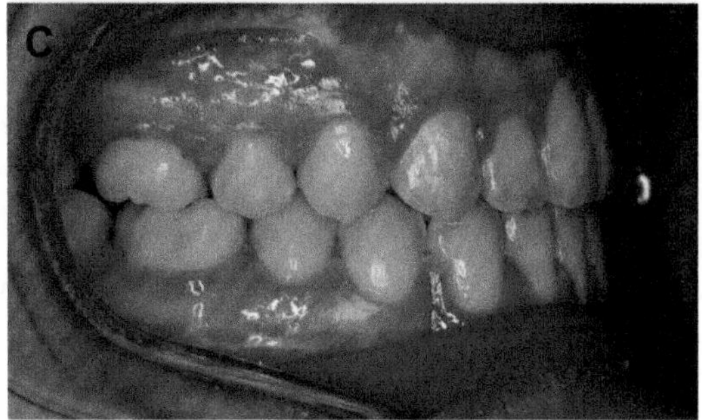

Fig. 11. (*A*) Class III surgical patient, (*B*) decompensated before orthognathic surgery, and (*C*) occlusion after two-jaw orthognathic surgical procedure.

and results in a more esthetic outcome postsurgery. Before orthognathic surgery, the surgeon and the orthodontist should collaborate to determine the desired amount of negative overjet that will allow the surgeon to obtain the optimal profile change.

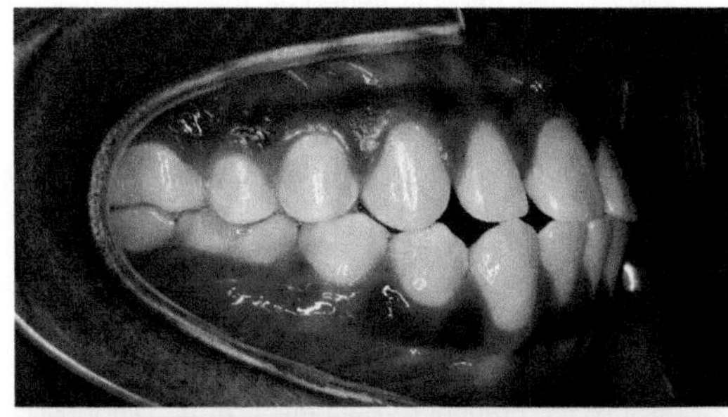

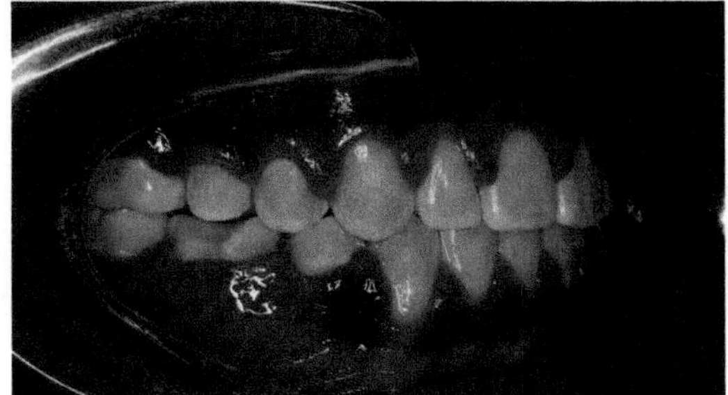

Fig. 10. A patient with a 100% Class III malocclusion treated with lower first premolar extractions.

SUMMARY

Although all dentofacial deformities involve deviation of skeletal and dental units that require correction, the timing and method of treatment can vary considerably (**Fig. 12**). Because some dentofacial deformities can effectively be managed by growth modification, the clinician must constantly make an effort to evaluate growth and determine appropriate management strategies. Having a firm understanding of the role of growth and dentofacial orthopedics is especially important for the oral and maxillofacial surgeon, who may encounter growing patients with dentofacial deformities that could benefit from interceptive dentofacial orthopedics.

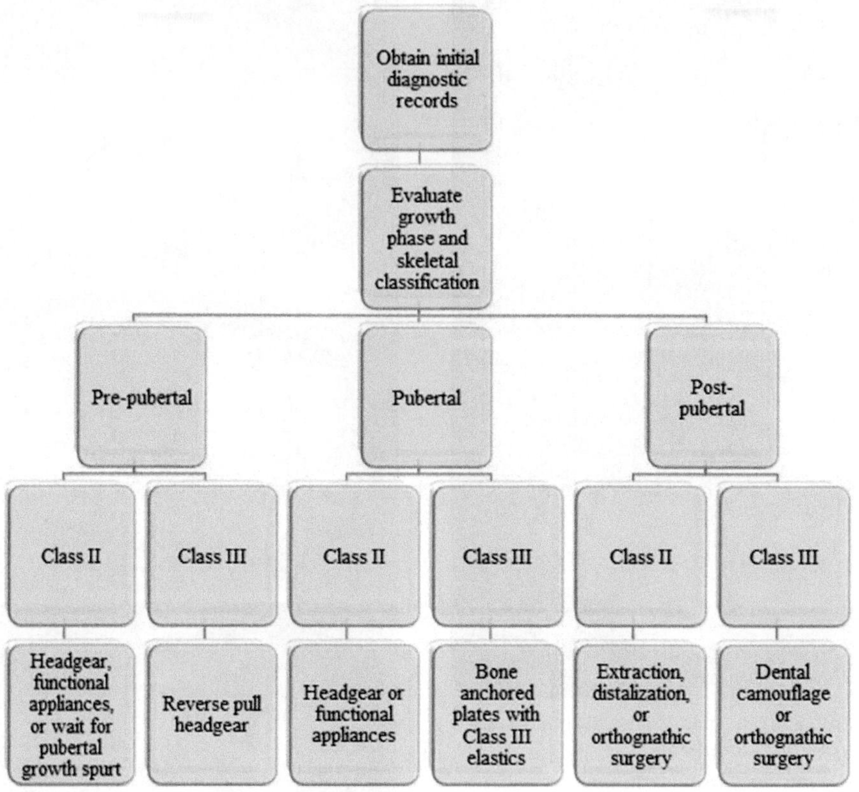

Fig. 12. Evaluating growth phase and treatment options for Class II and Class III patients.

REFERENCES

1. Bailey LJ, Phillips C, Proffit WR. Long-term outcome of surgical Class III correction as a function of age at surgery. Am J Orthod Dentofacial Orthop 2008; 133(3):365–70.
2. Grave KC. Timing of facial growth: a study of relations with stature and ossification in the hand around puberty. Am J Orthod 1874;65(3):320.
3. Perinetti G, Westphalen GH, Biasotto M, et al. The diagnostic performance of dental maturity for identification of the circumpubertal growth phases: a meta-analysis. Prog Orthod 2013;14(1):8.
4. Abdel-Kader HM. The reliability of dental x-ray film in assessment of MP3 stages of the pubertal growth spurt. Am J Orthod Dentofacial Orthop 1998; 114(4):427–9.
5. Rajagopal R, Kansal S. A comparison of modified MP3 stages and the vervial vertebrae as growth indicators. J Clin Orthod 2002;36(7):398–406.
6. Perinetti G, Primozic J, Franchi L, et al. Cervical vertebral maturation method: growth timing versus growth amount. Eur J Orthod 2016;38(1): 111–2.
7. Nestman TS, Marshall SD, Qian F, et al. Cervical vertebrae maturation method morphologic criteria: poor reproducibility. Am J Orthod Dentofacial Orthop 2011;140(2):182–8.
8. Predko-Engel A, Kaminek M, Langova K, et al. Reliability of the cervical vertebrae maturation (CVM) method. Bratisl Lek Listy 2015;116(04):222–6.
9. Bjork A, Helm S. Prediction of the age of maximum puberal growth in body height. Angle Orthod 1967; 37:134–43.
10. Demirjian A, Goldstein H, Tanner J. A new system of dental age assessment. Hum Biol 1973;45:211–27.
11. Hägg U, Taranger J. Maturation indicators and the pubertal growth spurt. Am J Orthod 1982;82(4): 299–309.
12. Tassi NGG, Franchi L, Baccetti T, et al. Diagnostic performance study on the relationship between the exfoliation of the deciduous second molars and the pubertal growth spurt. Am J Orthod Dentofacial Orthop 2007;131(6):769–71.
13. Franchi L, Baccetti T, De Toffol L, et al. Phases of the dentition for the assessment of skeletal maturity: a diagnostic performance study. Am J Orthod Dentofacial Orthop 2008;133(3):395–400.
14. Bishara SE, Jamison JE, Peterson LC, et al. Longitudinal changes in standing height and mandibular parameters between the ages of 8 and 17 years. Am J Orthod 1981;80(2):115–35.

15. Perinetti G, Baccetti T, Contardo L, et al. Gingival crevicular fluid alkaline phosphatase activity as a non-invasive biomarker of skeletal maturation: GCF ALP activity and skeletal maturation. Orthod Craniofac Res 2011;14(1):44–50.
16. Perinetti G, Franchi L, Castaldo A, et al. Gingival crevicular fluid protein content and alkaline phosphatase activity in relation to pubertal growth phase. Angle Orthod 2012;82(6):1047–52.
17. Masoud MI, Marghalani HYA, Masoud IM, et al. Prospective longitudinal evaluation of the relationship between changes in mandibular length and bloodspot IGF-1 measurements. Am J Orthod Dentofacial Orthop 2012;141(6):694–704.
18. Jain N, Tripathi T, Gupta SK, et al. Serum IGF-1, IGFBP-3 and their ratio: potential biochemical growth maturity indicators. Prog Orthod 2017; 18(1):11.
19. Kaban L, Cisneros G, Heyman S, et al. Assessment of mandibular growth by skeletal scintigraphy. J Oral Maxillofac Surg 1982;40(1):18–22.
20. Beirne O, Leake D. Technetium 99m pyrophosphate uptake in a case of unilateral condylar hyperplasia. J Oral Surg 1980;38(5):385–6.
21. Hodder SC, Rees JIS, Oliver TB, et al. SPECT bone scintigraphy in the diagnosis and management of mandibular condylar hyperplasia. Br J Oral Maxillofac Surg 2000;38(2):87–93.
22. Pripatnanont P, Vittayakittipong P, Markmanee U, et al. The use of SPECT to evaluate growth cessation of the mandible in unilateral condylar hyperplasia. Int J Oral Maxillofac Surg 2005; 34(4):364–8.
23. Melsen B. Palatal growth studied on human autopsy material. Am J Orthod 1975;68(1):42–54.
24. Melsen B, Melsen F. The postnatal development of the palatomaxillary region studied on human autopsy material. Am J Orthod 1982;82(4):329–39.
25. Handelman CS, Wang L, BeGole EA, et al. Nonsurgical rapid maxillary expansion in adults: report on 47 cases using the Haas expander. Angle Orthod 2000;70(2):16.
26. Cantarella D, Dominguez-Mompell R, Mallya SM, et al. Changes in the midpalatal and pterygopalatine sutures induced by micro-implant-supported skeletal expander, analyzed with a novel 3D method based on CBCT imaging. Prog Orthod 2017;18(1):34.
27. Cantarella D, Dominguez-Mompell R, Moschik C, et al. Midfacial changes in the coronal plane induced by microimplant-supported skeletal expander, studied with cone-beam computed tomography images. Am J Orthod Dentofacial Orthop 2018;154(3):337–45.
28. Angelieri F, Cevidanes LHS, Franchi L, et al. Midpalatal suture maturation: classification method for individual assessment before rapid maxillary expansion. Am J Orthod Dentofacial Orthop 2013;144(5):759–69.
29. Angelieri F, Franchi L, Cevidanes LHS, et al. Cone beam computed tomography evaluation of midpalatal suture maturation in adults. Int J Oral Maxillofac Surg 2017;46(12):1557–61.
30. Abo Samra D, Hadad R. Midpalatal suture: evaluation of the morphological maturation stages via bone density. Prog Orthod 2018;19(1):29.
31. Ghoneima A, Abdel-Fattah E, Hartsfield J, et al. Effects of rapid maxillary expansion on the cranial and circummaxillary sutures. Am J Orthod Dentofacial Orthop 2011;140(4):510–9.
32. Martina R, Cioffi I, Farella M, et al. Transverse changes determined by rapid and slow maxillary expansion - a low-dose CT-based randomized controlled trial: rapid vs. slow maxillary expansion. Orthod Craniofac Res 2012;15(3):159–68.
33. Zhou Y, Long H, Ye N, et al. The effectiveness of non-surgical maxillary expansion: a meta-analysis. Eur J Orthod 2014;36(2):233–42.
34. Pereira JDS, Jacob HB, Locks A, et al. Evaluation of the rapid and slow maxillary expansion using cone-beam computed tomography: a randomized clinical trial. Dental Press J Orthod 2017;22(2):61–8.
35. Baccetti T, Franchi L, Cameron CG, et al. Treatment timing for rapid maxillary expansion. Angle Orthod 2001;71(5):8.
36. Geran RG, McNamara JA, Baccetti T, et al. A prospective long-term study on the effects of rapid maxillary expansion in the early mixed dentition. Am J Orthod Dentofacial Orthop 2006;129(5): 631–40.
37. Mohan CN, Araujo EA, Oliver DR, et al. Long-term stability of rapid palatal expansion in the mixed dentition vs the permanent dentition. Am J Orthod Dentofacial Orthop 2016;149(6):856–62.
38. Seif-Eldin NF, Elkordy SA, Fayed MS, et al. Transverse skeletal effects of rapid maxillary expansion in pre and post pubertal subjects: a systematic review. Open Access Maced J Med Sci 2019;7. https://doi.org/10.3889/oamjms.2019.080.
39. Proffit WR, Fields HW Jr, Moray LJ. Prevalence of malocclusion and orthodontic treatment need in the United States: estimates from the NHANES III survey. Int J Adult Orthodon Orthognath Surg 1998;13(2):97–106.
40. Baccetti T, Franchi L, Toth LR, et al. Treatment timing for twin-block therapy. Am J Orthod Dentofacial Orthop 2000;118(2):159–70.
41. Tulloch JFC, Proffit WR, Phillips C. Outcomes in a 2-phase randomized clinical trial of early class II treatment. Am J Orthod Dentofacial Orthop 2004;125(6): 657–67.
42. Dolce C, McGorray SP, Brazeau L, et al. Timing of Class II treatment: skeletal changes comparing 1-phase and 2-phase treatment. Am J Orthod

Dentofacial Orthop 2007;132(4):481–9. https://doi.org/10.1016/j.ajodo.2005.08.046.
43. Franchi L, Pavoni C, Faltin K, et al. Long-term skeletal and dental effects and treatment timing for functional appliances in Class II malocclusion. Angle Orthod 2013;83(2):334–40.
44. Huanca Ghislanzoni LT, Baccetti T, Toll D, et al. Treatment timing of MARA and fixed appliance therapy of Class II malocclusion. Eur J Orthod 2013; 35(3):394–400.
45. Perinetti G, Primožič J, Franchi L, et al. Treatment effects of removable functional appliances in prepubertal and pubertal class II patients: a systematic review and meta-analysis of controlled studies. PLoS One 2015;10(10):e0141198.
46. Pavoni C, Lombardo EC, Lione R, et al. Treatment timing for functional jaw orthopaedics followed by fixed appliances: a controlled long-term study. Eur J Orthod 2018;40(4):430–6.
47. Thiruvenkatachari B, Harrison J, Worthington H, et al. Early orthodontic treatment for Class II malocclusion reduces the chance of incisal trauma: results of a Cochrane systematic review. Am J Orthod Dentofacial Orthop 2015;148(1):47–59.
48. Maspero C, Galbiati G, Giannini L, et al. Class II division 1 malocclusions: comparisons between one- and two-step treatment. Eur J Paediatr Dent 2018;(4):295–9.
49. Frye L, Diedrich PR, Kinzinger GSM. Class II treatment with fixed functional orthodontic appliances before and after the pubertal growth peak: a cephalometric study to evaluate differential therapeutic effects. J Orofac Orthop 2009;70(6):511–27.
50. Papageorgiou SN, Kutschera E, Memmert S, et al. Effectiveness of early orthopaedic treatment with headgear: a systematic review and meta-analysis. Eur J Orthod 2017;39(2):176–87.
51. Siqueira DF, de Almeira RR, Janson G, et al. Dentoskeletal and soft-tissue changes with cervical headgear and mandibular protraction appliance therapy in the treatment of Class II malocclusions. Am J Orthod Dentofacial Orthop 2007;131(4):447.e21-30.
52. Woodside DG, Metaxas A, Altuna G. The influence of functional appliance therapy on glenoid fossa remodeling. Am J Orthod Dentofacial Orthop 1987; 92(3):181–98.
53. Voudouris JC, Woodside DG, Altuna G, et al. Condyle-fossa modifications and muscle interactions during Herbst treatment. Part 2. Results and conclusions. Am J Orthod Dentofacial Orthop 2003;124(1):13–29.
54. Ivorra-Carbonell L, Montiel-Company J, Almerich-Silla J, et al. Impact of functional mandibular advancement appliances on the temporomandibular joint: a systematic review. Med Oral Patol Oral Cir Bucal 2016. https://doi.org/10.4317/medoral.21180.
55. Zymperdikas VF, Koretsi V, Papageorgiou SN, et al. Treatment effects of fixed functional appliances in patients with Class II malocclusion: a systematic review and meta-analysis. Eur J Orthod 2016;38(2): 113–26.
56. Jakobsone G, Latkauskiene D, McNamara JA Jr. Mechanisms of Class II correction induced by the crown Herbst appliance as a single-phase Class II therapy: 1 year follow-up. Prog Orthod 2013;14(1). https://doi.org/10.1186/2196-1042-14-27.
57. Janson G, Sathler R, Fernandes TMF, et al. Correction of Class II malocclusion with Class II elastics: a systematic review. Am J Orthod Dentofacial Orthop 2013;143(3):383–92.
58. Ruf S, Pancherz H. Orthognathic surgery and dentofacial orthopedics in adult Class II Division 1 treatment: mandibular sagittal split osteotomy versus Herbst appliance. Am J Orthod Dentofacial Orthop 2004;126(2):140–52.
59. Kapust AJ, Sinclair PM, Turley PK. Cephalometric effects of face mask/expansion therapy in Class III children: a comparison of three age groups. Am J Orthod Dentofacial Orthop 1998;113(2):204–12.
60. Mandall NA, Cousley R, DiBiase A, et al. Is early class III protraction facemask treatment effective? A multicentre, randomized, controlled trial: 3-year follow-up. J Orthod 2012;39:176–85.
61. Cordasco G, Matarese G, Rustico L, et al. Efficacy of orthopedic treatment with protraction face mask on skeletal Class III malocclusion: a systematic review and meta-analysis. Orthod Craniofac Res 2014;17: 133–43.
62. Foersch M, Jacobs C, Wriedt S, et al. Effectiveness of maxillary protraction using facemask with or without maxillary expansion: a systematic review and meta-analysis. Clin Oral Investig 2015;19(6): 1181–92.
63. Woon SC, Thiruvenkatachari B. Early orthodontic treatment for Class III malocclusion: a systematic review and meta-analysis. Am J Orthod Dentofacial Orthop 2017;151(1):28–52.
64. Menéndez-Díaz I, Muriel J, Cobo JL, et al. Early treatment of Class III malocclusion with facemask therapy. Clin Exp Dent Res 2018;4(6):279–83.
65. Hägg U, Tse A, Bendeus M, et al. Long-term follow-up of early treatment with reverse headgear. Am J Orthod Dentofacial Orthop 2003; 123(5):95–102.
66. Westwood PV, McNamara JA, Baccetti T, et al. Long-term effects of Class III treatment with rapid maxillary expansion and facemask therapy followed by fixed appliances. Am J Orthod Dentofacial Orthop 2003;123(3):306–20.
67. Masucci C, Franchi L, Defraia E, et al. Stability of rapid maxillary expansion and facemask therapy: a long-term controlled study. Am J Orthod Dentofacial Orthop 2011;140(4):493–500.

68. Mandall N, Cousley R, DiBiase A, et al. Early class III protraction facemask treatment reduces the need for orthognathic surgery: a multi-centre, two-arm parallel randomized, controlled trial. J Orthod 2016;43(3):164–75.
69. Pangrazio-Kulbersh V, Berger JL, Janisse FN, et al. Long-term stability of Class III treatment: rapid palatal expansion and protraction facemask vs Le-Fort I maxillary advancement osteotomy. Am J Orthod Dentofacial Orthop 2007;131(1):7.e9-19.
70. Pavoni C, Gazzani F, Franchi L, et al. Soft tissue facial profile in Class III malocclusion: long-term post-pubertal effects produced by the Face Mask Protocol. Eur J Orthod 2019.

Surgical/Orthodontic Correction of Transverse Maxillary Discrepancies

Johan P. Reyneke, MChD, FCOMFS (SA), PhD[a,b,c,d,e,*],
Richard Scott Conley, DMD[f]

KEYWORDS

• Orthodontic maxillary expansion • Rapid palatal expansion • Surgical assisted palatal expansion • Surgical segmental palatal expansion

KEY POINTS

1. The maxillary arch in the primary dentition may be expanded by means of an orthodontic appliance and will involve tooth movement alone.
2. In the adolescent the patient the maxillary dental arch width may be increased by means of rapid palatal expansion involving bone and teeth movement.
3. In the post adolescent individual, skeletal expansion of the maxillary arch may be achieved by means of surgical assisted expansion.
4. A surgical assisted approach to expand the upper dental arch maybe by means of a bone borne, or tooth borne appliance.
5. Surgical expansion of the maxilla by segmentation of the maxilla on a Le Fort I level are often utilized as part of the correction of other dentofacial deformities.

The transverse dimension is often the most critical yet least recognized plane of space for the surgical-orthodontic patient. Patients will frequently come to the office fully aware and concerned about the vertical dimension with chief concerns such as "My teeth don't meet in the front" or "I have a big overbite." In the sagittal plane of space, patients will remark "I don't like to position of my chin," which could include both the skeletal Class II or the Class III malocclusion. Due to more limited visibility of the posterior dimension, patients will commonly be unaware of the transverse components of their malocclusion.

The article focuses on the diagnosis and treatment planning of the patient with transverse maxillary deficiency. Specific considerations regarding the effect of the transverse dimension on the simultaneous correction of the sagittal and vertical dimensions are presented.

SKELETALLY IMMATURE PATIENTS (CHILDREN AND EARLY ADOLESCENTS)

Orthodontic expansion of the maxillary dental arch in children and adolescents has been discussed for more than a century with the earliest

[a] Private Practice, Mediclinic, Mediclinic Cape Town, 21 Hof Street, Oranjezicht, Cape Town 8000, South Africa; [b] Department of Oral and Maxillofacial Surgery, Faculty of Health Sciences, University of the Western Cape, Cape Town, South Africa; [c] Department of Oral and Maxillofacial Surgery, University of Oklahoma, Oklahoma City, OK, USA; [d] Department of Oral and Maxillofacial Surgery, University of Florida College of Dentistry, Gainesville, FL, USA; [e] Department of Oral and Maxillofacial Surgery, VNAI Faculty of Dentistry, Universidad Nacional Autonoma de Mexico, San Salvador, Mexico; [f] Private Practice of Orthodontics, Washington, Pennsylvania
* Corresponding author.
E-mail address: johanrey@worldonline.co.za

Oral Maxillofacial Surg Clin N Am 32 (2020) 53–69
https://doi.org/10.1016/j.coms.2019.08.007

oralmaxsurgery.theclinics.com

reports by Angell[1] and later by Angle and others.[2] Modern approaches to expansion in the United States began in the late 1950s when Korkhaus[3] reintroduced the technique which was then popularized by Haas[4,5] and others. Techniques vary from slow expansion, rapid expansion, alternating expansion and constriction, arch wire expansion, and more recently temporary anchorage device–supported expansion. The biological and clinical justifications for each technique are discussed.

DENTAL EXPANSION

Many different approaches can be used to widen the dental arch; however, one must consider that there are limits to the amount one can widen the teeth without also widening the basal bone. Among dental expansion devices, orthodontic brackets with a wide arch wire can be among the simplest approaches. Other approaches include transpalatal arches (TPA), quad helix, and cross-arch elastics (**Fig. 1**).

ORTHOPEDIC EXPANSION

Part of the rationale for every child to have an initial orthodontic examination at the age of 7 years is to facilitate the correction of maxillary transverse deficiency. Other reasons include early recognition of severe skeletal malocclusion, such as Class II patients with >7 mm of overjet or Class III patients with <−1 mm of overjet. Both Severe Class II and Class III patients can have a component of maxillary transverse deficiency.

Early recognition and correction of transverse deficiency has many benefits. First, orthopedic expansion can prevent asymmetric growth in the case of bilateral crossbite with functional shift. Orthopedic expansion can also reduce or eliminate the need for later surgical correction. Secondary benefits can include additional arch perimeter for future alignment of the teeth,[4] mild improvement in the sagittal malocclusion, and possible improvement in airway.

Orthopedic expansion is most easily accomplished before closure of the cranial base and midfacial sutures. Previous research indicates that the

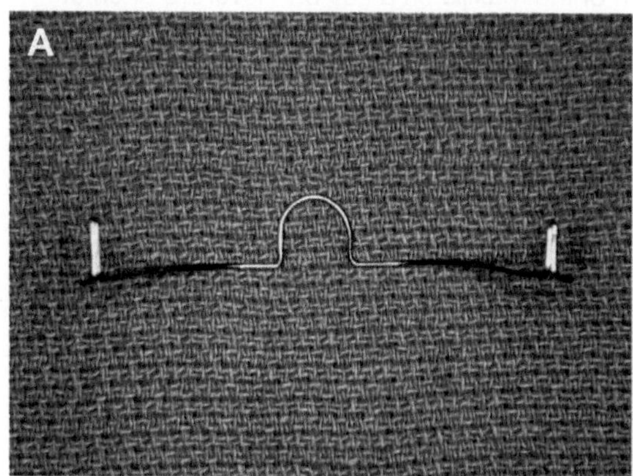

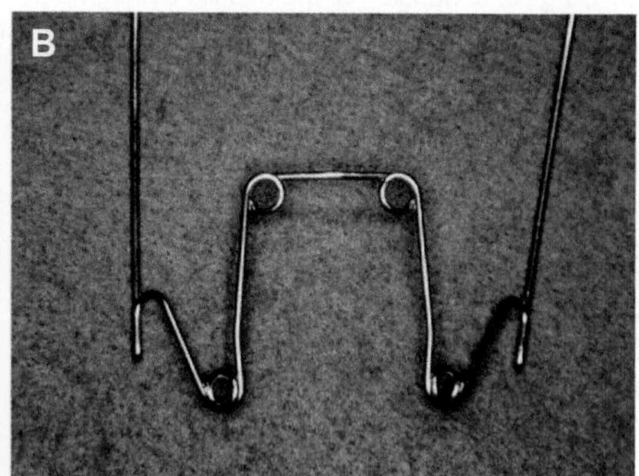

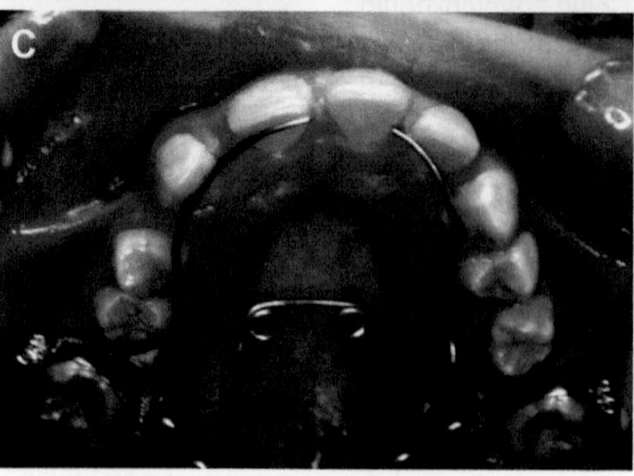

Fig. 1. (*A*) Transpalatal arch with a midline adjustment loop. The loop can start "closed" and be progressively "opened" to facilitate intermolar expansion. (*B*) Quad helix named for the 4 loops or helices. Each helix can be opened or closed to provide for expansion in the anterior, posterior, or both regions. (*C*) Clinical use of the quad helix.

transverse dimension is the first plane of space to cease growth, most notably at the inter-ethmoidal and inter-sphenoidal sutures. McNamara and colleagues[6] determined that both close before the age of 9 years. After their closure, increasing amounts of dental expansion and decreasing amounts of skeletal expansion are achieved until finally in late adolescence minimal to no skeletal expansion can be obtained.[7] The circum-maxillary sutures follow a similar pattern of increasing complexity and decreasing patency with increasing age. Various methods of assessing skeletal maturity have been advocated, including hand wrist radiographs, cervical vertebral maturation, and more recently a method of assessing maxillary sutural maturity using cone-beam computed tomography.[8]

Orthopedic expansion appliances generally fall into 2 types, tooth-borne hygienic rapid palatal expanders (Hyrax) or tooth plus tissue-borne expanders[9,10] (**Fig. 2**). Both types can be banded or bonded to the teeth. Research indicates that both are successful and conflict remains regarding which style produces more skeletal expansion. Activation protocols range from slow (1 turn every 2–3 days) to rapid (1–2 turns each day). According to Proffit and colleagues,[11] at the end of the expansion period, similar dental or skeletal expansion occurs (**Fig. 3**).

INDICATIONS FOR ORTHOPEDIC SKELETAL EXPANSION

1. Presence of cross bite
2. Class II patients with narrow maxillae, particularly when the patient protrudes and a crossbite exists in Class I
3. Class III patients for whom simultaneous expansion and protraction is considered
4. *Growing* (ie, nonskeletally mature) patient

FABRICATION TECHNIQUE: BANDED APPLIANCE

- Place separators for 7 to 14 days proximal to the teeth to be banded (**Fig. 4**). This typically involves the maxillary first molars ± the first premolars. In younger patients, some advocate use of the maxillary second primary molars.
- Remove separators to place orthodontic bands on the desired teeth. When using 4 teeth, it is helpful to have each band be slightly larger (1 size) to facilitate path of draw.
- Obtain a maxillary impression and remove the bands.
- Seat and stabilize the bands in the impression.
- Fabricate the expansion appliance either in office or send to the laboratory.
- If done digitally, a 3-dimensional digital scan can be sent to the commercial laboratory along with the bands and a digital photo of the band on the teeth.

FABRICATION TECHNIQUE: BONDED APPLIANCE

- Obtain a maxillary impression, mandibular counter-impression, and bite (**Fig. 5**).
- Send to the laboratory or make in house.
- If done digitally, a 3-dimensional digital scan can be sent to the commercial laboratory along with prescription.
- For a bonded Hyrax appliance, it is helpful to have a custom wire framework that surrounds the maxillary dentition. The framework can be soldered to the expansion screw to ensure a rigid appliance that will not come apart during expansion.

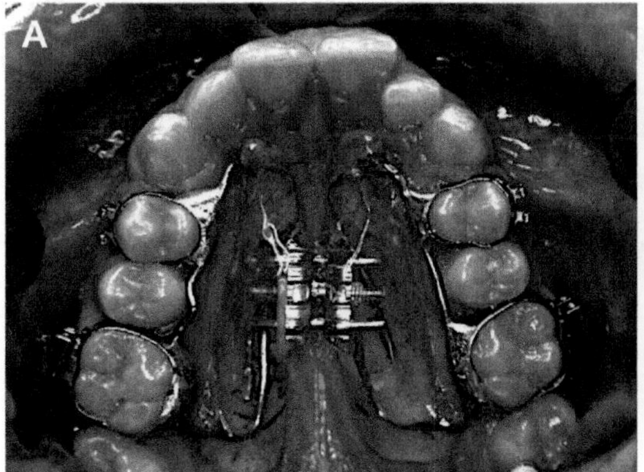

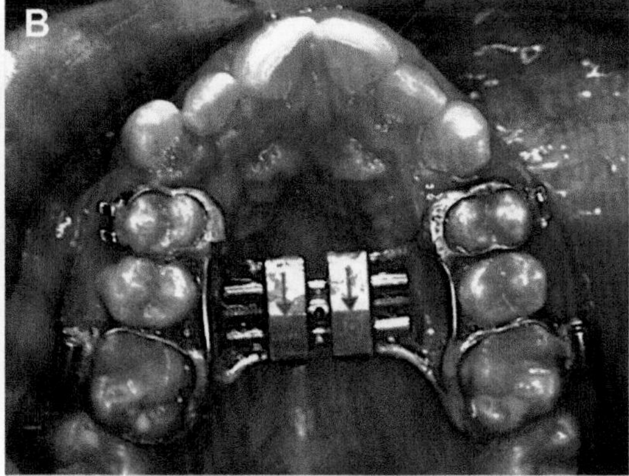

Fig. 2. (*A*) An example of a Haas expansion appliance. This appliance has both tooth and tissue-borne features. (*B*) An example of the Hyrax or hygienic appliance. The name results from the patient having the ability to clean all areas of the palate since acrylic does not contact the palate as it does in the Haas appliance.

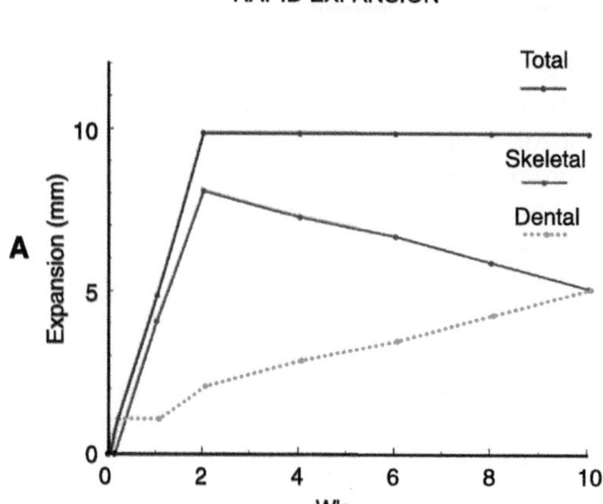

Fig. 3. Proffit and colleagues[11] describe similar expansion obtained from either rapid or slow expansion. During the rapid expansion, there is skeletal expansion that occurs first. As time progresses, some of the skeletal expansion is lost (relapse) yet the dentition is maintained resulting in dental expansion. (*Adapted from* Proffit WR, Fields HW, Sarver DM. Orthodontic treatment planning: limitations, controversies, and special problems. In: Contemporary orthodontics. 4th edition. St. Louis: Mosby Elsevier; 2007. p. 286; with permission.)

Other methods of expansion exist, including removable appliances, such as Frankel, Activator, or Bionator, although these have compliance challenges. Arch wire expansion is growing in popularity as self-ligating bracket systems continue to increase in the marketplace. Historically, most of the evidence indicates that arch wire expansion greater than 2 mm while possible has limited stability. The growing popularity of self-ligation brackets and lingual appliances have caused some members of the field to question the historical norms. Case reports demonstrate significant expansion being achieved, but no long-term data have been generated and imaging has not documented bone apposition on the buccal aspect.

In patients approaching skeletal maturity, some investigators have advocated for alternating expansion and constriction (Alt-RAMEC). Wang and colleagues[12] support this method as a way of enhancing the amount of skeletal protraction in Class III patients due to the greater mobilization of the circum-maxillary sutures resulting from the cycles of expansion and constriction.

Recently Lee and others[13,14] have advocated for temporary anchorage device supported expansion appliances. These vary considerable in implant type, location, patient age, and appliance style. Each offer promise and early reports indicate

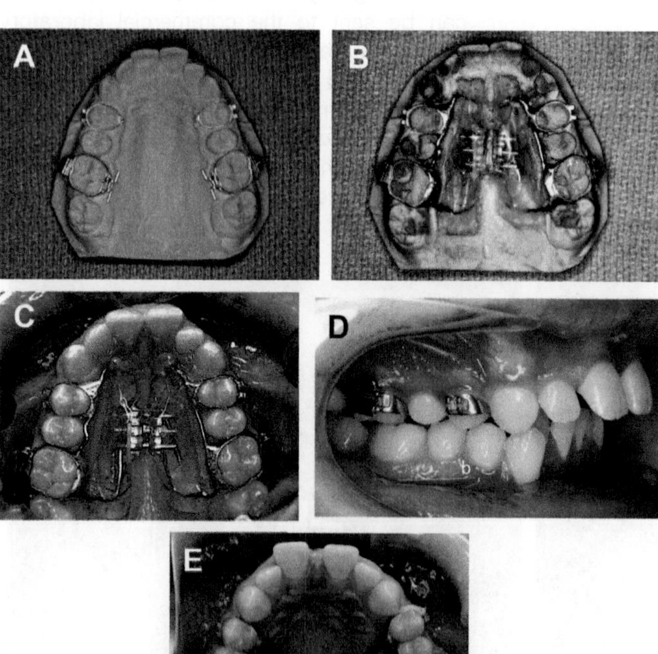

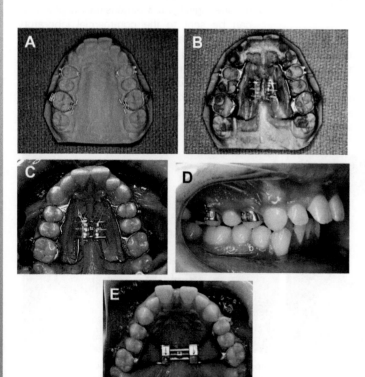

Fig. 4. Fabrication of a banded Haas expander. (*A*) Bands are placed on the patient with an impression (or digital scan) obtained. (*B*) A rigid framework is fabricated and then cold cure acrylic is placed in the palate to provide the tissue support. (*C*) Clinical application of the banded Haas appliance. (*D*) A rigid framework is fabricated. Clinical application of the banded Haas appliance. (*E*) No cold cure acrylic is placed enabling the patient to maintain oral hygiene.

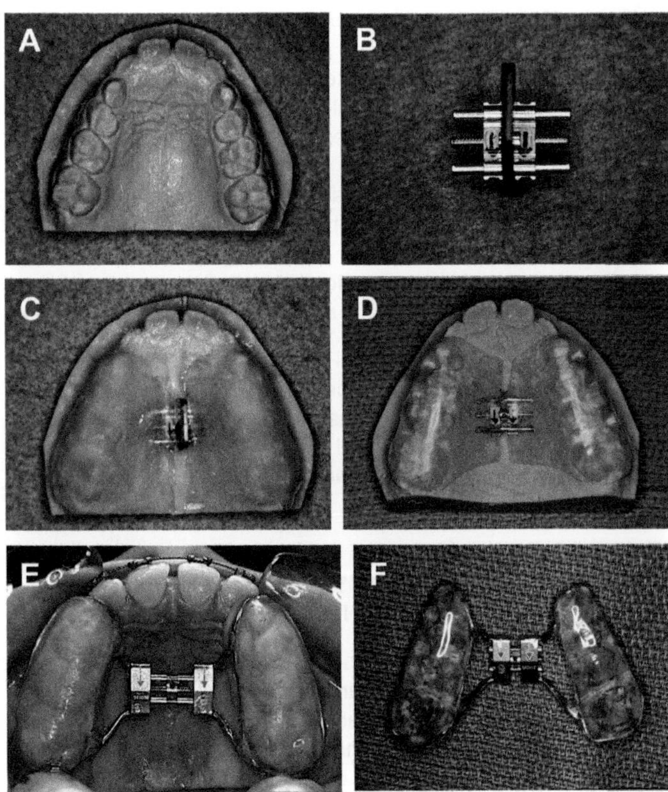

Fig. 5. Fabrication of a bonded Hyrax expander. (*A*) With an all acrylic appliance, only a maxillary impression is required. (*B*) The expansion screw is placed in the midline. (*C*) Acrylic is applied and cured, and (*D*) trimmed. (*E*) A rigid stainless steel framework is created to accept the acrylic. (*F*) The framework is soldered to the expansion screw to prevent appliance from coming apart.

a range of efficacy. Long-term results for temporary anchorage device-supported expanders have not yet become available, and the authors currently recommend caution until proper investigations are reported.

SKELETALLY MATURE PATIENTS (ADULTS AND LATE ADOLESCENTS)

Orthodontic expansion of the maxillary dental arch in the mature patient is limited to dental movement. Expansion in adult patients with skeletal transverse deficiency may require tooth movement beyond the maxillary alveolar bony base and may lead to tipping of the anchor teeth[15], extrusion,[16] root resorption,[17,18] relapse, and periodontal problems.[19]

The skeletal transverse dimension of the maxilla can, however, be altered by surgically assisted orthodontic palatal expansion (SARPE) or by surgical segmental surgery.

SURGICALLY ASSISTED PALATAL EXPANSION

The main area of resistance to orthodontic expansion was considered to be the midpalatal suture and consequently, the first reports of surgery to assist orthodontic palatal expansion involved surgical midpalatal splitting.

However, Lines in 1975,[20] and Bell and Epker[21] in 1976 concluded that the main area of resistance to maxillary expansion was not the midpalatine suture but the thick bone in the zygomaticomaxillary, zygomaticotemporal, and zygomaticofrontal suture areas. Wertz[22] was even of the opinion that the resistance was attributable to the zygomatic arches. The identification of various areas of resistance to skeletal maxillary expansion has led to the design and development of various osteotomies by which these areas could be weakened to allow for expansion.[23]

Transverse skeletal deficiency rarely occurs without coexisting vertical and/or sagittal discrepancies. When correction of a constricted maxilla is the only objective, distraction should be considered. Widening of the maxillary arch may, however, form part of a treatment plan also requiring several other corrective orthognathic surgical procedures. In cases in which a Le Fort I maxillary procedure is contemplated as part of on orthognathic treatment plan, expansion by surgical segmental surgery should be considered. SARPE, which is usually indicated in the early stages of treatment, will be followed by a Le Fort I procedure as a definitive surgical procedure. This will subject the patient to 2 surgeries.

There is controversy regarding the relative risks and benefits of planning to perform SARPE first followed by a 1-piece Le Fort I later in 2 stages as opposed to a single-stage, multipiece segmental maxillary osteotomy. The following are considered advantages and disadvantages of the 2 approaches:

- The transverse stability following SARPE exceeds the postoperative stability following segmental surgery.
- SARPE increases the arch length early in the orthodontic treatment creating both new bone and space for use in leveling and alignment that may facilitate nonextraction orthodontic care.
- SARPE allows for a greater degree of transverse expansion.
- Performing a single-piece Le Fort I osteotomy is less cumbersome with a lower complication rate than a multipiece Le Fort I osteotomy.
- Following segmental surgery, surgical splints must be left in place postoperatively for several weeks, thereby increasing postoperative discomfort for the patient.
- Impacted third molars can be removed at the same time as performing the SARPE surgery.
- Apart from clinical advantages and disadvantages, several factors, such as financial issues, time off work or school, and the psychological impact of surgery, should be taken into account.

According to Perciaccante and Bays,[24] the 2-stage approach is most often used and maxillary segmental expansion and is reserved for 2 specific case scenarios. In their opinion, segmental surgery should be reserved for cases in which there are different occlusal planes in the maxillary arch that cannot be addressed orthodontically, or for patients who have undergone orthodontic treatment for months or years before referral for a surgical option and the dentition has reached maximum limit of movement.

INDICATIONS FOR SURGICALLY ASSISTED MAXILLARY EXPANSION

1. When an increase in arch length is required to accommodate all the teeth, that is, the first or second bicuspids had been removed for orthodontic reasons; however, anchorage loss resulted in loss of the extraction spaces with severe crowding.
2. When palatal expansion is required in an adult patient and no other orthognathic procedures are contemplated in the maxilla.
3. When unilateral expansion is required.
4. When a transverse increase of more than 7 mm is required.
5. When space is required to accommodate an unerupted tooth that is an unerupted canine.
6. For patients whose previous orthodontic palatal expansion has failed.
7. Correction of a severe cross bite (scissors bite).

As with all surgical-orthodontic treatments, proper communication between the surgeon and the orthodontist is mandatory regarding the indications, timing, and sequencing of the previously mentioned approaches.

ORTHODONTIC CONSIDERATIONS FOR SURGICALLY ASSISTED ORTHODONTIC PALATAL EXPANSION

For many patients, it is immediately clear that large amounts of expansion (>7 mm) are required. If a tooth-borne expander is to be used, the orthodontist must have the appliance in place before the patient goes to the operating room. The steps listed in the fabrication can assist in understanding the timeline necessary.

For other patients, the magnitude of the transverse deficiency may not be obvious. A close examination of the Curve of Wilson in the mandibular arch and Curve of Monson in the maxillary arch, as well as other diagnostic aids, such as an occlusogram, can be beneficial. Where uncertainly remains, a useful approach is to place full fixed mandibular orthodontic appliances to level and upright the Curve of Wilson. Once accomplished, new models (or digital scans) can be obtained to reassess the transverse deficiency to make sure the full extent of correction is planned.

Other confounding variables include significant Class II or Class III deformities. The models should always be examined in the final anticipated sagittal occlusion so that the true transverse discrepancy is visualized.

Once SARPE has been determined to be the most appropriate course of care, the following items can dramatically assist the smooth progression of the case. The roots of the teeth adjacent to the osteotomy should either have clear divergence or the orthodontist should actively diverge the roots to facilitate the surgical cut. This can be accomplished quite simply either through subtle bends in the arch wire (**Fig. 6**A), or by adjusting the bracket orientation during initial bonding. Whichever approach is selected, the orthodontist

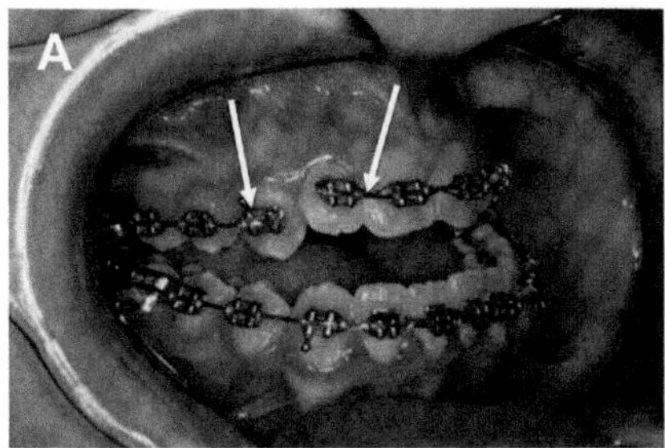

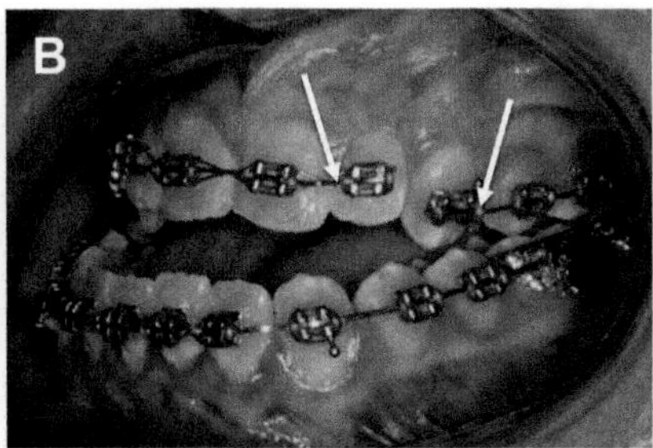

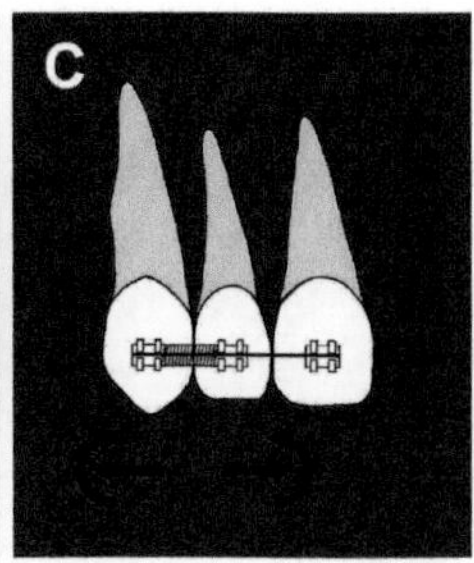

Fig. 6. (*A*) and (*B*) Subtle bends can be placed in the arch wire (between the central and lateral incisor and between the maxillary canine and first premolar bilaterally. There is a natural root divergence between the lateral incisor and canine making this site an efficient location for maxillary segmentation. (*C*) The force diagram from an open coil spring showing that root convergence occurs as the crowns separate. This should be avoided so that the orthodontist does not make the surgeon's job more difficult. [Fig 6C (*From* Conley RS, Legan HL. Biomechanical factors in surgical orthodontics. In: Nanda R, editor. Esthetics and biomechanics in orthodontics. St. Louis: Saunders; 2015. p. 483; with permission.)]

should be careful NOT to perform any maxillary expansion, merely work to create root separation. A final note of caution is to remember that it is inter-radicular space that is most important not space between the crowns. As a result, open coil spring should be avoided, as it tends to create greater root convergence (**Fig. 6**B). Once the necessary divergence has been created, the arch wire should be removed entirely the day of surgery or sectioned before or during the SARPE so that the 2 hemi-maxillae and the respective dentition is free of resistance to expansion.

SURGICAL TECHNIQUE

Tooth-Borne Appliance

Several surgical techniques exist based on where the treatment team believes the major points of resistance will be and in which area the maximum palatal expansion is required. The authors prefer to perform a 2-piece Le Fort I osteotomy without down-fracture, under general anesthesia through endotracheal intubation in an operating room setting. In **Fig. 7**, the expansion of the maxilla by means of a 3-piece segmentation and the use of a tooth-borne expansion appliance is demonstrated. The appliance is fabricated by the orthodontist and placed a few days before surgery.

1. Ten minutes before surgery the area of dissection is infiltrated with local anesthetic containing 1:100,00 adrenaline.
2. An upper buccal mucosal and periosteal incision is performed from the second bicuspid on the one side to the second bicuspid on the opposite side.
3. Start the submucosal dissection at the piriform aperture on the one side and carry it backward to the pterygomaxillary junction. Complete the dissection on the contralateral side.
4. The left and right linear osteotomies are now performed from the pterygomaxillary junction to the piriform aperture using a reciprocating saw. Keep these osteotomies straight, horizontal, and perpendicular the palatal plane. An osteotomy performed at an angle may resist horizontal movement of the segments (**Fig. 8**A [i]).
5. Dissect the nasal mucosa off the nasal floor.
6. Separate the nasal septum using a nasal septal osteotome. This will avoid postoperative nasal deviation because the septum will remain attached to one of the 2 maxillary segments (see **Fig. 8**A [iv]).
7. Mark the roots of the incisor teeth and draw the proposed interdental osteotomy directly on the bone (see **Fig. 8**A [ii]).
8. Use a #701 burr and score a line as marked on the labial cortex between the upper central incisor teeth and complete the interdental osteotomy using piezo surgery or a spatula osteotome (see **Fig. 8**A [iii]).
9. Complete the interdental osteotomy with a piezo surgical blade.
10. Separate the pterygomaxillary junctures on both sides using the pterygomaxillary osteotome (see **Fig. 8**B).
11. Place a thin 5-mm osteotome between the incisors in the osteotomy line while the surgeons index finger palpates the palatal mucosa feeling the osteotome as it is tapped by the assistant, posteriorly to complete the palatal osteotomy (**Fig. 8**C).
12. The expansion appliance is then activated to ensure adequate mobility of the halves of the maxilla.

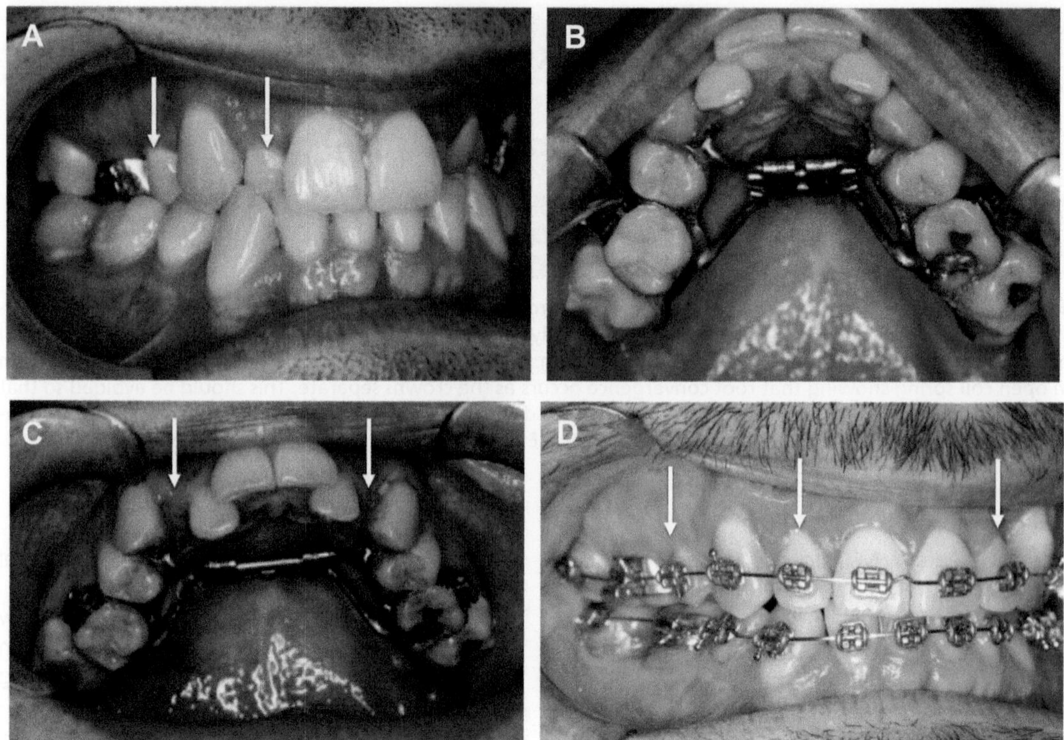

Fig. 7. (*A*) The pretreatment Class I occlusion with severe crowding requiring tooth-borne SARPE. The first bicuspids have been removed during orthodontic treatment at a young age. The treatment plan consisted of SARPE followed by orthodontic correction of the malocclusion. (*B*) A tooth-borne expansion appliance was placed before surgery. (*C*) Interdental osteotomies were performed between the lateral incisor and canine teeth and combined with a midpalatal osteotomy. Note the spaces created distal to the lateral incisors (*arrows*). (*D*) The additional space created was utilized to align the dentition (*arrows*).

13. The incisions are then sutured using resorbable sutures.
14. The same principle as for distraction osteogenesis apply. A latency period of 5 days after surgery will allow some soft tissue healing and the formation of a fibrovascular bridge to support bone formation in the distraction gap.
15. The expansion device is activated after 5 days and turned according to specific instructions (usually each turn represents 0.25 mm and it should be turned twice daily).
16. After 2 to 3 days of activation it is recommended to obtain an anterior occlusal radiograph to confirm bone separation.
17. Once the desired expansion has been achieved based on the treatment requirements the distraction is stopped and the device locked.
18. A consolidation period of 8 to 12 weeks is usually sufficient.

The SARPE osteotomy line(s) may be modified in cases in which widening of isolated maxillary segments are required. The selected interdental osteotomy is then connected to the midline palatal osteotomy (see **Fig. 7**).

Bone-Borne Appliance

Expanding the maxilla by means of SARPE requires the application of lateral forces to the maxillary segments. Using a dental expansion appliance as distractor, these forces are applied to the teeth, which is the same as with an appliance used for rapid maxillary expansion (RPE). The disadvantages of using a dental appliance for RPE expansion are well documented.[15–19] If the forces could be applied directly to the maxillary bone, several of the unfavorable effects could be avoided. Mommaerts[25] in 1999 introduced the Trans Palatal Expander (TPD) device, which could be directly attached to the bone on the palatal aspects of the maxilla. He found that by placing the distractor in the premolar area more expansion could be achieved in the canine region than in the posterior palatal region at a rate of 3:2. By moving the distracter

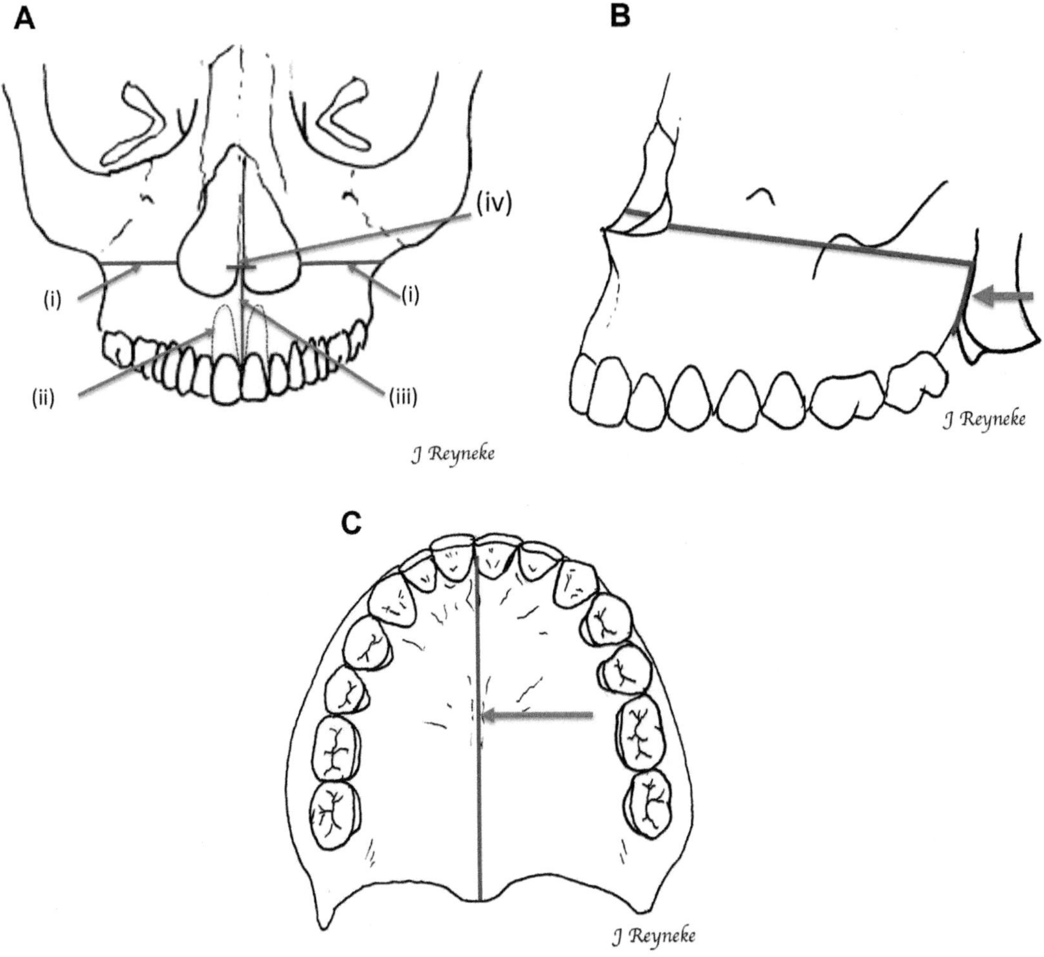

Fig. 8. (*A*) Use a reciprocating saw to perform the left and right lateral wall osteotomies from the pterygomaxillary junctions to the piriform rims (i). Draw the outline of the tooth roots adjacent to the interdental osteotomy (ii). Score the interdental osteotomy only through the labial cortex by using a 701 fissure bur (iii). (iv) Separate the nasal septum from the maxilla. (*B*) Separate the pterygomaxillary junctions using a pterygoid osteotome (*arrow*). (*C*) The interdental osteotomy is now completed by means of a piezo surgical blade and the midline palatal osteotomy performed using a small osteotome.

posteriorly and combine it with pterygoid disjunctures the distraction distance was found to be equal in the anterior and posterior palate. Since 1999, several bone-borne distractors with various designs have been developed and include: the Magdenburg palatal distractor,[26] Martin Rapid Palatal Expander (KLS Martin Group, Jacksonville, FL), the Rotterdam palatal distractor,[27] and the MDO-R device (Orthognathics, Ltd, Zurich, Switzerland).

Koudstaal and colleagues,[28] in a randomized trial, compared the posttreatment stability and relapse between 23 bone-borne cases versus 19 tooth-borne surgically assisted cases. They reported no significant difference in stability between the 2 groups.

The maxillary osteotomies performed does not differ from a tooth-borne distractor when a bone-borne distractor is used. However, some additional aspects should be addressed:

1. The surgeon should select a device that he or she is familiar with.
2. There are numerous distraction devices available and most of the designs offer several sizes to conform to the different palatal widths of patients. An appropriate size distractor should be selected by using the preoperative dental model.
3. The surgical/orthodontic team should plan the ideal positioning of the device in the palate indicated by the area in which the distraction force will be required for the specific case.

Surgical Technique

- Once the maxillary osteotomies are completed the selected distractor is again tested for size and position in the patient's palate.
- The planned positions of the footplates are marked on the mucosa.
- An incision ±6 mm long is now made bilaterally and the muco-periosteum reflected to accommodate the footplates of the device.
- Insert the footplates and secure them by using an appropriate length screws.
- To allow the footplates of the distractor to seat against the bone, secure the one side first and then turn the distractor once or twice before the second screw is placed.
- Once the distractor is secured in place it should be activated with a few turns to ensure the mobility of the maxillary segments.
- After a latent period of 5 days, the distractor is activated and turned twice daily. For most distractors, each turn would represent 0.25 mm. It is, however, important to follow the manufacturer's guidelines.
- Once the planned expansion has been achieved, the distractor can be locked and left in position for 4 to 8 weeks to act as a retainer.

Bilateral distraction with a midline palatal osteotomy between the central incisors are demonstrated in **Fig. 9**. In **Fig. 10** a unilateral distraction was performed to correct a severe scissors bite.

CORRECTION OF MAXILLARY TRANSVERSE DISCREPANCIES BY SEGMENTAL MAXILLARY SURGERY

The Le Fort I maxillary osteotomy is currently a routine procedure for the correction of dentofacial deformities and can be performed in one or multiple segments. Segmentation of the maxilla allows for differential repositioning of the bone segments of the maxilla, thereby enabling the surgeon to level occlusal curves, close open bites, close interdental spaces, and widen or narrow the maxillary dental arch. In a study by Venugoplan and colleagues[29] it was found that maxillary segmentation is the most frequent orthognathic procedure performed in the United States involving 45.8% of the cases.

Segmentation of the maxilla is certainly a versatile technique and 2 or more segments can be used. The interdental osteotomies are usually performed in 3 different sites: between the central incisor teeth, between the lateral incisor and canine teeth, and between the canine and bicuspids (with

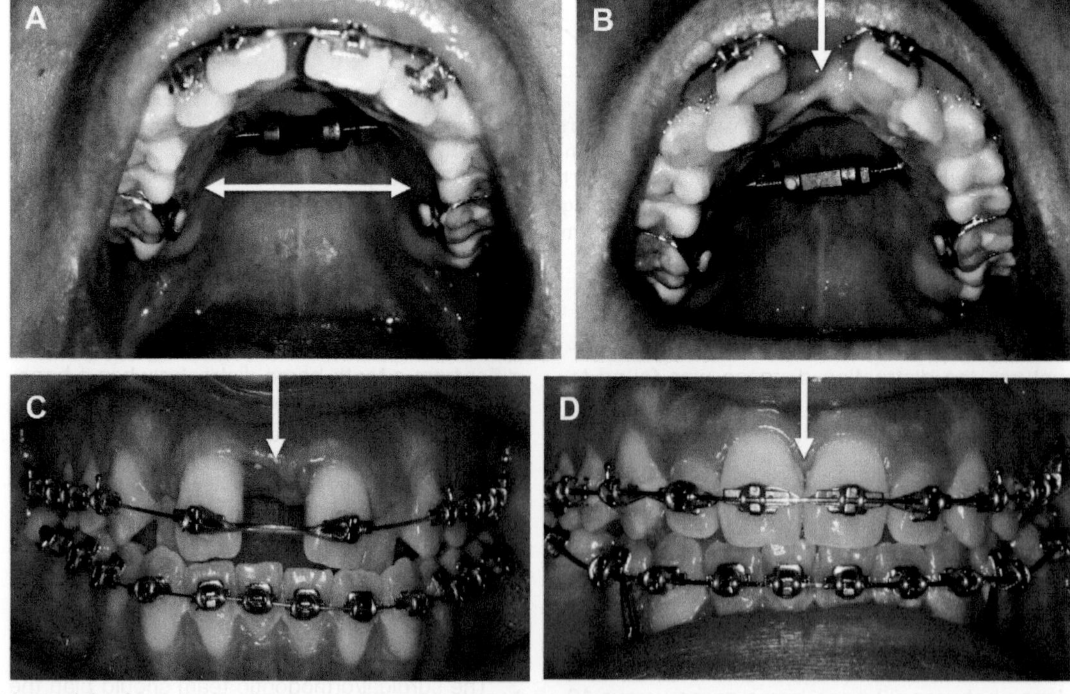

Fig. 9. (*A*) A bone-borne distraction appliance. (*B*) Note the diastema developing 3 days after activation and (*C*) 7 days after activation. (*C*) The dentition during the consolidation phase and an 8 mm expansion. The expander was locked and acted as a retainer for 4 to 8 weeks. (*D*) Following the consolidation phase, the orthodontist used the additional space to close the space and align the teeth.

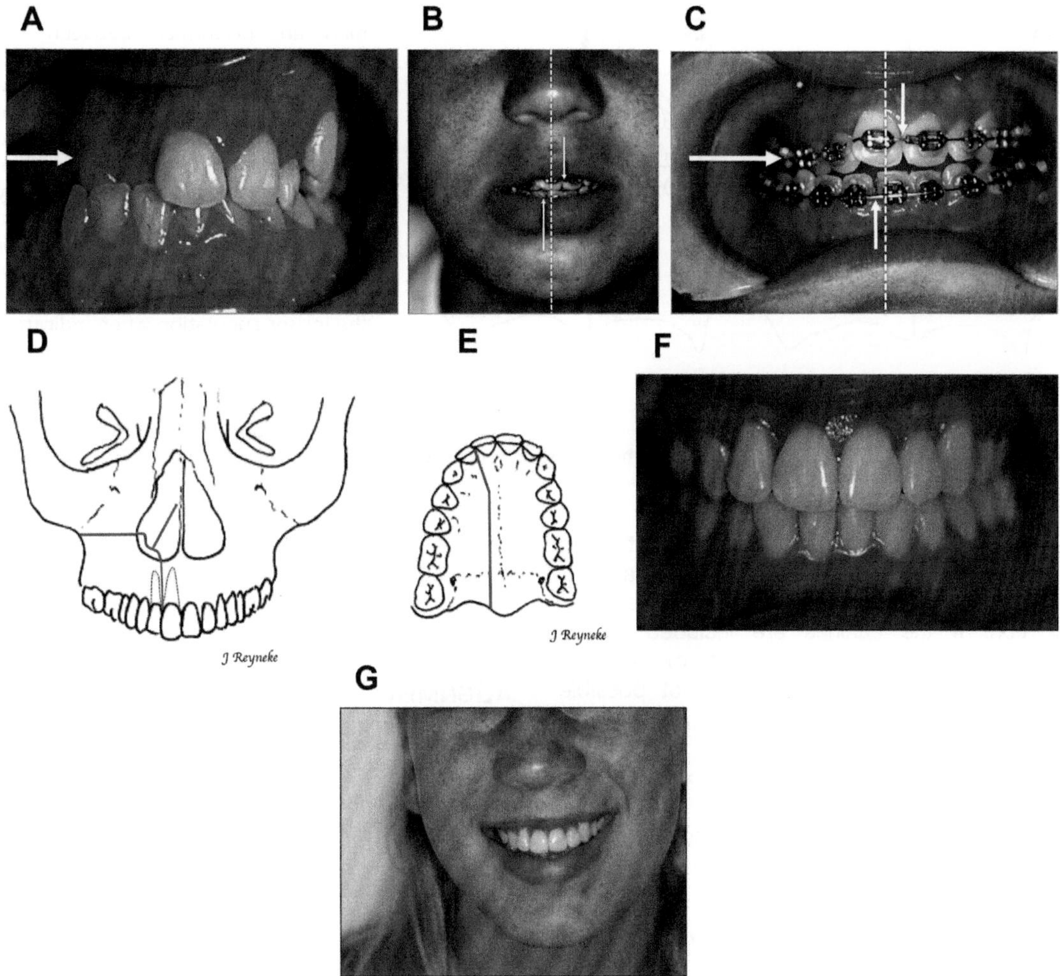

Fig. 10. (*A*) A pretreatment malocclusion with severe crowding and a scissors bite on the right side (*arrow*). (*B*) The upper dental midline is asymmetric to the left (*arrow*) and lower dental midline to the right (*arrow*) of the patient's facial midline (*dotted line*). (*C*) The upper dental arch was orthodontically aligned in 2 segments in preparation for a unilateral SARPE of the right maxillary segment (*arrow*). (*D*) The unilateral osteotomy design is demonstrated with the interdental osteotomy between the right upper lateral incisor and central incisor. (*E*) The palatal osteotomy was performed on the right side. (*F*) The posttreatment occlusion and (*G*) frontal view. (*Courtesy of* Johan Reyneke, B.Ch.D, M.Ch.D, FCOMFS (SA), PhD., Cape Town, South Africa).

or without bicuspid extraction). The malocclusion may however, in some cases require only unilateral segmentation that is, a unilateral scissors bite.

The positioning of interdental osteotomies is planned according to the presurgical orthodontic requirements and alignment of the segments; however, the authors prefer to perform most the interdental osteotomies between the lateral incisors and the canine teeth because it has specific advantages[30–32]:

Advantages

- It allows the surgeon to manage the intercanine width. If the interdental osteotomy is performed between the central incisors, or the canine and bicuspid teeth the control of the intercanine width is limited and torque control of the posterior segments harder to implement (**Fig. 11**).
- The alveolar bone is thin between the lateral and canine teeth and easy to section.
- The surgical area is anterior in the mouth and more accessible with better vision and orientation.
- A natural distal canine root inclination exists in many cases facilitating minimal orthodontic root divergence between the lateral and canine roots (**Fig. 12**).
- Minimal orthodontic root angle correction is required after surgery.

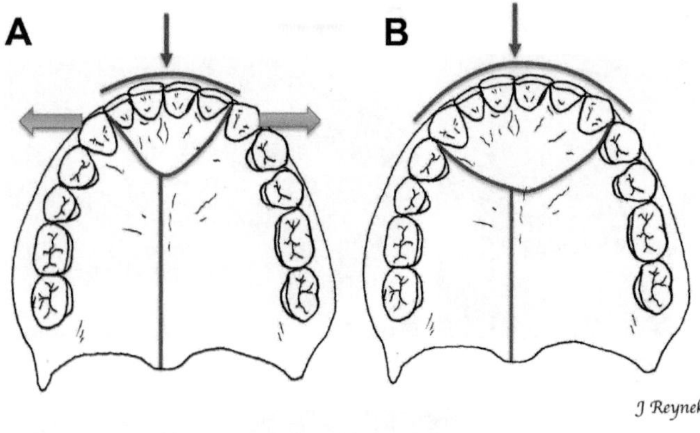

Fig. 11. (*A*) The interdental osteotomies are performed between the lateral incisor and canine teeth and allows for surgical control of the intercanine width (*arrows*), while with the interdental osteotomies between the canines and bicuspids (*B*) the control is lost. Note, the mid palatal osteotomy is performed slightly off the midpalatal raphe (*arrows*). In (*A*), the 4 incisor teeth form a near straight line (*arrow*), which will allow the surgeon to correct the incisor angulation when indicated. In (*B*) the canine teeth are included in the anterior segment forming a curve (*arrow*), which would not allow for the correction of the angulation of the incisors without lifting the canines out of the occlusion. (*Courtesy of* Johan Reyneke, B.Ch.D, M.Ch.D, FCOMFS (SA), PhD., Cape Town, South Africa).

- The arch-form including the 4 incisor teeth is nearly a straight line allowing for surgical management if the buccolingual incisor angulation. If the canines are included in the anterior segment the arch-form is more convex and surgical change not possible without lifting the canines out of occlusion (see **Fig. 11**).
- By leaving a small interdental space distal to the lateral incisors during surgery a Bolton tooth size discrepancy can be managed.

Presurgical Orthodontic Considerations for Maxillary Segmental Surgery

Patients requiring smaller amounts of expansion (<7 mm) who also need sagittal and/or vertical movements are excellent candidates for maxillary segmental surgery. However, this introduces some significant challenges for the orthodontist.

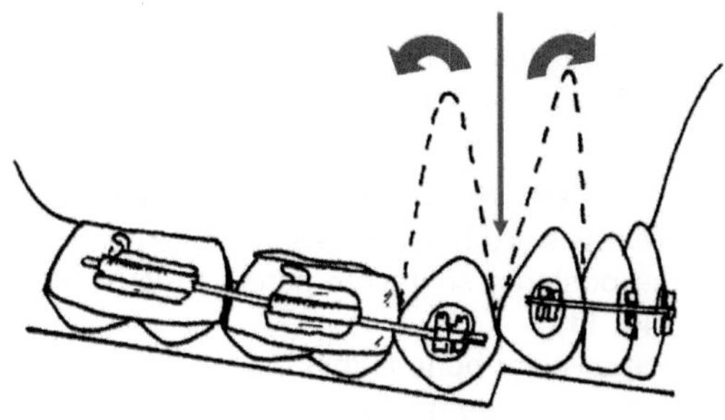

Fig. 12. Deviation of the roots of the teeth in the cases planned for an interdental osteotomy between the canine and bicuspid will require mesial tipping of the canine root (*arrow*). Following the surgery, the root will need to be tipped distally through the osteotomy line. This will add to orthodontic treatment time. (*Courtesy of* Johan Reyneke, B.Ch.D, M.Ch.D, FCOMFS (SA), PhD., Cape Town, South Africa).

ALIGNMENT

The ideal patient will have either spacing or minimal crowding. Spacing enables the orthodontist to align the teeth prior to the expansion. Minimal crowding can often be addressed through interproximal reduction (IPR). When the natural contact points are accessible, IPR can be done before alignment, which offers the smallest chance of dental expansion. If inaccessible, the teeth can be aligned first, then IPR performed afterward to remove any unintended expansion that occurred. The primary goal must be obtaining ideal alignment so that the teeth will fit the opposing arch after segmentation but not expanding the dental arch.

With crowded dental arches, the orthodontist needs space that is not available to align the teeth. Because expansion is to be avoided, significantly crowded dental arches may require dental extraction to create the space necessary to align the teeth. While adding time to the presurgical orthodontic phase, this is the most ideal approach and the space generated can be used not only to align the teeth but also to create the desired presurgical sagittal occlusion. In addition, the spaces can be used to facilitate the inter-radicular space for the segmental osteotomy(ies).

SEGMENTATION AND ROOT DIVERGENCE

In both the crossed and noncrowded occlusion an efficient approach is to use segmented maxillary arch wires. The orthodontist can perform the typical arch coordination and then segment the maxillary arch wire(s) in the anticipated osteotomy site(s) before ligating the wires in place. Segmentation also allows the orthodontist to adjust the root angulation at the osteotomy site(s) by either adjusting the bracket orientation or placing a "tip" bend at the end of each segment.

Surgical Technique

- Perform the soft tissue incisions and osteotomies as for a Le Fort I procedure described previously from 1 to 7.
- Carefully and patiently dissect the nasal mucosa from the nasal floor, the septum, and lateral nasal walls. A tear in the nasal mucosa should be carefully sutured to prevent the possible development of an oro-nasal communication later (see palatal soft tissue incision).
- Use a lateral nasal osteotome to bilaterally separate the lateral nasal walls while protecting the nasal mucosa.
- A delicate detachment of the buccal mucosa in the interdental osteotomy region is necessary, between the roots of the teeth (central incisors, lateral incisors, and canines or bicuspid and canines). It is not necessary to carry the dissection right down to the alveolar bone margin and interdental papilla.
- The authors prefer to perform the initial part of the interdental osteotomy before the maxillary is down fractured because, the maxilla is still stable at this stage the accurate orientation for the interdental osteotomy is easier for the surgeon. The root of the canine is often visible as a bulge on the buccal bone, which will act as a guide to safely perform the interdental osteotomies.
- First score a line through the cortex of the buccal bone where the interdental osteotomy is planned. Then use a piezo surgical blade to perforate the bone between the teeth into the palate and nasal floor. A spatula osteotome may also be used to complete the interdental osteotomy while supporting the palatal mucosa detecting the perforation of the bone digitally.
- The maxilla is now down fractured.
- Where the interdental osteotomy is performed between the central incisors, the interdental osteotomy is now identified in the nasal floor and the osteotomy can be completed posteriorly in the palate using either piezo surgery of a 701 fissure burr.
- Where the interdental osteotomies are performed between lateral incisor and canine or canine and bicuspid, Identify the interdental cuts on the nasal floor and connect them by using piezo surgery or a 701 fissure burr.
- Perform a paramedian palatal osteotomy(s) starting from posterior and connect it to the anterior interdental osteotomies. The authors prefer to perform the palatal osteotomy(s) just lateral to the midline (nasal septum line) because the palatal bone is thinner in this region. The palatal osteotomy can be performed according to the design of the treatment plan.
- For large expansions (>6 mm) bilateral paramedian incisions of the palatal mucosa can be performed between the central raphe and the palatine artery extending from the first molar to the canine. These incisions ensure that the mucoperiosteum of the palate is detached from the mucoperiosteum of the maxillary alveolar processes. Angle a #15 blade at 45°, which will create a slight overlap and enhance soft tissue healing. Ensure that the soft tissue incisions do not coinside with the palatal osteotomies. To prevent the development of a oro-nasal fistula later, it is also important to suture any small tears in the nasal mucosa as mentioned previously.
- Palatal soft tissue release is obviously nor necessary when the maxillary arch is surgically narrowed.
- At this time the segments are mobilized.
- The clinician may prefer to use a palatal splint in addition to an intermaxillary splint. Insert both the splints and ensure that the that the segments and teeth fit into the splint without excessive force. Apply intermaxillary fixation.
- The authors prefer to place an interdental wire around the brackets of the teeth next to the interdental osteotomies at the time of surgery to form a continuation of the arch wire (**Fig. 13**).
- For large maxillary expansions consideration to reenforcing the final splint to ensure that the splint is rigid and does not get distorted.
- Finally, internal rigid fixation is placed using 2.0 titanium plates and screws. The maxilla should be positioned passively and free from bone interferences according to the treatment plan.
- Bone defects can now be grafted using autogenous bone.
- Remove the interdental splint and examine the occlusion in centric relation.
- The incisions are sutured and light intermaxillary elastics placed.

Fig. 14 demonstrates the utilization of surgical segmenting the maxilla for the correction of an open bite dentofacial deformity. The maxilla required 3-dimensional correction: transverse

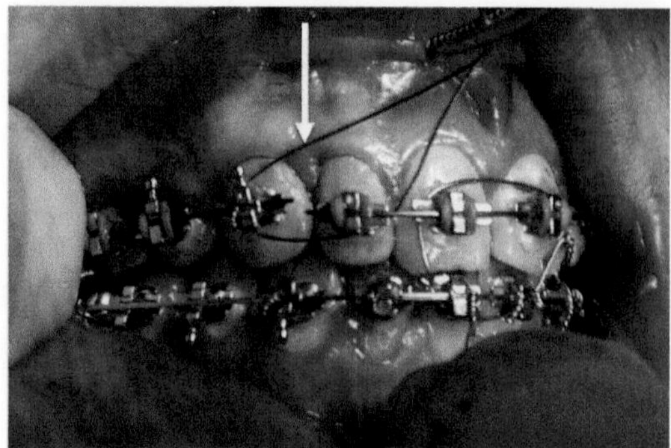

Fig. 13. Once the intermaxillary fixation is placed with the teeth into the final occlusion (with or without a final surgical splint), and interdental wire (014-inch) is placed around the brackets of the teeth adjacent to the osteotomy (*arrow*). (*Courtesy of* Johan Reyneke, B.Ch.D, M.Ch.D, FCOMFS (SA), PhD., Cape Town, South Africa).

expansion and superior repositioning of the posterior maxilla, and advancement of the maxilla and autorotation of the mandible.

POSTOPERATIVE ORTHODONTIC TREATMENT

Postoperative orthodontics should not begin until the patient is cleared by oral and maxillofacial surgery (OMFS). When segmental procedures are performed, the return to orthodontics may not occur for approximately 6 weeks due to the extended presence of the maxillary splint. Six weeks allows for hard callus formation and primary stability, but the segments remain mobile.

Ideally, the day the splint is removed by OMFS, the patient will return to the orthodontist for a heavy continuous stainless steel arch wire (17 × 25 in and 18 slot; 19 × 25 or 21 × 25 in for 22 slot). An efficient approach is to conform the wire to the arch-form created during the segmental model surgery. With plaster model surgery, this is quite simple; with digital model surgery, either the digital models can be 3-dimensionally printed, or the orthodontist can use the splint itself.

STABILIZING EXPANSION

Other useful aids in maintaining the arch width during the finishing orthodontics is use of passive TPAs or buccal stabilizing wires (**Fig. 15**). Regardless of the orthodontists preferred approach the wire should be passive in the transverse plane of space. No additional expansion should be placed and care must be taken to avoid inadvertently constricting the dental arches.

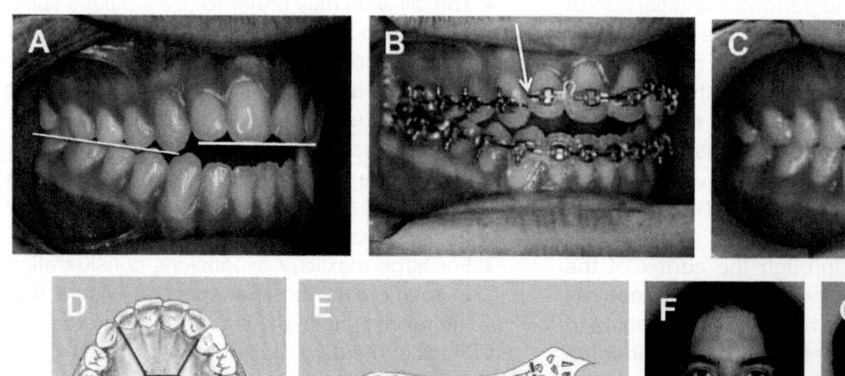

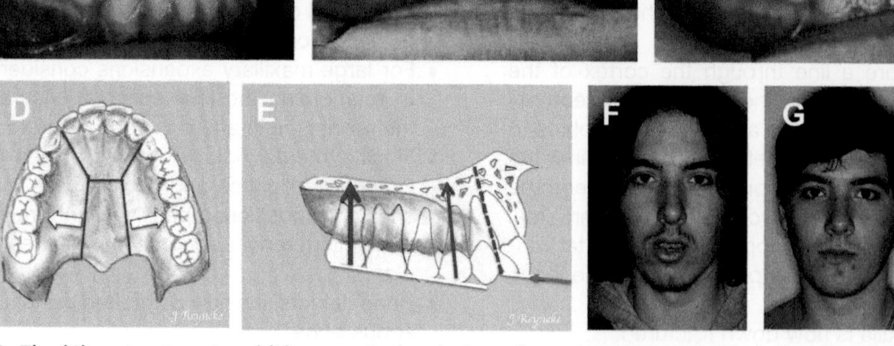

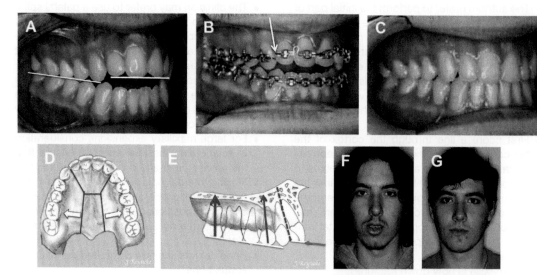

Fig. 14. The (*A*) pretreatment and (*B*) presurgical occlusion of a patient who presented with an anterior open bite dentofacial deformity, posterior vertical maxillary excess and bilateral cross bites. (*C*) The posterior maxilla was transversely deficient however vertically excessive and required segmental surgery to expand and superior repositioning of the posterior segments. (*F*) The patient's lower facial height was excessive, whereas his upper incisor/lip relationship proved to be normal. (*D*) The upper dental arch was orthodontically aligned into 3 segments. Note: the segmentation of the arch wire at the intended interdental osteotomies as well as the bend in the arch wire to achieve root deviation (*arrow*). The surgical plan involved a 4-piece Le Fort I maxillary osteotomy, (*D*) expanding and (*E*) superior repositioning the posterior segment while maintaining the height of the anterior segment (*arrows*). The improved occlusion (*C*) and aesthetic change is demonstrated in (*F*) and (*G*). (*Courtesy of* Johan Reyneke, B.Ch.D, M.Ch.D, FCOMFS (SA), PhD., Cape Town, South Africa).

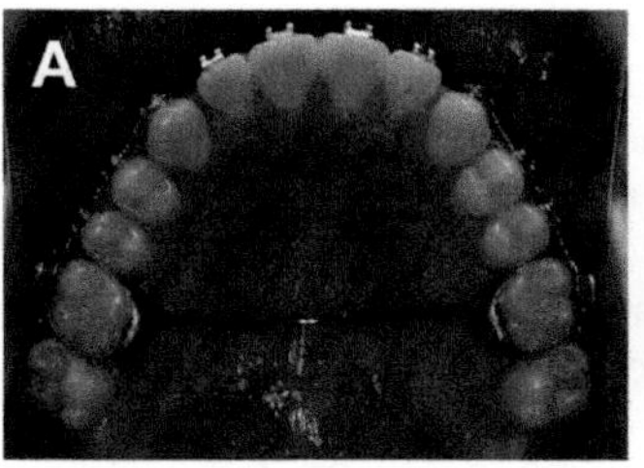
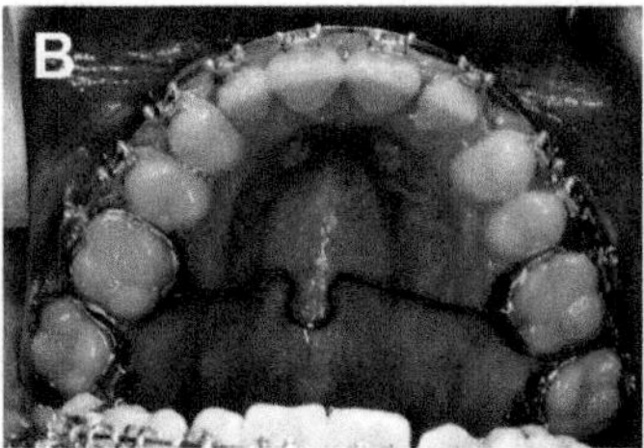

Fig. 15. TPA for stabilization. (*A*) The version without a loop is more rigid. (*B*) Using a loop adds more wire length, which adds greater flexibility minimizing the efficacy for stabilization. (*Courtesy of* Johan Reyneke, B.Ch.D, M.Ch.D, FCOMFS (SA), PhD., Cape Town, South Africa).

The final item is correcting the angulation of the teeth adjacent to the osteotomy site. If bends were previously used, the bends can be incrementally reduced to obtain root parallelism. If bracket orientation was altered during the initial bonding phase, either the brackets can be removed and rebounded in the ideal position/angulation or new bends can be placed to adjust to remove the root divergence.

RETENTION

Full-coverage palatal acrylic can be particularly beneficial in retaining the segmented maxillary expansion. Patients should be informed that there is greater relapse tendency with segmental maxillary surgery than with SARPE. Ideally patients should be prepared to wear the retainers full time for at least 6 months and nightly for as long as possible. No form of retention is perfect and compliance is critical. Failure to comply with retention immediately following care can have rapid and unfortunate effects not only on the transverse dimension but also the vertical. For patients who relapse transversely, the overbite will get shallower as cuspal inclines articulate against one another rather than the preferred cusp/fossa relationships.?

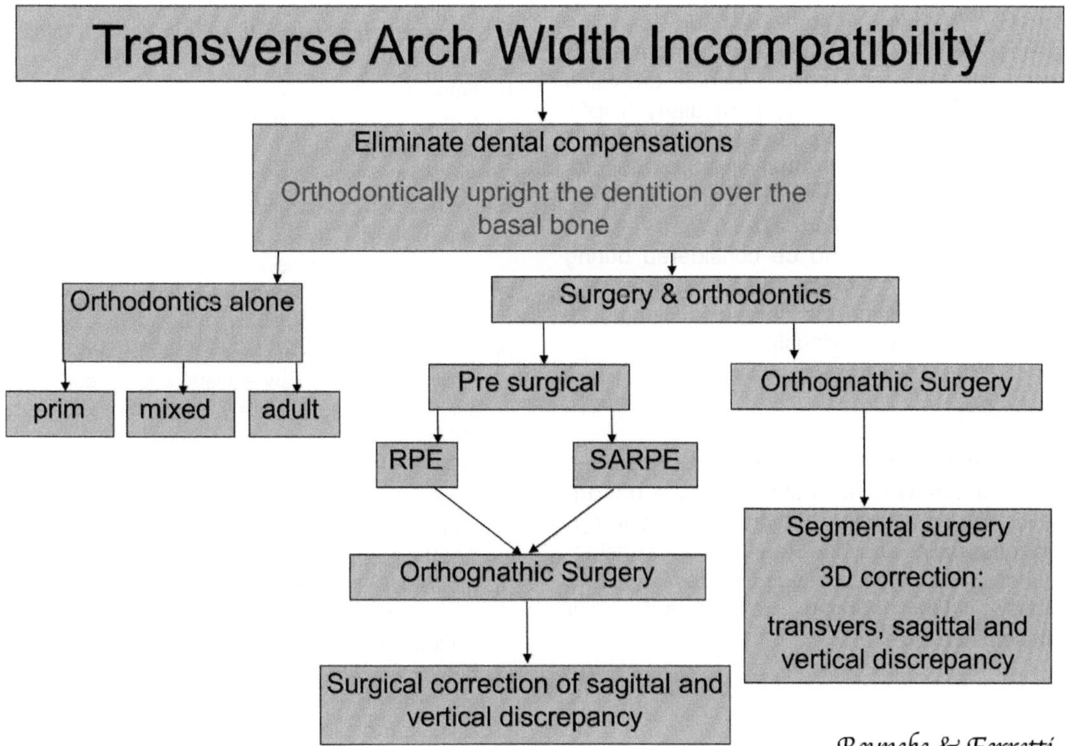

Fig. 16. The flowchart demonstrates the surgical and orthodontic decision-making processes as described in this article. (*Courtesy of* Johan Reyneke, B.Ch.D, M.Ch.D, FCOMFS (SA), PhD., Cape Town, South Africa).

DISCUSSION

Stability

In a review of postoperative stability following various orthognathic surgical procedures, Proffit and colleagues[33] in 1996, found that maxillary expansion by means of segmental surgery proved to be the least stable of all maxillary procedures. The surgical technique and postoperative orthodontic control to improve transverse stability has certainly been adapted during the following 22 years. The same authors published improved results and extensions in an update following rigid fixation in 2007.[33,34]

Marchetti and colleagues[35] in 2009, compared the postoperative stability following surgically assisted palatal expansion and segmental maxillary surgery after 2 years. They found that segmental surgery proved to be more stable.

PROS AND CONS OF DIFFERENT TREATMENT APPROACHES

As previously described, both SARPE and multisegment Le Fort osteotomies are effective in addressing the transverse dimension. During treatment planning one must consider the patient's needs and fears. If the expansion is limited and other planes of space need to be corrected, the multisegment Le Fort can be preferred (Fig. 14). For patients with larger transverse deficiency and severe dental crowding SARPE is preferred. This is particularly helpful when other planes of space need not be corrected. If a true 3-dimensional skeletal malocclusion with large transverse deficiency must be corrected, while unfortunate, the 2-stage approach is preferred to be considered during treatment planning? In **Fig. 16** a flowchart is presented demonstrating the decision-making process as discussed previously.

SUMMARY

The transverse dimension is a critical component of the comprehensive treatment of the orthognathic surgery patient. Several treatment approaches exist and the team must consider the individual patient's needs, desires, and limitations when working to correct their malocclusion.

REFERENCES

1. Angell EC. Treatment of irregularities of the permanent or adult tooth. Dental Cosmos 1860;1:540–4, 599-601.
2. Babcock JH. The screw expansion plate. The Dental Record 1911;31:588–90, 596-599.
3. Korkhaus G. Discussion of report: a review of orthodontic research (1946-1950), Internat. Dent J 1959; 33:356.
4. Haas AJ. Palatal expansion: just the beginning of dentofacial orthopedics. Am J Orthop 1970;57(3): 219–55.
5. Adkins MD, Nanda RS, Currier GF. Arch perimeter changes on rapid palatal expansion. Am J Orthod Dentofacial Orthop 1990;97(3):194–9.
6. McNamara JA Jr, Riolo ML, Enlow DH. Growth of the maxillary complex in the rhesus monkey (Macaca mulatta). Am J Phys Anthropol 1976; 44(1):15–26.
7. Baccetti T, Franchi L, Cameron CG, et al. Treatment timing for rapid maxillary expansion. Angle Orthod 2001;71(5):343–50.
8. Angelieri F, Franchi L, Cevidanes LHS, et al. Cone beam computed tomography evaluation of midpalatal suture maturation in adults. Int J Oral Maxillofac Surg 2017;46(12):1557–61.
9. Haas A. Rapid palatal expansion of the maxillary dental arch and nasal cavity by opening the midpalatal suture. Angle Orthod 1961;31:73–90.
10. Haas A. The treatment of maxillary deficiency by opening the midpalatal suture. Angle Orthod 1965; 35:200–17.
11. Proffit WR, Fields HW Jr, Sarver DM. Contemporary orthodontics. 4th edition. St. Louis (MO): Mosby Elsevier; 2007.
12. Wang YC, Chang PM, Liou EJ. Opening of circum maxillary sutures by alternate rapid maxillary expansions and constrictions. Angle Orthod 2009;79(2): 230–4.
13. Lee RJ, Moon W, Hong C. Effects of monocortical and bicortical mini-implant anchorage on bone-borne palatal expansion using finite element analysis. Am J Orthod Dentofacial Orthop 2016;151(5): 887–97.
14. Vassar JW, Karydix A, Trojan T, et al. Dentoskeletal effects of a temporary skeletal anchorage device supported rapid maxillary expansion appliance (TSADRME): A pilot study. Angle Orthod 2016; 86(2):241–9.
15. Timms DJ. A study of basal movement with rapid maxillary expansion. Am J Orthod 1980; 77:500–7.
16. Isaacson R, Murphy T. Some effects of rapid maxillary expansion in cleft lip and palate patients. Angle Orthod 1964;34:143–54.
17. Barber A, Simms M. Rapid maxillary expansion and external root resorption I man: a scanning electron microscope study. Am J Orthod 1980;79: 630–52.
18. Langford SR. Root resorption extremes resulting from clinical RME. Am J Orthod 1982;81:371–7.

19. Greenbaum KR, Zachrisson BU. The effect of palatal expansion therapy on the periodontal tissues. Am J Orthod 1982;81:12–21.
20. Lines P. Adult rapid maxillary expansion with corticotomy. Am J Orthod 1975;67:44–56.
21. Bell WH, Epker B. Surgical-orthodontic expansion of the maxilla. Am J Orthod 1976;705:17–28.
22. Wertz R. Skeletal and dental changes accompanying rapid midpalatal suture opening. Am J Orthod 1970;58:41–66.
23. Suri L, Taneja P. Surgically assisted rapid palatal expansion: a literature review. Am J Orthod Dentofacial Orthop 2008;133:290–302.
24. Perciaccante VJ, Bays RA. Principles of maxillary orthognathic surgery. In: Miloro M, editor. Peterson's principles of oral and maxillofacial surgery, vol. 2. Schelton, (CT): People Med Publ. House; 2012. Ch 58.
25. Mommaerts MY. Transpalatal distraction as a method of maxillary expansion. Br J Oral Maxillofac Surg 1999;37:268–72.
26. Gerlach K, Zahl C. Transversal palatal expansion using a palatal distractor. J Orofac Orthop 2003;64: 443–9.
27. Koudstaal M, Van Der Wal K. The rotterdam palatal distractor; introduction of the new bone-borne device and report of the pilot study. Int J Oral Maxillofac Surg 2006;35:31–4.
28. Koudstaal MJ, Wolvius EB, Shulten AJM, et al. Stability, tipping and relapse of bone-borne versus tooth-borne surgically assisted rapid palatal maxillary expansion; a prospective randomized patient trial. Int J Oral Maxillofac Surg 2009;38:308–15.
29. Venugoplan SR, Nanda V, Turkistani K, et al. Discharge patterns of orthognathic surgeries in the United States. J Oral Maxillofac Surg 2012;70(1): 77–86.
30. Reyneke JP. Essentials of orthognathic surgery. Chicago: Quintessence; 2010.
31. Wolford M, Alexander CM, Stevago ELL, et al. Orthodontics for orthognathic surgery. In: Ghali GE, Larsen PE, Waite PD, editors. Principles of oral and maxillofacial surgery. 4th edition. Shelton, (CT): People's Medical Publishing House; 2012. p. 1263–4.
32. Esteves LS, dos Santos JN, Sullivan SM, et al. Why segment the maxilla between laterals and canines? Dental Press J Orthod 2016;21(1):110–25.
33. Proffit WR, Turvey TA, Phillips C. Orthognathic surgery: a hierarchy of stability. Int J Adult Orthodon Orthognath Surg 1996;11:191–204.
34. Proffit WR, Turvey TA, Phillips C. The hierarchy of stability and predictability in orthognathic surgery with rigid fixation: an update and extension. Head Face Med 2007;30:3, 21.
35. Marchetti C, Pironi M, Bianchi A, et al. Surgically assisted rapid palatal expansion vs. segmental Le Fort I osteotomy: transverse stability over a 2-year period. J Craniomaxillofac Surg 2009;37(2):372–8.

Orthognathic Surgery and Orthodontics

Inadequate Planning Leading to Complications or Unfavorable Results

Katherine P. Klein, DMD, MS[a,*], Leonard B. Kaban, DMD, MD[a], Mohamed I. Masoud, BDS, DMSc[b]

KEYWORDS

• Orthodontics • Orthognathic surgery • Complications • Unfavorable results

KEY POINTS

- Overall goals and a coordinated surgical/orthodontic plan should be developed and agreed upon by the orthodontist/surgeon team and approved by the patient before the start of treatment.
- Continuous communication between the orthodontist and surgeon through all phases of treatment is essential to minimize complications or unfavorable outcomes.
- Preoperative orthodontic treatment progress should be monitored by the surgeon every 4 to 6 months and discussed with the orthodontist.
- Frequent progress models to assess tooth position and arch compatibility are recommended.
- Inadequate preoperative planning may necessitate delay or alteration of the ideal surgical plan.

INTRODUCTION

Inadequate and inappropriate presurgical treatment planning are commonly the source of unfavorable outcomes or complications in patients undergoing orthognathic surgery.[1–5] It is critical that the patient's chief complaint, treatment goals, and expectations are established and understood by the clinicians. The diagnosis, orthodontic, and surgical goals and the overall plan should be discussed and agreed upon by the surgeon and orthodontist before beginning treatment.[1–5] When possible, the need for orthognathic surgery should be determined before any tooth movement has been started so that orthodontic treatment can be accomplished as efficiently and effectively as possible.[1–5] Miscommunication between providers can result in improper or insufficient dental decompensation, increased treatment time, delay, or potentially an increase in magnitude of the operation (eg, turning what could be a single-jaw into a 2-jaw procedure).[6–8]

Identifying common pitfalls in orthognathic surgical cases[6–27] and developing a systematic approach to address potential missteps are essential for treatment success. Most errors can be classified into 4 general categories:

1. Complications related to treatment planning
2. Complications related to inadequate dental decompensation
3. Complications related to appliances
4. Complications related to postsurgical orthodontic care

When orthodontists and surgeons work together to formulate a proper diagnosis and treatment

[a] Massachusetts General Hospital, OMFS Academic Offices, Warren 1201, 55 Fruit Street, Boston, MA 02114, USA; [b] Department of Developmental Biology, Harvard School of Dental Medicine, 188 Longwood Avenue, Boston, MA 02115, USA
* Corresponding author.
E-mail address: Kklein1@mgh.harvard.edu

Oral Maxillofacial Surg Clin N Am 32 (2020) 71–82
https://doi.org/10.1016/j.coms.2019.08.008
1042-3699/20/

plan, monitor and give feedback to each other throughout the preoperative orthodontic process, and agree on the use of appropriate appliances and postsurgical treatment strategies, patients will have the best chance for a successful outcome.[1–5]

COMPLICATIONS RELATED TO TREATMENT PLANNING

Before treatment begins, the patient, orthodontist, and surgeon should all agree on the dental and skeletal diagnosis and a conceptual surgical and orthodontic plan. The orthodontist and surgeon should feel comfortable that the patient has an understanding of the goals and reasonable expectations regarding the predicted esthetic and functional outcomes. The Orthognathic Surgical Team at Massachusetts General Hospital (MGH) meets once each week for initial case presentations, progress evaluations as necessary, assessment of immediate postoperative outcomes, discussion of complications, and long-term follow-up evaluations. There is a standardized format for presentation and a systematic process to evaluate each patient. The authors review a checklist to mitigate the risk of overlooking an important diagnostic or treatment detail (**Table 1**).

When treatment goals are not clear, tooth movement may be carried out in the wrong direction. For example, if an orthodontist attempts to further compensate the teeth to "minimize the magnitude" of the operation, this may have to be reversed to accomplish the desired anatomic or esthetic outcome. Orthodontic treatment time will be extended; the operative plan may have to be changed, or the outcome may be less than ideal. Ultimately this will result in increased anxiety and frustration for all members of the treatment team and the patient.

COMPLICATIONS RELATED TO PRESURGICAL ORTHODONTIC TREATMENT

The objectives for presurgical orthodontic treatment are (1) to decompensate the teeth to make the magnitude of the dental discrepancy as close to the skeletal discrepancy as possible. This requires dental decompensation in the sagittal, vertical, and transverse planes; (2) to eliminate dental interferences that would prevent achieving the desired final occlusion; and (3) to address tooth-size discrepancies that would prevent interdigitation at the desired postoperative overjet and overbite.

Table 1
Massachusetts General Hospital surgical orthodontic patient pretreatment checklist

✓ Has the patient's chief complaint been identified?
✓ Are the names and contact information of the patient's treatment team (oral and maxillofacial surgeon, orthodontist, dentist) in the chart?
✓ Have pretreatment records been analyzed?
✓ Are there any dental pathologic conditions (caries and similar) that need to be addressed immediately? Do third molars need to be extracted before the operation?
✓ Meet with the team and finalize the dental and skeletal diagnosis and global treatment plan (1 jaw vs 2 jaws, midline rotations, presurgical position of incisors). Has the final plan been documented in the chart and communicated to the patient?
✓ When does the patient want the operation? Is there a major life event/deadline that we must work around (wedding, pregnancy, patient moving, insurance expiring, and so forth)?
✓ What orthodontic appliances will be used (metal braces, clear braces, clear aligners, and so forth)? What downstream implications will this have for the presurgery setup?
✓ Has the patient signed the informed consent?
✓ When will the other providers see the patient for follow-up appointments?

Developing a systematic process to evaluate and manage each surgical-orthodontic patient is key to effective and efficient treatment.

Complications Related to Inadequate Orthodontic Decompensation in the Sagittal Plane

Patients with class III malocclusions often have physiologic dental compensations in an attempt to improve function and occlusal intercuspation. These compensations result in proclined upper incisors (tongue function), retroclined lower incisors (orbicularis), and lingually tipped lower posterior teeth (buccinator). The anterior crossbite is therefore significantly smaller than the skeletal deformity in the sagittal plane, and the transverse discrepancy may be masked. The presurgical orthodontic objective is usually to procline the lower incisors, upright the mandibular posterior teeth, and retrocline the upper incisors. This often involves treating a crowded lower arch without extractions (**Fig. 1**). The position of the lower lip and the lower incisors relative to the chin should be evaluated to avoid moving the lower incisors too far anteriorly, which may compromise their periodontal support and their relationship to the chin (too far forward). If this cannot be avoided, an advancement genioplasty may be required to achieve the desired facial esthetics.

The maxillary arch, on the other hand, often requires extraction even in the absence of crowding to create space to decompensate the upper teeth. This may involve extraction of the upper premolars (**Fig. 2**) or distalizing into the space of the extracted third molars. Distalizing the upper buccal segments can be challenging and often involves temporary anchorage devices or fixed class II bite correctors if compliance with class II elastics is not optimal. The latter approach can only achieve a minimal amount of upper incisor retraction and is useful in cases where a smaller surgical movement is planned because the patient has petite features.

Care must be taken to avoid over-retroclining the upper incisors because that can lead to unsatisfactory seating of the buccal segments.[6–9] Upper incisor control can be achieved using larger wires with torque, accentuated curves, and torquing auxiliaries when necessary.

Patients with class II malocclusions often have retroclined upper incisors and proclined lower incisors that limit the magnitude of mandibular movement and prevent the achievement of an orthognathic profile. Orthodontic decompensation often involves proclination of the upper incisors and retroclination of the lower incisors to maximize the overjet, the surgical advancement of the mandible, and the improvement of chin projection relative to the lower lip. **Fig. 3** shows a case with mandibular hypoplasia and severe retroclination of the upper incisors. Despite the severe upper crowding, the upper arch was treated with proclination instead of extractions to improve the upper incisor inclination. The patient was treated with clear aligners, which are

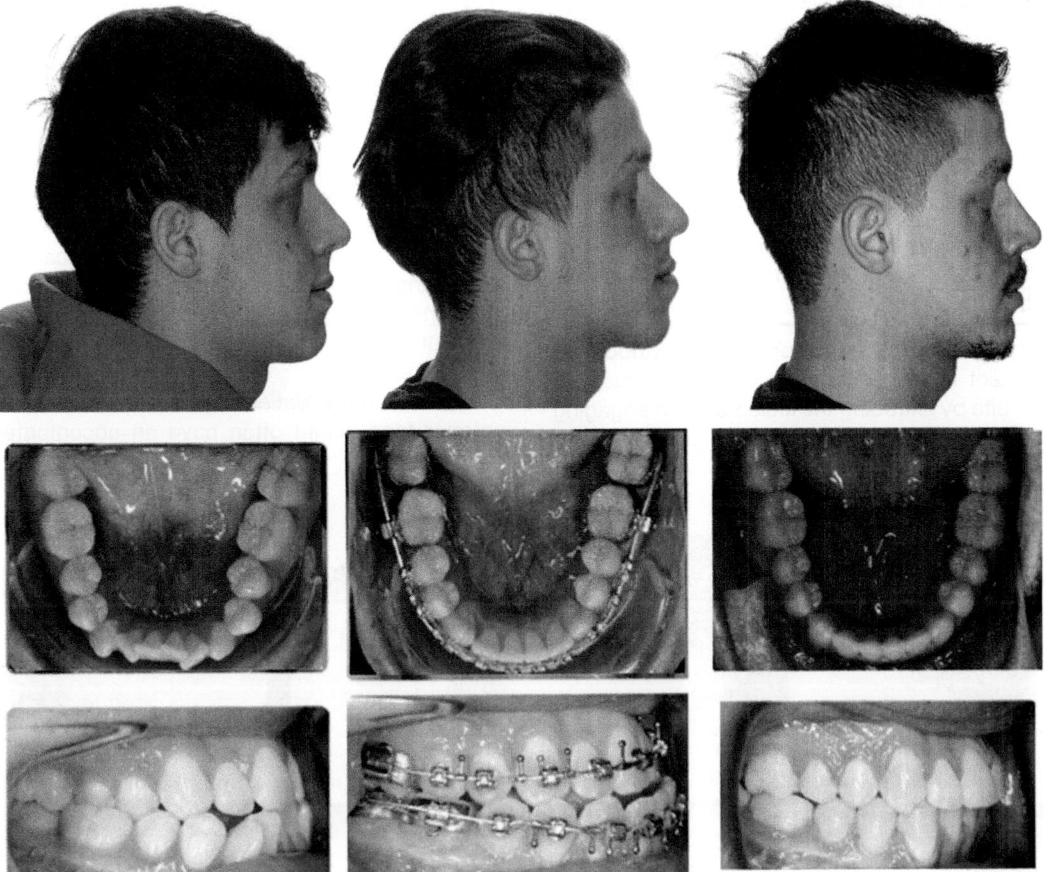

Fig. 1. The patient was planned for a Le Fort I maxillary advancement. Notice how the bite and lower lip position "worsen" as the teeth are aligned. Patients should be adequately prepared for the profile changes that are associated with orthodontic decompensation.

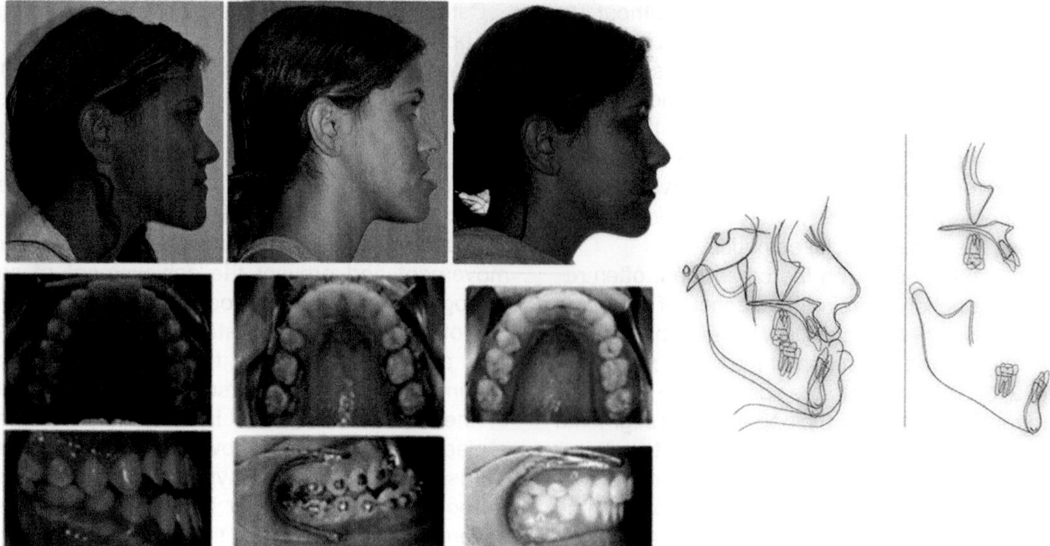

Fig. 2. The patient was planned for a Le Fort I maxillary advancement with extractions of 2 maxillary premolars. The maxillary arch required extraction of premolars even in the absence of crowding to create space to decompensate the upper teeth. In the cephalometric superimpositions, note the retroclination of the upper incisors and the proclination of the lower incisors. If teeth are not adequately decompensated, the desired postsurgical facial outcome cannot be achieved.

less effective than traditional braces at torquing the upper incisors. This resulted in only partial decompensation of their position and a less than ideal amount of mandibular advancement.

Complications Related to Inadequate Orthodontic Decompensation in the Vertical Plane

A common mistake during presurgical orthodontic treatment is to inadvertently close or reduce an open bite by extruding the incisors when engaging a continuous wire to level and align the arches (**Fig. 4**). The orthodontist should avoid any anterior elastics and use curved wires to maintain or exaggerate the initial open bite. If a biplanar occlusion is present and the surgeon is planning on segmenting the maxilla, segmental wires should be used instead of continuous wires. The anterior segmental may or not include the upper canines depending on whether the surgeon is planning to make the osteotomies between the lateral incisors and canines or between the canines and first premolars.

Hypodivergent patients with a short lower anterior face height often have an accentuated

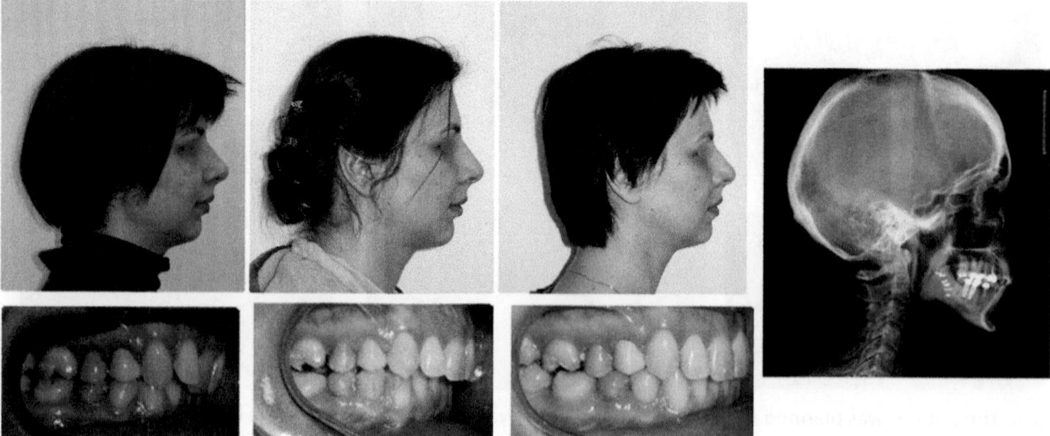

Fig. 3. When teeth are not fully decompensated before surgery, less mandibular advancement is possible.

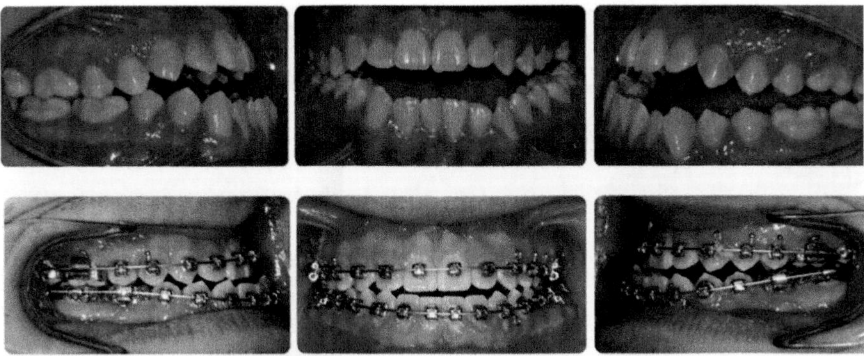

Fig. 4. A common presurgical orthodontic mistake is to level a biplanar maxillary dental malocclusion with a continuous archwire.

mandibular curve of Spee with a deep impinging overbite and a thick soft tissue chin button. Leveling the lower occlusal plane on these patients is another common mistake because it dentally opens the bite, reduces the vertical distance from the lower incisal edge to menton, and results in a straight horizontal mandibular advancement, making the chin too prominent and not increasing the lower anterior face height. In these cases, if the accentuated curve of Spee is maintained, during the preoperative orthodontic treatment, the mandible can be advanced and rotated in a clockwise rotation, thereby increasing the occlusal plane and the lower anterior face height. The patient may not need a maxillary osteotomy. Once the curve of Spee is leveled, the patient will be obligated to a maxillary operation to increase the occlusal plane and to allow clockwise rotation of the maxilla and mandible.

Maintaining the deep lower curve of Spee during presurgical orthodontics using curved wires and setting the patient in a tripoded occlusion can help avoid these issues. The curve of Spee can be leveled after surgery by allowing the premolars to erupt. **Fig. 5**A shows a patient with a hypoplastic mandible and a reduced lower anterior facial height. Because the upper incisors did not require decompensation and the lower arch naturally had a deep curve of Spee, it was a suitable case for surgery before orthodontic treatment. A surgical splint was provided to the surgeon to set the lower jaw in a tripod occlusion with 2 mm of overjet and overbite. After the operation, the acrylic opposing the premolars was trimmed and elastics to the lower premolars were used to extrude the lower premolars and level the lower curve of Spee while maintaining the distance from the lower incisal edges to the menton (**Fig. 5**B, C).

Complications Related to Inadequate Orthodontic Decompensation in the Transverse Plane

Patients with maxillary constrictions often have buccally flared upper molars and lingually inclined lower molars. If a 2-piece Le Fort I is planned, the presurgical orthodontic treatment should tip the crowns of the upper molars to the palatal and the crowns of the lower molars to the buccal. This will tend to create space in the lower arch and require space in the upper arch so this should be considered when assessing the crowding or spacing. If surgically assisted maxillary expansion is planned before orthodontic treatment, the expansion screw should be activated enough to put the molars in a buccal crossbite tendency. This is necessary to make up for normalizing the inclination of the molars as well as potential relapse of the procedure. The space created during surgically assisted expansion needs to be taken into consideration and can be used to help tip the crowns of the upper molars palatally and relieve existing crowding in the upper arch. Failure to overcorrect the posterior crossbite during surgically assisted maxillary expansion can result in recurrence of the posterior crossbite after the teeth are bonded, and the inclination of the molars is normalized. Some patients have significant maxillary constriction paired with a narrow mandible and no crossbite. These cases often require surgically assisted expansion of the maxilla and widening of the mandible by midline distraction osteogenesis. This is to avoid developing a buccal crossbite when the maxillary constriction is corrected. The space created in the mandible using surgically assisted expansion can often be sufficient to resolve even severe crowding in the lower arch (**Fig. 6**).

In patients with significant mandibular asymmetry, presurgical orthodontic treatment focuses on

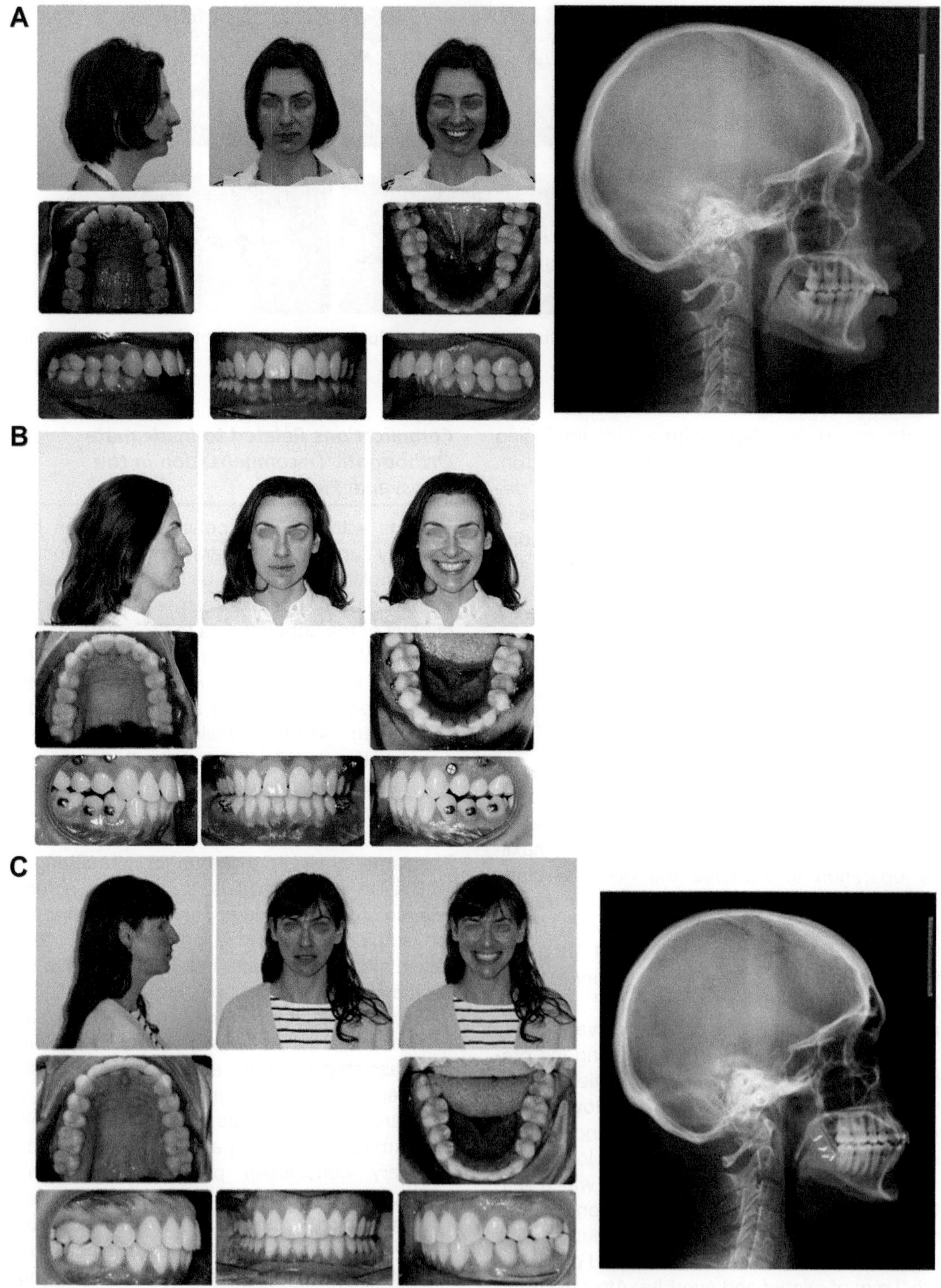

Fig. 5. (*A*) This individual has a hypoplastic mandible and a reduced lower anterior face height. Be-cause of the proclined lower incisors and already present curve of Spee, she was planned for surgery first. (*B*) Postsurgical result. Orthodontic treatment with clear aligners was initiated after surgery. Note the attachments and temporary anchorage devices used to extrude the man-dibular premolars and level the curve of Spee. (*C*) Final result after surgery first followed by orthodontic tre-atment.

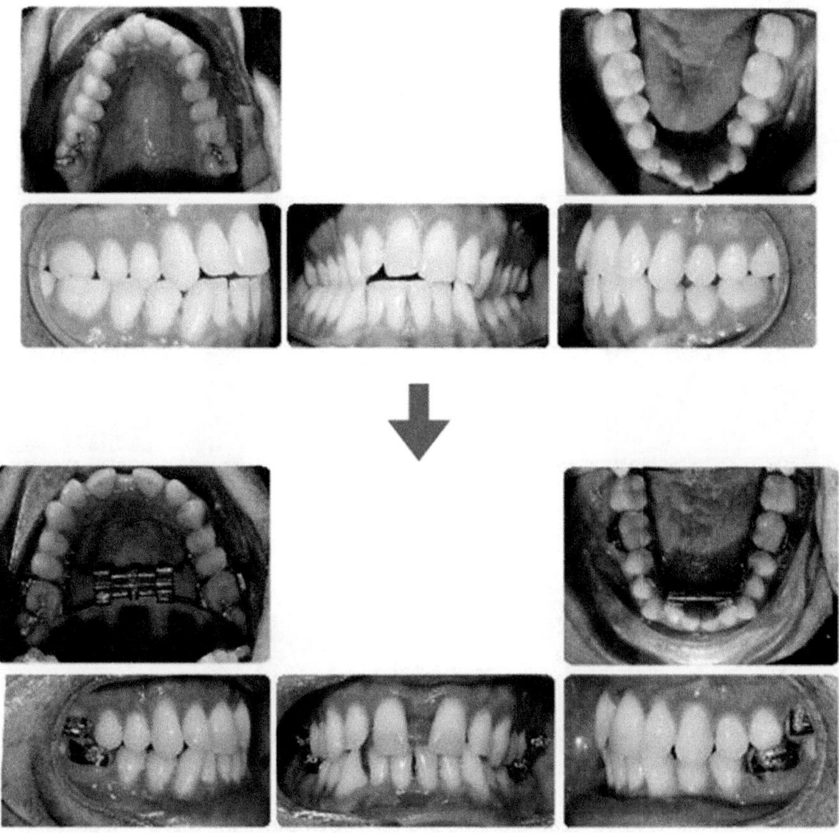

Fig. 6. This individual had a surgically assisted expansion of the maxilla and widening of the mandible by midline distraction. Note the large midline diastema and how mandibular crowding was alleviated.

decompensation in the axial or transverse plane to get the lower dental midline to be coincident with the chin point, exaggerating or creating a lingual crossbite on the shorter side of the mandible, and exaggerating or creating a buccal crossbite on the longer side of the mandible (**Fig. 7**). Failure to accomplish this decompensation will result in inadequate correction of the asymmetry when the anatomic position of the mandible is guided by the occlusion. Conversely, the occlusion will not fit correctly if the final surgical position is set to put the chin point coincident with the facial midline (**Fig. 8**).

The surgical correction of a skeletal III malocclusion by maxillary advancement and/or mandibular setback can often resolve a presurgical transverse discrepancy because the movement in the sagittal plane results in a wider part of the upper arch occluding with a narrower part of the lower arch. The greater the necessary sagittal surgical correction, the less likely surgical intervention will be needed to correct the transverse relationship. The case in **Fig. 2** had a crossbite before treatment and would have needed a 2-piece Le Fort I if the teeth were not sufficiently decompensated in the sagittal plane. Extracting the upper premolars allowed full decompensation of the upper incisors, creating a large anterior crossbite preoperatively. The posttreatment photographs show the molars set in a class II relationship with a normal anterior relationship and no posterior crossbite, despite the fact that the patient had a 1-piece maxillary osteotomy.

Likewise, the surgical sagittal correction of a class II malocclusion can often exaggerate a transverse skeletal discrepancy because it results in a wider part of the mandible occluding with a narrower part of the maxilla (**Fig. 9**).

Complications Related to Adequately Addressing Dental Interferences and Tooth Size Discrepancies

Surgical patients often spend years functioning out of an ideal occlusion and develop wear patterns that result in significant prematurities when the teeth are articulated in the desired postoperative position. During the final months of presurgical orthodontic treatment, impressions should be

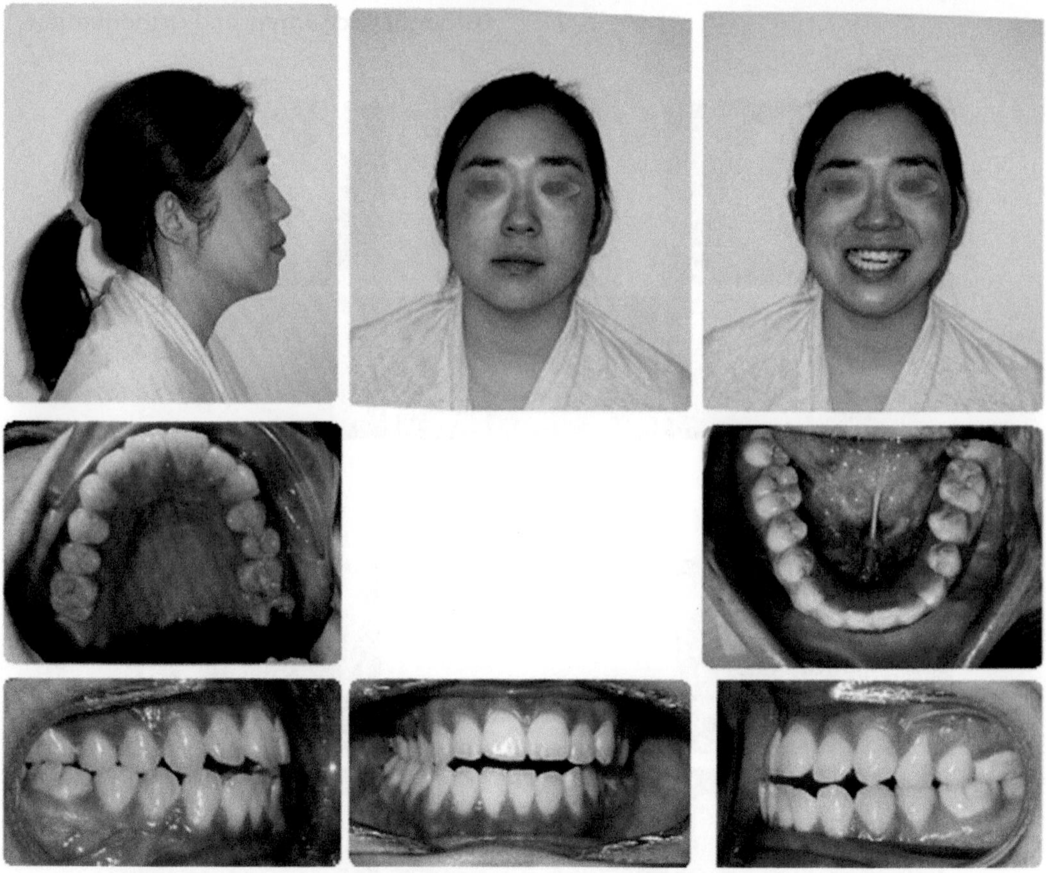

Fig. 7. This individual has significant mandibular asymmetry. To properly decompensate teeth in preparation for surgery, a lingual crossbite needs to be created on the shorter side of the mandible, and a buccal crossbite on the longer side of the mandible. The goal is to decompensate the teeth in the axial or transverse plane and get the lower dental midline to be coincident with the chin point.

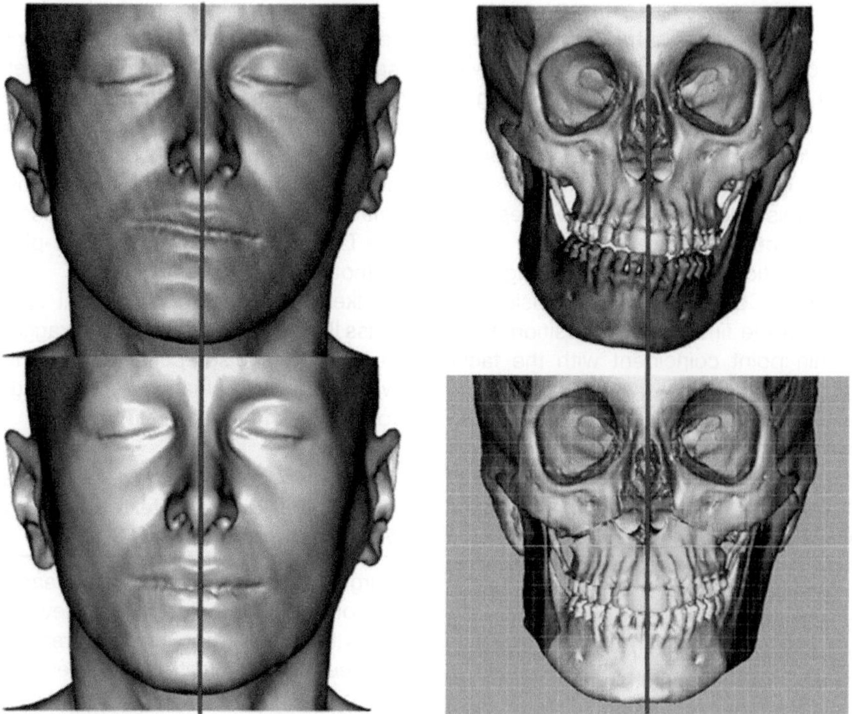

Fig. 8. This individual had inadequate orthodontic decompensation before surgery. Even after bimaxillary surgery, she needed a genioplasty to correctly align her chin with her facial midline.

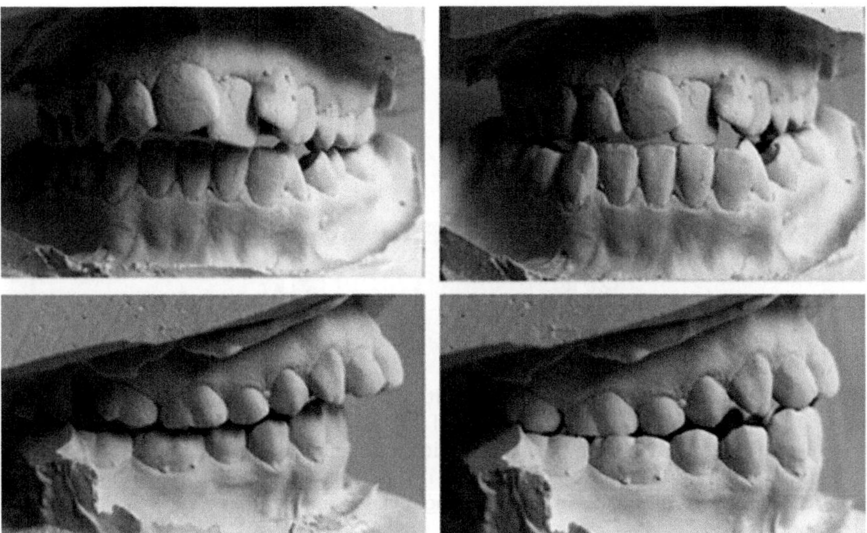

Fig. 9. Patients with a class II phenotype frequently also have a transverse maxillary deficiency. Note how models show a posterior crossbite when a class I canine and molar relationship is visualized. This diagnosis should ideally be noted before the start of orthodontic treatment so decisions can be made about appropriate appliance selection (palate expander) or surgical plan.

taken every visit to check the bite and perform the necessary detailing and occlusal adjustment to achieve a stable postoperative bite (**Fig. 10**).

Similarly, tooth size discrepancies like undersized upper lateral incisors or large lower anterior teeth need to be addressed before the surgical procedure because they prevent the buccal segments from seating at a normal overjet and overbite during the operation. This puts the surgeon in the difficult position of having to decide between setting the bite with an ideal canine relationship and little or no overjet or setting the bite at the correct overjet and class II buccal segments (**Fig. 11**).

These problems can be identified by performing a tooth size discrepancy analysis and checking the

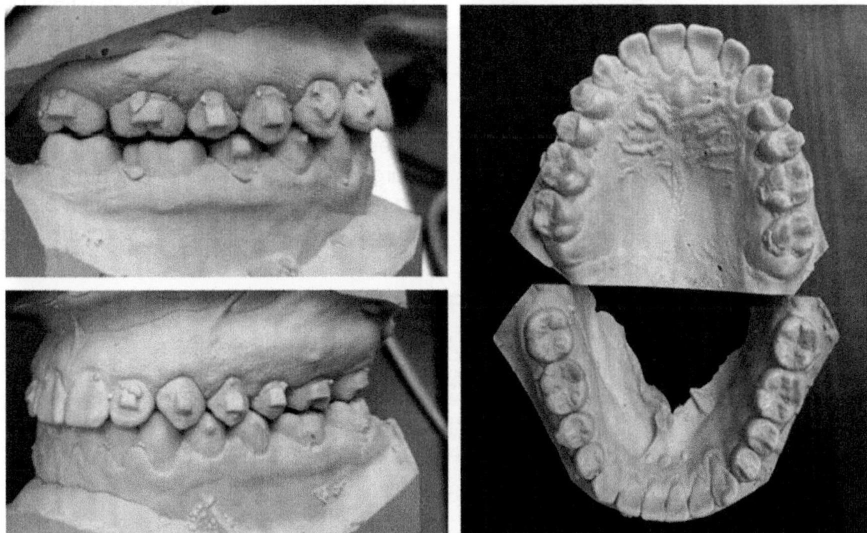

Fig. 10. When preparing an orthodontic patient for surgery, taking an adequate number study models is essential. Study models are often taken before every visit and serve as a powerful tool that allows the orthodontist to both modify wear facets from occlusal prematurities owing to years functioning out of the ideal occlusion, and detail and finish the bite. This careful presurgical preparation prevents the surgeon from needing to perform extensive occlusal adjustment during the operation.

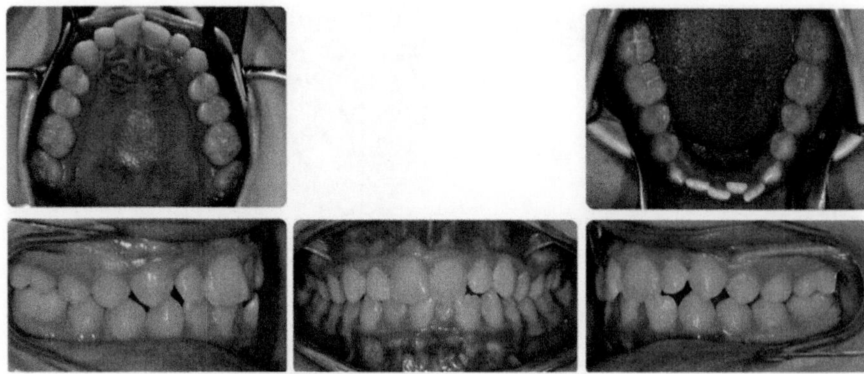

Fig. 11. During the pretreatment diagnostic workup, it was noted that this patient had a Bolton tooth size discrepancy in the maxillary anterior arch (small lateral incisors). Orthodontists should manage the tooth size discrepancy presurgically and either leave space for the ideal buildup or adjust the size of the teeth in the lower arch before the operation. When a tooth size analysis in not performed and the small tooth size is not taken into account, the buccal segments will not fit in an ideal Angle class I relationship.

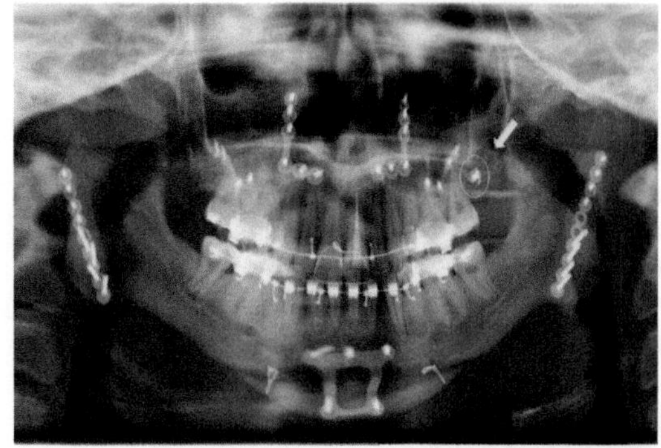

Fig. 12. During surgery, a bracket was broken off the maxillary second molar. The arrow points to the bracket which is in the wound. The patient required a second operation to retrieve the bracket.

presurgical models for fit. If the canines cannot be positioned in class I without the incisors being edge to edge or very shallow, lower incisor interproximal reduction should performed and/or spaces for upper lateral incisor build-ups should be opened.

COMPLICATIONS RELATED TO APPLIANCES

Orthodontists use a variety of appliances to align teeth in preparation for orthognathic surgery: traditional braces, lingual braces, and clear aligner systems. With traditional braces, the ideal presurgical orthognathic setup includes brackets on the facial surfaces of teeth tied with stainless steel ligatures; a full-dimension stainless steel arch wire, which has been inactive for 2 to 3 months; bands on the first and second molars; and surgical hooks between all teeth. This orthodontic setup gives the surgeon maximum flexibility in the operating room to use the orthodontic appliances to attach splints and accomplish necessary surgical movements.

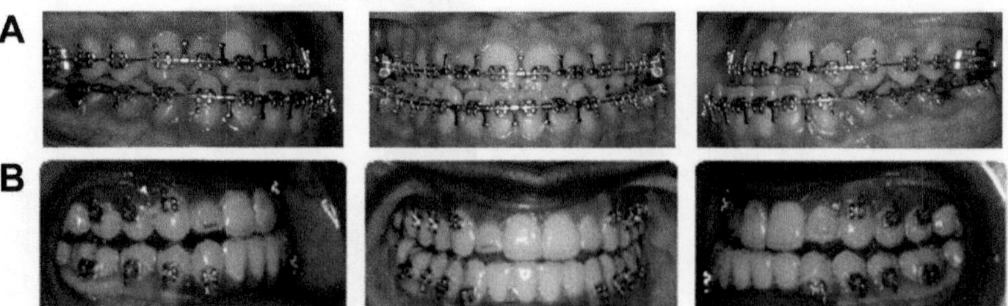

Fig. 13. (*A*) An ideal presurgical orthodontic setup in traditional braces includes full-dimension stainless steel arch wires, bands on first and second molars, ligature ties on all teeth, and surgical hooks. (*B*) An ideal presurgical orthodontic setup using clear aligners includes attachments on teeth that will need elastics after surgery. The authors' center prefers the use of metal buttons in case one is dislodged during the operation; it is easier to find with the use of radiographs.

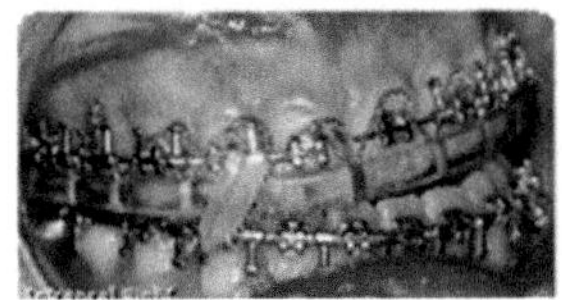
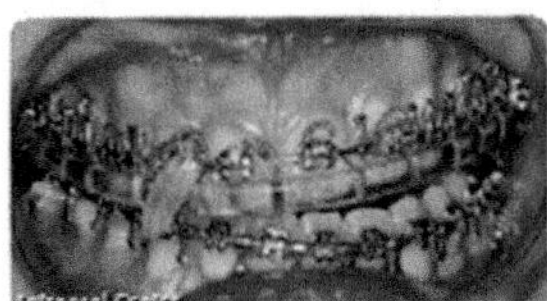
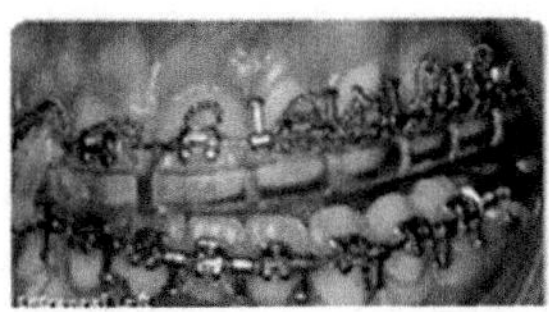

Fig. 14. This individual failed to return for appropriate postsurgical appointments with both the orthodontist and surgeon. During this 8-week period, she wore an anterior elastic on the right side only. Note the dental cant and open bite on the patient's left. Improper elastic wear can result in distortion of the dentoalveolar segments and jaw position, turning an excellent postsurgical outcome into a nonideal surgical result.

In a 2-piece Le Fort operation, surgeons fasten wires around the bands on the first molars and pull laterally to separate the maxilla. At the authors' institution, there is a higher incidence of brackets separating from the tooth than bands. When a distal bracket breaks during the operation, it can slide off the wire and disappear into the wound. Locating the bracket is difficult and takes additional time under anesthesia, or a second procedure to remove the lost bracket (**Fig. 12**). For this reason, bands are recommended on distal molars.

An increasing number of surgical orthodontic cases are now treated with clear aligners. When using clear aligners, it is important to provide the surgeon with enough attachments so that surgical splints may be placed, and so that postoperative guiding elastics can be used (**Fig. 13**).

Regardless of the specific material or appliance that is used, the following 3 guiding principles should be followed:

1. *No loose brackets or attachments.* Appliances need to be firmly attached to teeth to minimize intraoperative risk.
2. *No tooth movement immediately before surgery.* Teeth should be stabilized approximately 8 weeks before surgery with either a stainless steel arch wire or the final aligner. Surgical treatment plans are developed based on the location of the dentition. If dental changes occur before surgery, the dentition may not fit together as planned intraoperatively, resulting in a nonideal outcome.
3. *Ample surgical hooks.* Surgical hooks are used intraoperatively to aid in positioning the maxilla and/or the mandible and splint. Place ample surgical hooks (between all teeth) to give the surgeon maximum flexibility during the operation.

COMPLICATIONS RELATED TO POSTSURGICAL ORTHODONTIC CARE

Careful postsurgical orthodontics is essential for a successful outcome.[1–9] The length of postsurgical orthodontic care depends on a variety of factors, including how precise the presurgical orthodontic set up was to the desired result, how close the predicted surgical plan was to the achieved final surgical positioning of the jaw or jaws, and the patient's level of compliance with elastics after surgery.

At MGH, postoperative patients are followed closely by both the surgeon and the orthodontist to ensure that postoperative directions are being appropriately observed. Regular checks with both the surgeon and the orthodontist ensure that patients are complying with proper elastic wear. Unchecked elastic wear can result in distortion of the dentoalveolar segments and jaw position (**Fig. 14**).

SUMMARY

When orthodontists and surgeons work together to formulate an accurate diagnosis and treatment plan, monitor and give feedback to each other throughout the preoperative and postoperative orthodontic process, and agree on the use of appropriate appliances and postsurgical treatment strategies, patients will have the best chance for a successful outcome.[1–4] Miscommunication between providers can result in improper or insufficient dental decompensation, increased treatment time, delay or potentially an increase in magnitude of the operation (eg, turning what would could be a single-jaw into a 2-jaw procedure), and a less than satisfactory skeletal and esthetic result. The authors recommend developing a regular communication schedule between orthodontist and surgeon throughout the entire treatment process to avoid errors in treatment planning, inadequate preoperative dental decompensation of the teeth, complications related to inadequate or failed orthodontic appliances, and errors in immediate postoperative orthodontic management. The authors also recommend frequent progress dental casts to ensure proper decompensation of the teeth and adequacy of the occlusal fit preoperatively, regular communication regarding immediate surgical outcomes relative to planned surgical movements, frequent communication in the postoperative period to ensure correct elastic traction, and long-term follow-up to critically assess the outcomes over time.

REFERENCES

1. Kaban LB, Pogrel MA, Perrot DH. Complications in oral and maxillofacial surgery. WB Saunders Co; 1997.
2. Proffit WR, White RP, Sarver DM. Contemporary treatment of dentofacial deformity. St Louis (MO): Mosby; 2003.
3. Proffit WR, Fields HW, Sarver DM. Contemporary orthodontics. St Louis (MO): Mosby; 2007.
4. Posnick JC. Orthognathic surgery: principles & practice. St Louis (MO): Elsavier; 2014.
5. Larson BE. Orthodontic preparation for orthognathic surgery. Oral Maxillofac Clin North Am 2014;26: 441–58.
6. Potts B, Fields HW, Shanker S, et al. Dental and skeletal outcomes for class II surgical-orthodontic treatment: a comparison between novice and experienced clinicians. Am J Orthod Dentofacial Orthop 2011;139:305–15.
7. Troy BA, Shanker S, Fields HW, et al. Comparison of incisor inclination in patients with class III malocclusion treated with orthognathic surgery or orthodontic camouflage. Am J Orthod Dentofacial Orthop 2009; 135:146.e1-9.
8. Potts B, Shanker S, Fields HW, et al. Dental and skeletal changes associated with class II surgical-orthodontic treatment. Am J Orthod Dentofacial Orthop 2009;135:566.e1-7.
9. Chow LK, Singh B, Chiu WK, et al. Prevalence of postoperative complications after orthognathic surgery: a 15-year review. J Oral Maxillofac Surg 2007;65:984.
10. Ayoub AF, Lalani Z, Moos KF, et al. Complications following orthognathic surgery that required early surgical intervention: fifteen years'experience. Int J Adult Orthodon Orthognath Surg 2001;16:138.
11. Chen N, Neal CE, Lingenbrink P, et al. Neurosensory changes following orthognathic surgery. Int J Adult Orthodon Orthognath Surg 1999;14:259.
12. Cunningham SJ, Crean SJ, Hunt NP, et al. Preparation, perception and problem: a long-term follow-up of orthognathic surgery. Int J Adult Orthodon Orthognath Surg 1996;11:41.
13. Dimitroulis G. Complications of orthognathic surgery. Aust Orthod J 1996;14:158.
14. El Deeb M, Wolford L, Bevis R. Complications of orthognathic surgery. Clin Plast Surg 1989;16: 825.
15. Essik GK, Phillips C, Turvey TA, et al. Facial altered sensation and sensory impairment after orthognathic surgery. Int J Oral Maxillofac Surg 2007;36:577.
16. Waack D. Perioperative complication associated with Le Fort I osteotomies. J Oral Maxillofac Surg 1994;52(suppl 2):92.
17. Gunaseelan R, Anantanarayanan P, Veerabahu M, et al. Intraoperative and perioperative complications in anterior maxillary osteotomy: a retrospective evaluation of 103 patients. J Oral Maxillofac Surg 2009; 67:1269.
18. O'Ryan F. Complications of orthognathic surgery. Oral Maxillofac Surg Clin North Am 1990;2:602.
19. Patel PK, Morris DE, Gassman A. Complications of orthognathic surgery. J Craniofac Surg 2007;18:975.
20. Phillips C, Essik G, Blakey G III, et al. Relationship between patients' perceptions of postsurgical sequelae and altered sensations after bilateral sagittal split osteotomy. J Oral Maxillofac Surg 2007;65:597.
21. Tung TC, Chen YR, Bendor-Samuel R. Surgical complications of the Le Fort I osteotomy: a retrospective review of 146 cases. Changgeng Yi Xue Za Zhi 1995;18:102.
22. Turvey TA. Intraoperative complication of sagittal osteotomy of the mandibular ramus: incidence and management. J Oral Maxillofac Surg 1985;43:594.
23. August M, Marchona J, Donady J, et al. Neurosensory deficit and functional impairment after sagittal ramus osteotomy: a long-term follow-up study. J Oral Maxillofac Surg 1998;56:1231–5.
24. Raffaini M, Pisani C, Conti M. Orthognathic surgery "again" to correct aesthetic failure of primary surgery: report on outcomes and patient satisfaction in 70 consecutive cases. J Craniomaxillofac Surg 2018;46:1069–78.
25. Proffit WR, Phillips C, Douvartzidis N. A comparison of outcomes of orthodontic and surgical-orthodontic treatment of class II malocclusion in adults. Am J Orthod Dentofacial Orthop 1992;101:556–65.
26. Burden D, Johnston C, Kennedy D, et al. A cephalometric study of class II malocclusion treated with mandibular surgery. Am J Orthod Dentofacial Orthop 2007;131:7.e1-8.
27. Jang JC, Fields HW, Vig KWL, et al. Controversies in timing of orthodontic treatment. Semin Orthod 2005; 11:112–8.

Dentoalveolar Distraction Osteogenesis for Rapid Maxillary Canine Retraction

An Overview of Technique, Treatment, and Outcomes

Sumit Yadav, MDS, PhD[a], Michael R. Markiewicz, DDS, MPH, MD[b], Veerasathpurush Allareddy, BDS, PhD[c,*]

KEYWORDS

• Dentoalveolar distraction osteogenesis • Distraction osteogenesis • Rapid tooth movement • Canine retraction

KEY POINTS

- Maxillary first premolar extraction space closures by canine retractions are closed rapidly (in around 2 weeks) when compared with traditional orthodontic mechanics (around 6 months).
- First premolar extraction spaces are closed with minimal loss of posterior anchorage (mesialization of molars into extraction spaces).
- Space closure is accomplished by a combination of tipping and translation of canines.
- Current evidence suggests that there are no major adverse sequelae (eg, root resorption, pulp vitality) associated with rapid canine retraction through a dentoalveolar distraction osteogenesis procedure. However, there is a paucity of long-term clinical trials in this area.

BACKGROUND

Recent years have witnessed an increasing number of adults seeking orthodontic treatment.[1] Although this points to a positive trend for the specialty, increasingly orthodontists and patients are keen on having reduced treatment times.[2] A survey of orthodontists indicated that patients are willing to pay up to 20% increase in fees, and orthodontists are willing to pay up to 20% of their fees for companies that provide technologies to accelerate teeth movement.[2] Traditionally, orthodontic teeth movement is done through application of light, continuous, and controlled forces. Typically the duration of orthodontic treatment is around 24 months. This, however, depends on a multitude of patient- and treatment-related factors, such as patient compliance with treatment protocols, complexity of malocclusion, and extraction space closure. Dentoalveolar distraction (DAD) osteogenesis is one of several techniques that is used for rapid space closure.[3–9] Usually, the maxillary/mandibular canines are distracted distally into the extraction spaces of maxillary/mandibular first premolars within a

Disclosure Statement: The authors have nothing to disclose.

[a] Department of Craniofacial Sciences, University of Connecticut School of Dental Medicine, 263 Farmington Avenue, Farmington, CT 06030, USA; [b] Department of Oral & Maxillofacial Surgery, School of Dental Medicine, University at Buffalo, 112 Squire Hall, Buffalo, NY 14214, USA; [c] Department of Orthodontics, College of Dentistry, University of Illinois at Chicago, 801 South Paulina Street, 138AD (MC841), Chicago, IL 60612-7211, USA

* Corresponding author.
E-mail address: sath@uic.edu

Oral Maxillofacial Surg Clin N Am 32 (2020) 83–88
https://doi.org/10.1016/j.coms.2019.09.005
1042-3699/20/

2-week time frame. This article provides an overview of the DAD technique and associated outcomes.

HISTORY AND BIOLOGIC BASIS OF DISTRACTION OSTEOGENESIS

Distraction osteogenesis was incepted by Codivilla in 1905 and popularized by Illizarov as a procedure for lengthening the limbs.[10,11] McCarthy and colleagues[12] used distraction osteogenesis in craniofacial skeleton for the lengthening of the hypoplastic mandible. Dental periodontal ligament (PDL) distraction was first reported by Liou and Huang[4] in 1998, whereas Işeri and colleagues[8] described the DAD technique.

Alveolar bone is a dynamic mineralized tissue and it responds to any mechanical stimuli by resorbing bone (catabolic bone modeling) in the direction of applied load and forming bone in the direction opposite to applied load (anabolic bone modeling).[13,14] The cellular components in the alveolar bone interacts to carry out this complex mechanotransduction. The bone modeling and remodeling are essential aspects of orthodontic tooth movement. Any attempt to increase the rate of orthodontic tooth movement has to alter the rate of bone modeling and remodeling. Orthodontists using the principle of distraction osteogenesis have attempted to retract the canine at a faster rate to shorten the overall treatment time.

OVERVIEW OF RAPID CANINE RETRACTION USING DENTOALVEOLAR DISTRACTION

The primary indications for rapid canine retraction include:

1. Dentoalveolar bimaxillary protrusion cases
2. Anterior crowding (ie, blocked out lateral incisors) with maximum anchorage requirements
3. Class II div 1 malocclusion cases

Surgical Technique for Dentoalveolar Distraction

Horizontal mucosal incision is made parallel to the gingival margin of the canine and the premolar beyond the depth of the vestibule. Cortical holes are made in the alveolar bone around the canine (tooth to be distracted) with a small round carbide bur (**Fig. 1**A).[8] A thin tapered fissure bur is used to connect the holes and make a groove around the tooth to be distracted (**Fig. 1**B). Fine osteotomes are advanced in the coronal direction.[8] The first premolar is then extracted or similar cortical holes are made in the alveolar bone surrounding the premolar (**Fig. 1**C) and the buccal bone is removed between the outlined bone cut at the distal canine region anteriorly and the second premolar posteriorly (**Fig. 1**D). Additionally, osteotomes are used to mobilize the alveolar segment that includes the canine by fracturing the surrounding bone around its root off the lingual or palatal cortex. The buccal and apical bone through the extraction socket of premolar might be encountered during the distraction process. These should be eliminated or smoothed between the canine and the second premolar, preserving palatal or lingual cortical shelves. The palatal cortical and trabecular bone should be preserved to maintain the blood supply, but the apical bone near the sinus wall has to be removed, leaving the sinus membrane intact to avoid interferences during the active distraction process.[8] Osteotomes along the anterior aspect of the canine are used to split the surrounding bone around its root from the palatal or lingual cortex and neighboring teeth. The transport dentoalveolar segment that includes the canine also includes the buccal cortex, leaving an intact lingual or palatal cortical plate and the bone around the apex of the canine.[15]

Activation Protocol for Dentoalveolar Distraction

Distraction of the canine is typically initiated 3 to 4 days after surgery. This is the latency period during which time the blood clots consolidate. The distractor is typically teeth borne with anchorage obtained from canines and first molars. Canine and first molar teeth are banded and the distractor comprises an activating screw attached to the bands. The distractor rods should be positioned in such a manner to transmit the orthodontic forces through the center of resistance of canine during space closure. This enables translation

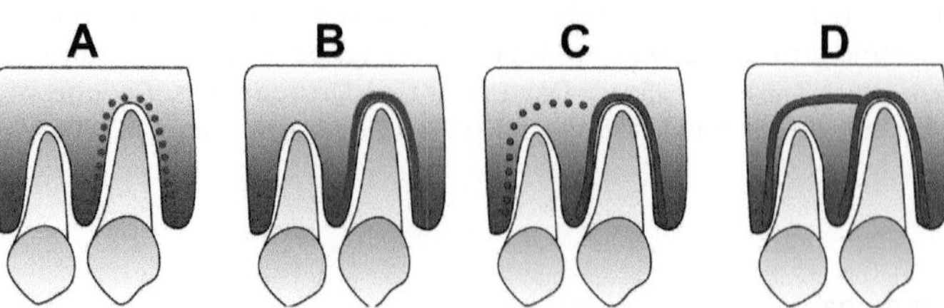

Fig. 1. Schematic of the surgical procedure. (*A*) Cortical holes around canine. (*B*) Connect cortical holes. (*C*) Cortical holes around first premolar. (*D*) Bone cut.

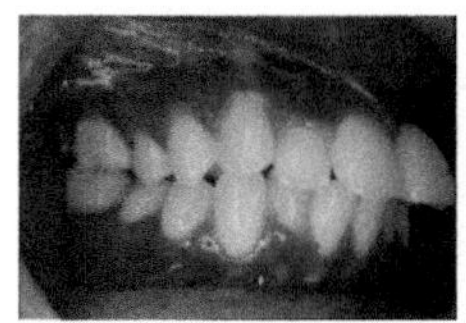
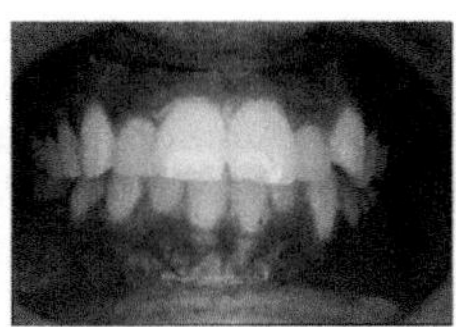
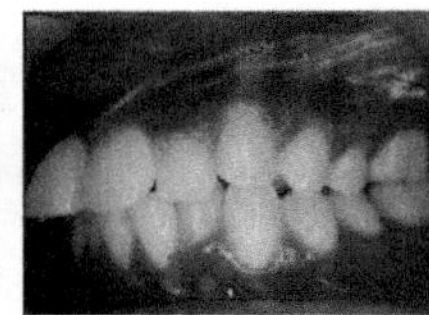

Fig. 2. Pretreatment intraoral pictures.

(bodily movement) of canines into the extraction spaces. However, the bulky nature of the distraction appliance and anatomic limitations with vestibule and position of cheek preclude an ideal placement of distractor screws. Consequently, one should expect some degree of tipping of canine as it is distalized into the extraction space of first premolar. The canine is usually distracted twice per day for a total of about 0.8 mm to 1 mm per day.[3–9,16] It has been reported in literature that up to 2 mm is distracted per day (four activations of 0.5 mm each).[16] The distracted canine should be consolidated with the other posterior teeth in the arch for 3 to 4 months with a stainless steel ligature to prevent the relapse of distracted canine.[4–9,12,15] This consolidation phase is essential for the bone to heal. Callus maturation into partial ossification usually takes 4 to 6 weeks. To shorten the overall treatment time, the orthodontic treatment should be initiated immediately after the canine is distracted because the bone distal to the lateral incisor is not mineralized and the maxillary incisors are retracted at a faster rate.

Case Report

We illustrate the previously mentioned procedure with a case that was treated by the primary author. An 18-year-old woman reported to the clinic with proclined upper and lower incisors and anterior crowding in the lower arch. She had end-on molar and canine relationship bilaterally (**Fig. 2**). The treatment goals were to obtain an ideal overjet and overbite, class I canine relationship, and class I molar relationship. The plan was to do a comprehensive phase of orthodontic treatment with extractions of maxillary first premolars and mandibular second premolars. The maxillary extraction spaces were closed by rapid retraction of maxillary canines aided by the DAD procedure followed by en-masse retraction of maxillary incisors immediately following complete distalization of maxillary canines. In the mandibular arch, the second premolar extraction spaces were closed by mesialization of molars. The detailed description of the DAD procedure (**Fig. 3**) is provided in the prior section. The maxillary canines were distracted 0.4 mm in the morning and 0.4 mm in the evening. The canine was completely distracted in 10 days (**Fig. 4**). The total treatment time for the patient was 14 months (**Fig. 5**).

PERIODONTAL LIGAMENT DISTRACTION OSTEOGENESIS

This technique was initially described by Liou and Huang in 1998.[4] This technique is based on the premise that during orthodontic tooth movement, the process of osteogenesis in the PDL is similar to that in the mid-palatal suture.[4,16] This surgical technique is usually performed under local anesthesia as an outpatient procedure. After the

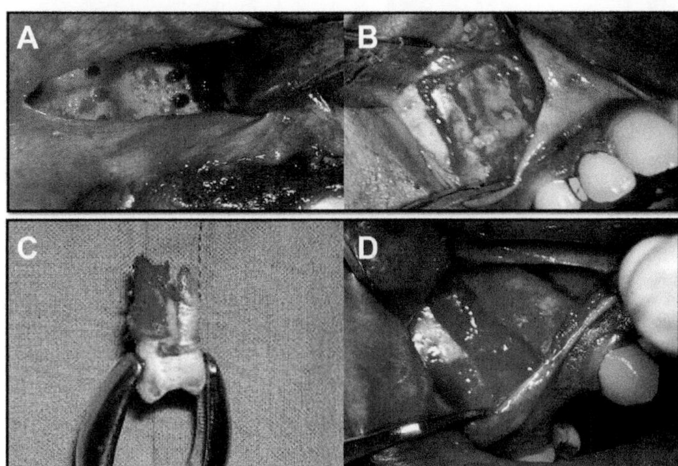

Fig. 3. Surgical procedure. (*A*) Round holes made in the alveolar bone surrounding the canine and the premolar. (*B*) Round holes connected with the straight fissure bur to form a groove. (*C*) The first premolar extracted along with the buccal cortical plate. (*D*) The socket of the premolar without the buccal cortical bone where the canine will be distracted.

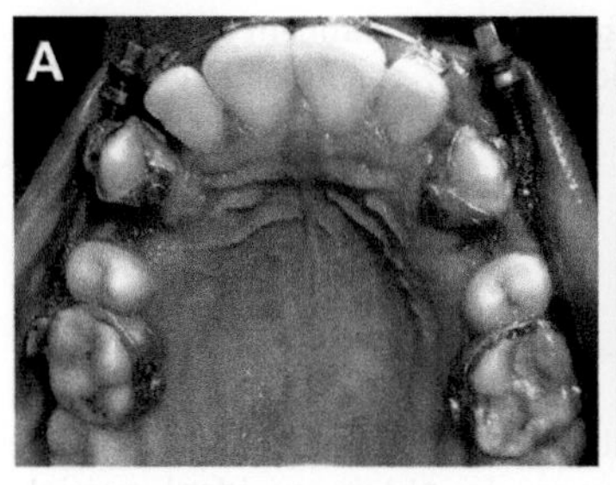

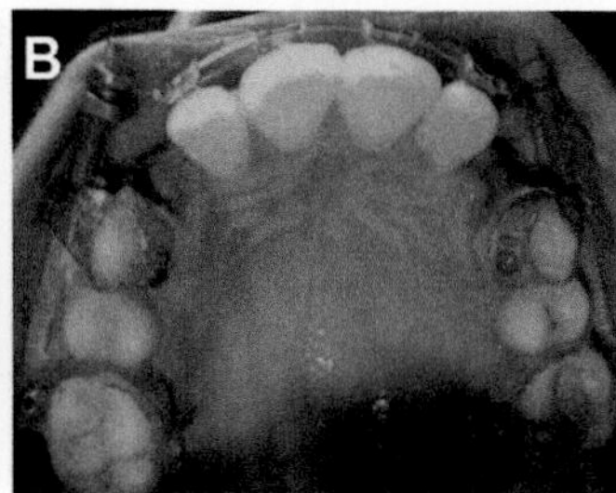

Fig. 4. Canine distraction. (*A*) Initiation of canine distraction. (*B*) Completion of canine distraction.

extraction of the first premolar, interseptal bone distal to canine is undermined and reduced in thickness. Because the socket depth of the premolar is less than that of canine so to achieve the bodily tooth movement, the depth of premolar socket is extended to the same depth as that of canine socket using a round carbide bur. After equaling the socket depth, the bone distal to canine is undermined and reduced in thickness to 1 to 2 mm. Undermining of the distal bone should be performed precisely with the aid of the radiograph and precaution should be taken not to severely traumatize the canine.[4]

REVIEW OF OUTCOMES FOLLOWING DENTOALVEOLAR AND PERIODONTAL LIGAMENT DISTRACTION OSTEOGENESIS

Are Canines that Are Retracted Rapidly by the Dentoalveolar Distraction or Periodontal Ligament Technique More Prone for Root Resorption?

Inflammatory root resorption is a dreaded sequela of prolonged orthodontic treatment. Inflammatory root resorption usually initiates 2 to 3 weeks after the orthodontic force application and root resorption may continue for the entire duration of the orthodontic treatment time. With the canine completely retracted in approximately 2 weeks with DAD procedure or PDL distraction osteogenesis the chances of root resorption are minimal. Liou and Huang[4] and Kumar and colleagues[17] have shown minimal to no inflammatory root resorption with PDL canine distraction. Similar findings were reported by several authors following DAD procedure.[5,8,18]

What Kind of Teeth Movement (Tipping or Translational) Is Accomplished Through Dentoalveolar Distraction and Periodontal Ligament Distractions?

Three-dimensional control of tooth movement is necessary to shorten the overall treatment time. The type of tooth movement with dental distraction depends on the initial position of the canine to be distracted. Liou and Huang[4] have reported bodily tooth movement of the canine with PDL

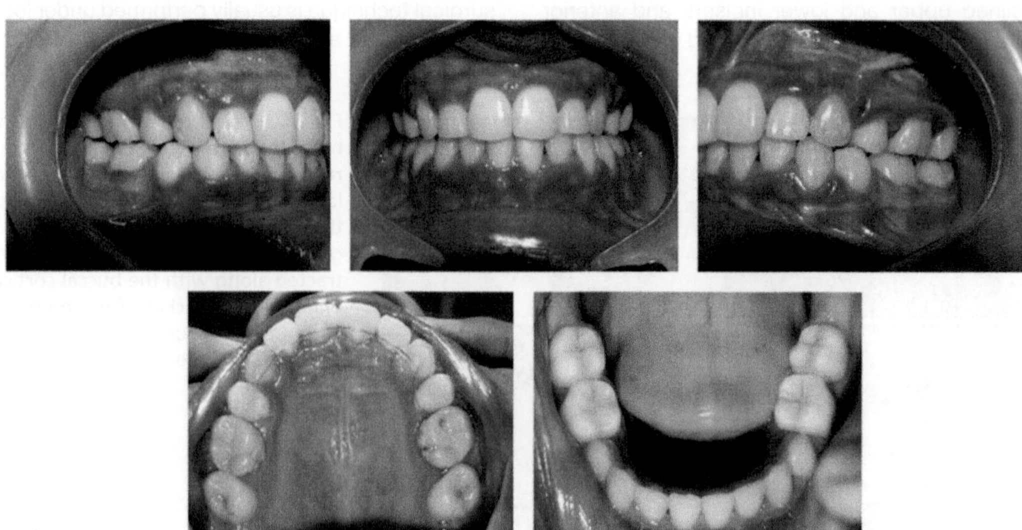

Fig. 5. Post-treatment intraoral pictures.

distraction, whereas Kumar and colleagues[17] reported tipping of canine approximately 16°. Similar findings of tipping of canine were reported by Kharkar and colleagues[15,16] with DAD of canine. The type of tooth movement of distracted canine is surgery sensitive. If the bone is removed precisely then the distracted canine tips less.

What Are Some Potential Surgical Complications Associated with Dentoalveolar Distraction?

Several studies have examined perioperative and postoperative surgical complications associated with DAD.[3,5–9,15,16,18] A review of the available literature on this topic suggests that DAD is a safe procedure with no serious morbidity. However, as with any surgical procedure one has to be mindful of local area inflammation, pain, infections, and so forth. The most often reported side effect is lack of patient tolerance because of the bulky nature of the appliance and its position in relation to the check and vestibule.

Can Teeth Get Devitalized Following Dentoalveolar Distractions?

Kumar and colleagues[5] examined pulp vitality following DAD in a cohort of seven patients (20 teeth that were subject to DAD procedure). They assessed pulp vitality by an electrical vitality test before and after 6 months following DAD and found that none of the 20 teeth reacted negatively to the test. No signs of discoloration or pulpal pain were observed in this sample. Kurt and colleagues[6] conducted a prospective clinical study of 19 patients (36 maxillary canines) to examine pulp vitality by thermal stimulation and electric pulp testing at 6 months before treatment with DAD, after fixed orthodontic treatment, and 6 months into retention. They did not observe any loss of vitality of maxillary canines that were subject to DAD treatment. Kurt and colleagues[9] reported on a 5-year follow-up of a class II malocclusion case in which maxillary canines were retracted distally into the extraction spaces of first premolars by the DAD procedure. They tested for pulp vitality by electronic and thermal pulp tester. They did not observe any loss of vitality of distracted teeth at end of DAD and at the 5-year follow-up period. Currently there is no empirical evidence to conclude DAD is associated with loss of pulp vitality of canines that were subject to DAD procedure. However, it should be noted that all studies that have examined DAD-associated outcomes are from single centers with limited sample numbers. Consequently, external validity and generalizability are questionable. More research on long-term outcomes needs to be conducted to document further evidence on the long-term impact of DAD procedure on pulp vitality.

Can There Be Loss of Anchorage (Molars Mesializing) During Dentoalveolar Distraction and Periodontal Ligament Distractions?

Anchorage loss in all three dimensions is a potential side effect of orthodontic mechanotherapy. The dental distraction was popularized because it can retract the canine in a short period of time and secondly prevents the mesial movement of the anchor teeth, thereby preserving anchorage. The published literature has only focused on anchorage loss in anterior-posterior direction. Liou and Huang[4] and Kumar and colleagues[17] have shown insignificant loss of anchorage (anterior-posterior) with PDL distraction. However, Kumar and colleagues[17] have reported 1 mm of molar extrusion (vertical loss of anchorage). Furthermore, Kisnisci and colleagues[18] have showed no loss of anchorage with DAD. However, there is a paucity of published reports on long-term evaluations of the dental distraction on anchorage loss.

SUMMARY

Maxillary canines are predictably distalized rapidly into the extraction spaces of first premolars. About 0.8 mm of space closure per day is accomplished. Tipping of canines during space closure is inevitable because it is difficult to place the orthodontic forces through the center of resistance of canines. Although current evidence suggests that adverse sequelae, such as root resorptions and pulp devitalization, are rare, prospective clinical studies that are adequately powered and documenting long-term follow-up of these outcomes are lacking.

REFERENCES

1. American Association of Orthodontists survey. The economics of orthodontics. Available at: https://www1.mylifemysmile.org/cms/wp-content/uploads/2015/07/Results-of-AAO-Patient-Census-Survey-2012.pdf. Accessed March 1, 2017.
2. Uribe F, Padala S, Allareddy V, et al. Patients', parents', and orthodontists' perceptions of the need for and costs of additional procedures to reduce treatment time. Am J Orthod Dentofacial Orthop 2014;145(4 Suppl):S65–73.
3. Kateel SK, Agarwal A, Kharae G, et al. A comparative study of canine retraction by distraction of the periodontal ligament and dentoalveolar

distraction methods. J Maxillofac Oral Surg 2016; 15(2):144–55.
4. Liou EJ, Huang CS. Rapid canine retraction through distraction of the periodontal ligament. Am J Orthod Dentofacial Orthop 1998;114(4):372–82.
5. Kumar N, Prashantha G, Raikar S, et al. Dento-alveolar distraction osteogenesis for rapid orthodontic canine retraction. J Int Oral Health 2013;5(6):31–41.
6. Kurt G, İşeri H, Kişnişçi R, et al. Rate of tooth movement and dentoskeletal effects of rapid canine retraction by dentoalveolar distraction osteogenesis: a prospective study. Am J Orthod Dentofacial Orthop 2017;152(2):204–13.
7. Nair A, Kumar JP, Venkataramana V, et al. Dento-alveolar distraction osteogenesis using rigid intra-oral tooth borne distraction device. J Int Oral Health 2014;6(2):106–13.
8. Işeri H, Kişnişci R, Bzizi N, et al. Rapid canine retraction and orthodontic treatment with dentoalveolar distraction osteogenesis. Am J Orthod Dentofacial Orthop 2005;127(5):533–41 [quiz: 625].
9. Kurt G, Işeri H, Kişnişci R. Rapid tooth movement and orthodontic treatment using dentoalveolar distraction (DAD). Long-term (5 years) follow-up of a Class II case. Angle Orthod 2010;80(3):597–606.
10. Codivilla A. The classic: on the means of lengthening, in the lower limbs, the muscles and tissues which are shortened through deformity. 1905. Clin Orthop Relat Res 2008;466(12):2903–9.
11. Codivilla A. On the means of lengthening, in the lower limbs, the muscles and tissues which are shortened through deformity. Clin Orthop Relat Res 1904;1994(301):4–9.
12. McCarthy JG, Schreiber J, Karp N, et al. Lengthening the human mandible by gradual distraction. Plast Reconstr Surg 1992;89(1):1–8 [discussion: 9–10].
13. Dutra EH, Ahmida A, Lima A, et al. The effects of alveolar decortications on orthodontic tooth movement and bone remodelling in rats. Eur J Orthod 2018;40(4):423–9.
14. Chang J, Chen PJ, Dutra EH, et al. The effect of the extent of surgical insult on orthodontic tooth movement. Eur J Orthod 2019. https://doi.org/10.1093/ejo/cjz006.
15. Kharkar VR, Kotrashetti SM. Transport dentoalveolar distraction osteogenesis-assisted rapid orthodontic canine retraction. Oral Surg Oral Med Oral Pathol Oral Radiol Endod 2010;109(5):687–93.
16. Kharkar VR, Kotrashetti SM, Kulkarni P. Comparative evaluation of dento-alveolar distraction and periodontal distraction assisted rapid retraction of the maxillary canine: a pilot study. Int J Oral Maxillofac Surg 2010;39(11):1074–9.
17. Kumar PS, Saxena R, Patil S, et al. Clinical investigation of periodontal ligament distraction osteogenesis for rapid orthodontic canine retraction. Aust Orthod J 2009;25(2):147–52.
18. Kisnisci RS, Iseri H, Tuz HH, et al. Dentoalveolar distraction osteogenesis for rapid orthodontic canine retraction. J Oral Maxillofac Surg 2002; 60(4):389–94.

Surgery-First Approach in the Orthognathic Patient

Flavio A. Uribe, DDS, MDentSc[a,*], Brian Farrell, DDS, MD[b,c]

KEYWORDS

- Surgery-first approach • Orthognathic surgery • Virtual surgical planning • Surgical orthodontics

KEY POINTS

- This article explains the rationale and indications for the surgery-first approach (SFA).
- This article illustrates step-by-step the sequence to implement SFA with virtual surgical planning.
- This article describes 2 case reports of patients treated with SFA.

Significant advances have occurred in the treatment of dentofacial deformities with orthognathic surgery since the start of this new millennium. One of the main advances has been with 3-dimensional (3D) virtual surgical planning, which has emerged as a more comprehensive and precise approach to treat these deformities and has become mainstream. Another change has been an alternative approach to the conventional 3-stage (presurgical orthodontics-surgery-postsurgical orthodontics) sequence. This new approach, commonly referred to as "surgery-first" bypasses the presurgical orthodontic phase by performing surgery without the conventional tooth decompensations, followed by a postsurgical orthodontics phase.

Although the concept of surgery-first had been applied in orthognathic surgery in the distant past, the 3-stage sequence known as the conventional approach became the most popular method to treat dentofacial deformity in the past 30 to 40 years, given that occlusal stability after surgery is more likely attained. However, in the past few years the rationale for surgery-first has been justified from the standpoint of improving the psychosocial well-being of patients with dentofacial dysmorphology because the skeletal problem can be corrected earlier on in treatment.[1,2] In the conventional approach, the presurgical orthodontics phase aims to eliminate dental compensations, which worsens the dentofacial deformity thereby violating our patient-centered objectives of treatment. With the psychosocial aspect and patient-centered approach, Behrman and Behrman[3] discussed the concept of building a house (osteotomies to move the bones) and then move the furniture (orthodontic tooth movement), and were the first authors to rationalize the benefits of the surgery-first approach.

Surgery-first was revived with the advent of skeletal anchorage provided by means of miniplates. Nagasaka and colleagues[4] published on the treatment of a Class III female patient who was treated without any presurgical orthodontics, with surgery performed less than a month after the orthodontic appliances were bonded. In this article, the advantages of a surgery-first approach were described, and the investigators highlighted a striking reduction in total treatment duration. The miniplates provide the assurance that the transitional malocclusion observed after surgery is corrected to an ideal occlusal outcome, even in the absence of a presurgical orthodontic phase.

Many reports support the reduction in treatment duration with the surgery-first approach.[5–8] With the conventional approach, many studies have

Disclosure: The authors have nothing to disclose.

[a] Division of Orthodontics, Department of Craniofacial Sciences, University of Connecticut, 263 Farmington Avenue, Farmington, CT 06030, USA; [b] Carolina Center for Oral and Facial Surgery, 411 Billingsley Road, #105, Charlotte, NC 28211, USA; [c] Department of Oral and Maxillofacial Surgery, Louisiana State University, School of Dentistry, New Orleans, LA, USA

* Corresponding author.

E-mail address: furibe@uchc.edu

Oral Maxillofacial Surg Clin N Am 32 (2020) 89–103

https://doi.org/10.1016/j.coms.2019.08.009

1042-3699/20/

oralmaxsurgery.theclinics.com

shown that the total mean treatment duration ranges from 27 months to 36 months.[9–11] More specifically, the presurgical phase typically lasted 15 to 24 months and the postsurgical phase from 5 to 12 months. On the other hand, the initial publications reported a 10-month average treatment duration with the surgery-first approach.[5,8] However, a recent systematic review evaluating studies where the conventional approach was compared with the surgery-first approach by the same surgical teams implementing both techniques found a much smaller difference in treatment duration between both groups.[12] Rather than a twofold reduction, a 5-month reduction to treatment duration was reported, a stark contrast to what had been previously reported. Interestingly, the groups reported a longer time than typically reported for surgery-first and a shorter time than typically reported for the conventional approach.

From a patient-centered treatment approach, the psychosocial advantage of surgery-first has recently been evaluated.[1,2] The findings of a study comparing the surgery-first approach with the conventional approach using Oral Health Impact Profile-short version and Orthognathic Quality-of-Life Questionnaires as the measurement tools, highlighted that patients undergoing surgery-first had better scores.[1] This is an expected outcome, as it has been reported that the aspect with the least patient satisfaction in orthognathic surgery is the orthodontic component,[13] especially considering that it is the presurgical phase, which is responsible for worsening of the facial profile.

One important advantage of the surgery-first approach for the orthodontist is that patients obtain insurance approval for the surgical procedure without having started the typical decompensation presurgical phase where the deformity is accentuated. It is problematic for an orthodontist that has committed to surgery to find out that the patient has lost insurance coverage and will not be able to have the planned surgical procedure. Camouflaging the skeletal deformity then is complicated, especially if teeth had been extracted as part of this presurgical orthodontic phase. With surgery-first, the surgical procedure occurs once the insurance approval is obtained and therefore this is not a concern.

One final advantage in the surgery-first approach is the possibility of overcorrection. Because the occlusion after surgery-first approach is usually not perfect, slight accentuation of the surgical movements can be executed. For example, a patient with a Class II malocclusion will be brought into a slightly Class III canine relationship. On the other hand, a patient with a Class III malocclusion is brought into a slight Class II canine relationship. Typically, patients tend to slightly relapse in the few months after surgery and fall into a good occlusal relationship. If this slight relapse is not observed, intermaxillary elastics to revert the overcorrection at the occlusal level are effective since the magnitude of the overcorrection is not large.

INDICATIONS FOR SURGERY-FIRST

Although most patients with dentofacial deformity could be treated with the surgery-first approach, there are clear indications for the technique. Typically, a nonextraction orthodontic treatment is performed in surgery-first. Therefore, a patient with mild to moderate crowding in the maxilla and in the mandible is a good candidate for this approach. In addition, the maxillary incisor inclination has to be near normal. Together, the minimal to moderate amount of crowding and the close to normal inclination of the maxillary incisor allows for orthodontic anteroposterior angular control of this tooth without the need of extractions. For example, if the maxillary incisors are slightly proclined and some crowding is present, distalization of the molars after surgery by means of skeletal anchorage allows for maintaining or reducing the labial inclination of the maxillary incisors while addressing the crowded arch.

Another important indication for the surgery-first approach is the presence of an adequate transverse relationship of the dental arches once the anteroposterior relationship is corrected. This can be easily assessed by occluding the initial dental models in a Class I canine relationship. Minor transverse discrepancies can be managed with the archwires after surgery. In the presence of a major transverse discrepancy, maxillary arch expansion could be approached before surgery with surgically assisted rapid palatal expansion (SARPE) or MARPE (miniscrew-assisted rapid palatal expansion). The MARPE approach is typically indicated in patients no older than the third decade of life because higher success with this procedure is noted up until this age.[14] Alternatively, the transverse correction can be also achieved through a segmental maxillary osteotomy (2-piece or 3-piece maxilla) with the surgery-first procedure, but this results in more complex surgical procedure that, although not contraindicated, it should be approached by a more experienced surgery-first team.

Patients with temporomandibular joint (TMJ) conditions, syndromes, and multiple missing teeth are not typical candidates for surgery-first. However, this surgical approach could still be applied on these patients. Perhaps the patient with TMJ problems requiring joint replacement could be the patient that would likely be excluded due to the instability of the joint and likely difficulty to achieve a good occlusion after surgery. The same applies to patients with multiple missing teeth in whom posterior occlusion cannot be achieved, excluding them from the ideal candidates for this surgical approach.

One medical condition in which surgery-first may be primarily indicated is in patients with obstructive sleep apnea. Patients with obstructive sleep apnea may benefit from an immediate resolution of their functional airway problem through maxillomandibular advancement through the surgery-first approach. A lengthy presurgical orthodontic phase is not in the best interest of patient suffering from this particular medical condition. The medical urgency takes precedence over the occlusal objectives that the typical patient undergoing orthognathic surgery requires. With surgery-first, the functional problem can be resolved expeditiously and then followed by some minimal orthodontic treatment to refine the occlusion.

Box 1
Treatment planning considerations in surgery-first

Step 1. Occlude pretreatment dental models in the vicinity of Class I occlusion

Step 2. Evaluation of overbite; ensure at least 1 mm of incisor overlap

Step 3. Evaluation of molar openbite at second M level

Step 4. Evaluation of the transverse dimension

Step 5. Evaluation of maxillary crowding

Step 6. Positioning of the maxillary incisors vertically, anteroposteriorly, and transversely in space

Step 7. Evaluation of the inclination of the maxillary incisors

Step 8. Evaluation of the occlusal plane as it relates to facial convexity

Step 9. Evaluation of need for genioplasty

TREATMENT PLANNING THE SURGERY-FIRST PATIENT

There are 2 major aspects that need to be considered in the patient undergoing orthognathic surgery with surgery-first. These 2 elements are esthetics and occlusion. These 2 aspects are not different from those to be considered in the patient having the conventional 3-stage surgical approach. Most often, resolving the skeletal dysmorphology will resolve the malocclusion. For example, a patient with a significant mandibular deficiency will likely have a Class II malocclusion with a large overjet. In this hypothetical patient, advancing the mandible will likely resolve the unfavorable occlusal traits while maximizing the esthetics though proper mandibular projection.

The specific process of treatment planning the patient undergoing surgery-first is as follows (**Box 1**). The first step is to occlude the dental models to evaluate the possible occlusal relationship once the anteroposterior skeletal discrepancy is normalized. Special attention in this step is placed on the overbite, canine relationship, and buccal occlusion. The orthodontist will need to anticipate the postsurgical movement of the maxillary teeth. Vertically, it is important to obtain an adequate overbite, especially in patients who have an open bite. If the overbite is not deep enough, a clockwise rotation of the maxilla resulting in a slight open bite on the second M usually allows for enough interincisal coverage. However, it is important to limit the magnitude of the open bite at the level of the second M, as extruding these teeth into occlusion after surgery can be a difficult orthodontic movement. Approximately 2 mm of open bite is an adequate magnitude that can be corrected with extrusion after surgery.

In some instances, it may be necessary to assess the transverse and vertical changes of the maxilla when a 3-piece maxilla is planned. This is typically the case when a patient is dolichofacial. Typically, these patients have excessive vertical dimension with a steep mandibular plane angle and excessive maxillary vertical height that includes gingival maxillary excess posteriorly. There is also an anterior open bite with normal or slightly excessive incisor display. These patients benefit from a segmented maxilla in 3 pieces in which the differential impaction of the posterior 2 pieces in comparison with the anterior pieces can be accomplished. Typically, the anterior segment is left in place (depending of the relationship of tooth to lip show) and the posterior segments are impacted 3 to 4 mm, which levels the occlusal plane, expands the arch, and allows the mandible to rotate into an ideal occlusal relationship.

From an esthetic aspect, the positioning of the maxillary central incisors vertically and anteroposteriorly is the first step. A clinical evaluation of the amount of tooth display at smile and nasolabial angle are important elements in determining this position. In addition, the anteroposterior inclination of this tooth is important for the orthodontist, as it is this member of the team who has the best control of changing this angle. Once the maxillary incisor position is determined in space, the crowding in the arch and the amount of correction of the inclination of the maxillary incisor needs to be considered. If the inclination is close to normal and the maxillary crowding is mild to moderate (3–6 mm) the orthodontic treatment would likely not require extraction of teeth and distalization of the maxillary teeth after surgery would be able to obtain a well-aligned arch and proper positioning of the maxillary incisors. The transverse dimension needs to be addressed as the relationship between the maxilla and mandible is normalized anteroposteriorly. In the patient with a Class III malocclusion, the normalization of the overjet results in improving any posterior crossbite tendencies in the original malocclusion. On the other hand, a Class II relationship with adequate initial relationship may require transverse expansion of the maxilla either surgically or orthodontically.

The last aspect in the planning of the maxilla is to evaluate the occlusal plane. In this step, occlusal plane rotation maximizes the anteroposterior change. For example, a large mandibular advancement of 15 mm can be managed by advancement of the mandible in conjunction with a counterclockwise rotation of the maxilla. Once the maxilla is positioned, the mandible will follow. As a result, a projection of the chin is significantly advanced in comparison with a straight advancement along the occlusal plane. The orthodontic postsurgical treatment relies on aligning and leveling the mandibular arch, which is achieved by extruding the premolars into the new occlusal plane.

Similarly, the occlusal plane rotation can be obtained in a counterclockwise manner. This is usually recommended for the patient with mandibular prognathism, maxillary deficiency, flat occlusal plane, and normal to short lower facial height.[15] In these patients the smile arc is usually improved with the rotation of the occlusal plane, the mandibular projection is reduced and maxillary projection is evidenced.

The final step is no different from the virtual 3D planning for orthognathic surgery, which is the genioplasty. This step allows to increase or decrease the amount of mandibular projection. Also, vertical control can be achieved by vertically displacing the chin with this procedure. Finally, any mild to moderate asymmetry can also be addressed with this step.

EXECUTING THE SURGERY-FIRST APPROACH

Once the patient has been planned 2-dimensionally through a digital software planner, a cone-beam computed tomography (CBCT) scan of the patient is acquired. Typically, this visit is 2 weeks before the surgical procedure to ensure that enough time is available for the manufacturing of the surgical splints. In this appointment, a preliminary plan is already in place that will be refined after obtaining a CBCT. When this scan is acquired, the patient has all the bands and brackets cemented and bonded to the teeth, but no archwire in place. Hooks are preferred on the molar and premolar brackets because intermaxillary elastic wear is very important after the surgical procedure with the surgery-first approach.

The CBCT scans with the models scanned to the finalized occlusion are sent to the company for the planning of the specific surgical movements. The steps in the planning are no different from those in the conventional approach at this step, because the final occlusion has been determined. Overall, based on the 2D plans, the movements are incorporated into the 3D plan, but on this occasion, paying particular attention to symmetry. This is done by determining the maxillary midline and maxillary left to right inclination. The vertical and anteroposterior movements are confirmed in the 3D plan. Finally, the precise position of the chin for symmetry is accomplished in this step.

The day before the surgery, the surgical wire is placed. This wire is typically a 0.016 x 0.022 nickel titanium (NiTi) or braided stainless steel wire. If the amount of crowding is moderate, a 0.016 NiTi wire or braided stainless steel wire is placed in the mandible. Surgical hooks are placed from canine to canine in both arches on each interproximal space. In some instances, only 3 hooks are placed in the mandible due to the anterior crowding that reduces the space available for hook placement. In this situation, the surgical hooks are placed in the midline and between the lateral incisors and canines.

The surgery is performed according to plan and the patient returns to the orthodontist approximately 2 weeks after surgery to start the tooth movement. Patients who receive a segmented maxilla are seen approximately 5 weeks after surgery. These patients also will maintain the surgical splint until this visit, where the orthodontist typically removes the splint. At this time the patient has been wearing intermaxillary elastics after surgery to maintain the occlusal result. The archwires are changed to 0.016 x 0.022 NiTi wires and vertical elastics are worn to maintain the occlusal relationship achieved with surgery. Because the patients are often overcorrected, this postsurgical interim occlusal relationship will be noted and should be maintained for 2 months of monitoring for any relapse tendencies. After 2 months, if no relapse is observed, intermaxillary elastics are worn with a Class II or Class III vector, depending on the direction needed to normalize the occlusion. However, it is often observed that after 2 months the anteroposterior occlusal relationship has normalized on its own. After 3 to 5 months it is often observed that the occlusion is almost ideal in the simpler cases of surgery-first (those that do not involve distalization or maxillary segmentation) and at this point the refinement phase can start.

CASE REPORTS

Patient 1

The following case report illustrates the typical treatment planning process in a patient in whom all of the ideal parameters for a surgery-first approach were observed. Specifically, this 17-year-old female patient had a minor facial concavity with slight mandibular prognathism and slight maxillary deficiency (**Fig. 1**A–C). A slight mandibular asymmetry was noted with the chin point deviated approximately 3 mm to the left. The incisor display at rest and smile was very close to normal. The vertical facial proportions were also close to normal. At the occlusal level, the patient presented with negative overjet and Class III molar and canine relationships (**Fig. 1**D–F). The lower midline was deviated to the left reflecting the mandibular asymmetry. Because of this asymmetry, a more severe Class III occlusal relationship can be noted on the right (full cusp) compared with the left (half cusp). The maxillary arch had an hour-glass shape (**Fig. 1**G), which resulted in a crossbite on the right side in the premolar region. The mandibular premolars had a lingual tip (**Fig. 1**H). When the models were articulated into the vicinity of a Class I malocclusion, the transverse relationship was normal with a crossbite tendency on the right premolars and slightly increased buccal overjet on the left premolars. Based on this, no maxillary expansion was deemed necessary for this patient. On evaluation of the lateral cephalogram, the maxillary incisor inclination was close to ideal (**Fig. 1**I). The vertical proportions were adequate, as well as the occlusal plane inclination. The panoramic

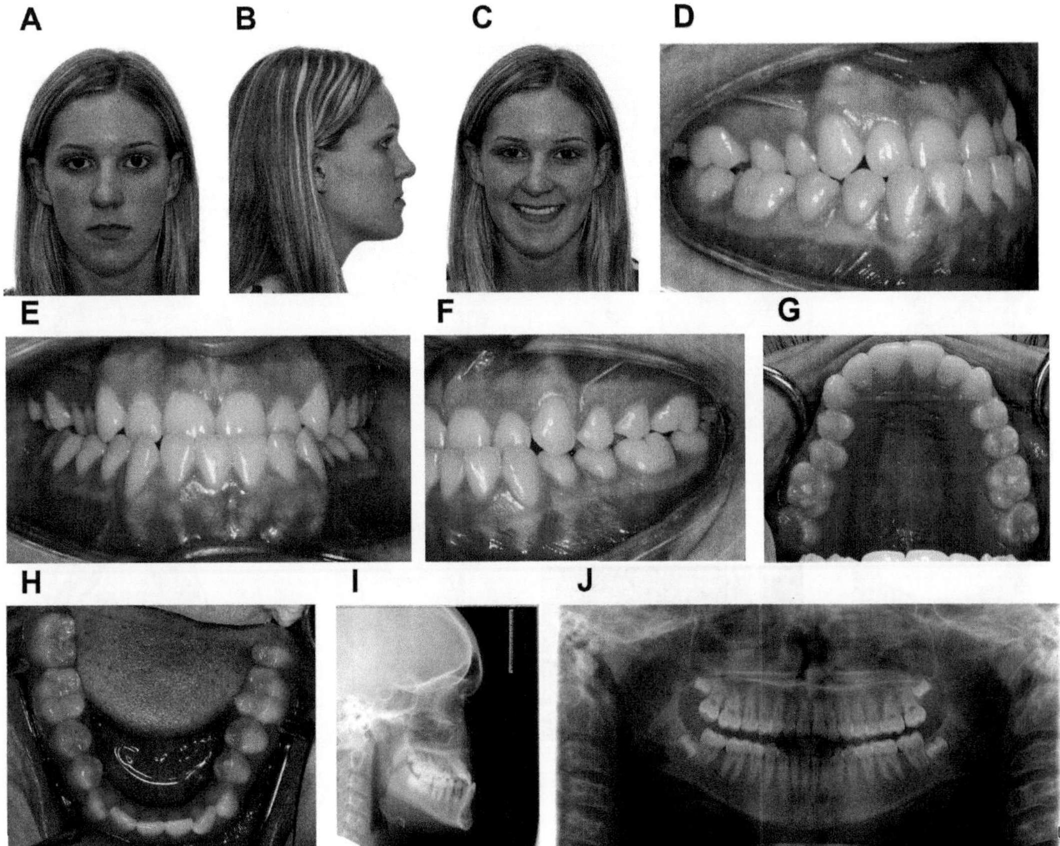

Fig. 1. Pretreatment records of patient 1. (*A*) Frontal, (*B*) profile, and (*C*) smile photographs. (*D*) Right buccal occlusion, (*E*) frontal occlusion, (*F*) left buccal occlusion, (*G*) maxillary occlusal arch, (*H*) mandibular occlusal arch, (*I*) lateral cephalogram, (*J*) panoramic radiograph.

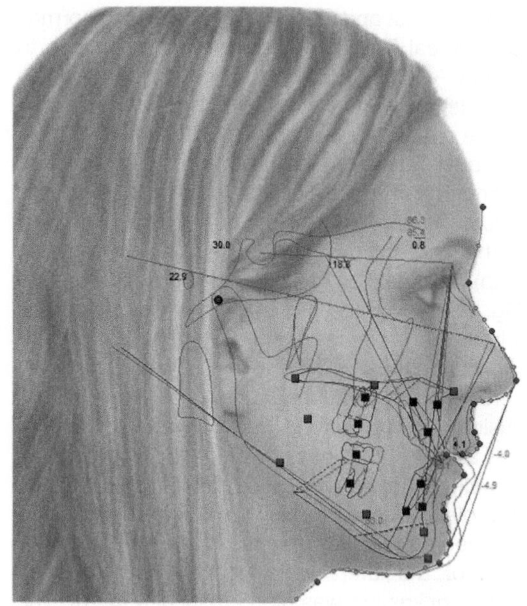

Fig. 2. Two-dimensional surgically planned movements.

radiograph revealed third molars with only the crown formed at that point (**Fig. 1**J).

Because the maxillary arch and the mandibular arch had minimal crowding and the maxillary incisor inclination was close to ideal, it was decided to proceed with a nonextraction approach without maxillary distalization. The archform for both arches was to be established through the archwires after surgery and this step would also address the minimal amount of crowding in both arches. From a 2D approach, it was decided to advance the maxilla approximately 3 mm and set back the mandible by the same amount (**Fig. 2**). Anteroposteriorly at the occlusal level, slight overcorrection of the malocclusion into a slight Class II occlusal relationship of the buccal segments was planned. This step is usually adopted when the magnitude of the movements is larger to account for any relapse tendencies. It is important to state that in this step the orthodontist plays a critical role in determining the postsurgical occlusion that he or she feels comfortable in correcting after surgery. As

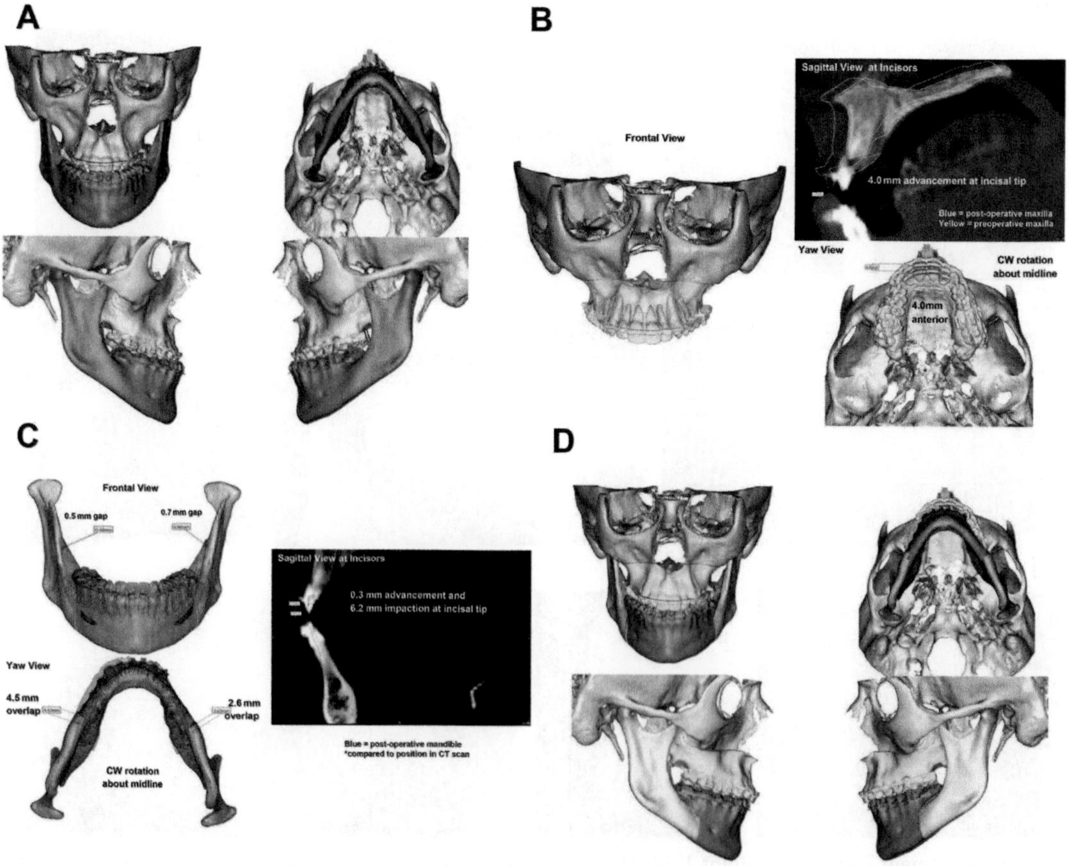

Fig. 3. Three-dimensional surgically planned movements. (*A*) Pretreatment CBCT, (*B*) maxillary surgical movements, (*C*) mandibular surgical movements, and (*D*) final predicted outcomes with all osteotomies.

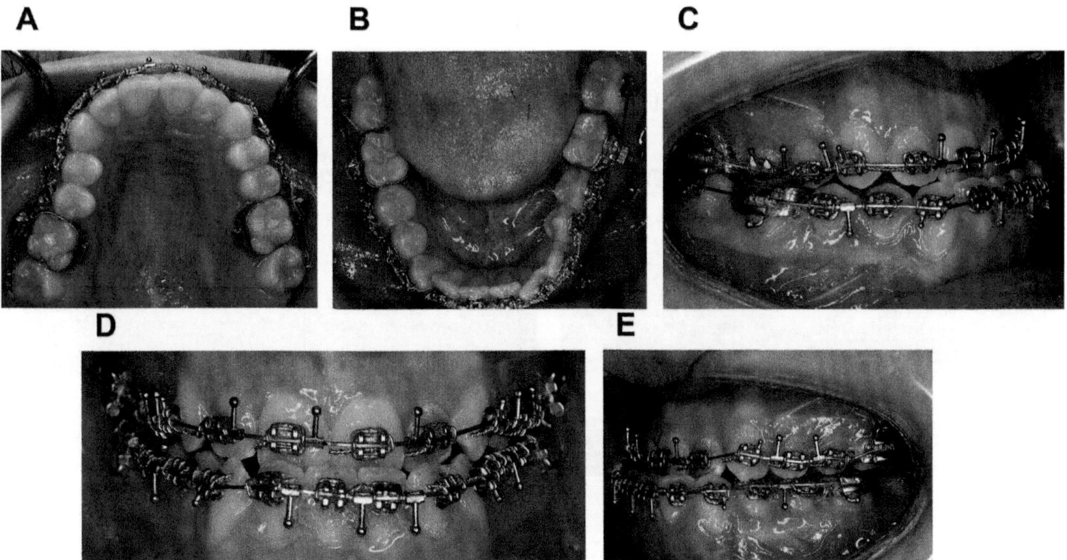

Fig. 4. Presurgical orthodontic wires. (*A*) Maxillary occlusal view. (*B*) Mandibular occlusal view. (*C*), Right buccal view. (*D*) Frontal view. (*E*) Left buccal view.

mentioned previously, in some instances the correction of the malocclusion may require the use of temporary anchorage devices (TADs) to accomplish the desired outcome.

In the 3D plan, the surgical movements planned in 2D were incorporated (**Fig. 3**). It was observed that the patient had a slight maxillary cant and therefore a maxillary impaction of 2 mm was planned on the right side at the first molar level. The maxilla was advanced 4 mm anteriorly along the same occlusal plane inclination. The mandible was brought to the new maxillary position. Due to the mandibular asymmetry, a significant yaw movement was observed in the mandible when it was coupled to the maxilla in the appropriate occlusal relationship. Because facial symmetry was observed with the mandibular movement, a genioplasty was not necessary.

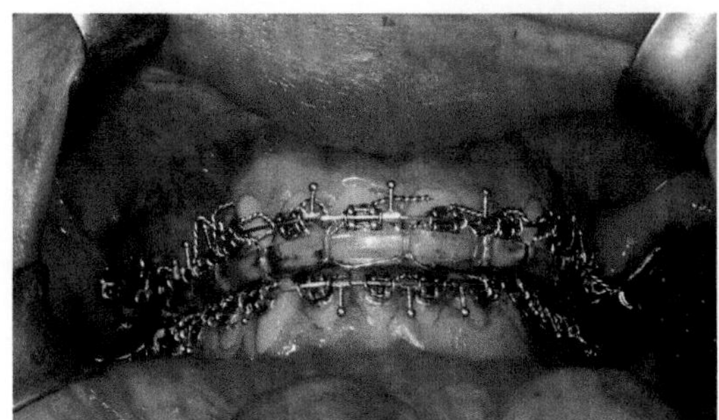

Fig. 5. Occlusal relationship with final splint at the end of surgical procedure.

The day before surgery 0.016 x 0.022-inch NiTi wires were placed in both the maxilla and mandible with surgical hooks in the anterior region (**Fig. 4**). Surgical hooks were placed in the posterior region; however, these are not necessary because the brackets had hooks attached. The patient had the planned surgical procedure (**Fig 5**) and returned 2 weeks later to remove the surgical wires and start the orthodontic movement. The patient had been wearing straight vertical, interocclusal elastics full-time after the surgical procedure. A 0.016 x 0.022-inch and a 0.016-inch NiTi wires were placed on the maxilla and mandible, respectively (**Fig. 6**).

Two months after surgery, the occlusion and alignment were progressing well (**Fig. 7**). The major occlusal goal at this point was to address the buccal overjet in the premolar region on the right side. For this, cross elastics from the lingual of the right mandibular premolars were prescribed as the archwires increased in dimension and stiffness. Ten months after surgery, the patient was debonded. A mandibular anterior bonded retainer from canine to canine was placed. The patient wore a maxillary vacuum-formed Essix retainer at night. Excellent esthetic and occlusal outcomes were observed with treatment (**Fig. 8**). The facial convexity was normalized and the asymmetry corrected. The panoramic radiograph showed good root parallelism. Follow-up records 5 years after debond show very stable results in the occlusion and in the facial esthetics (**Fig. 9**).

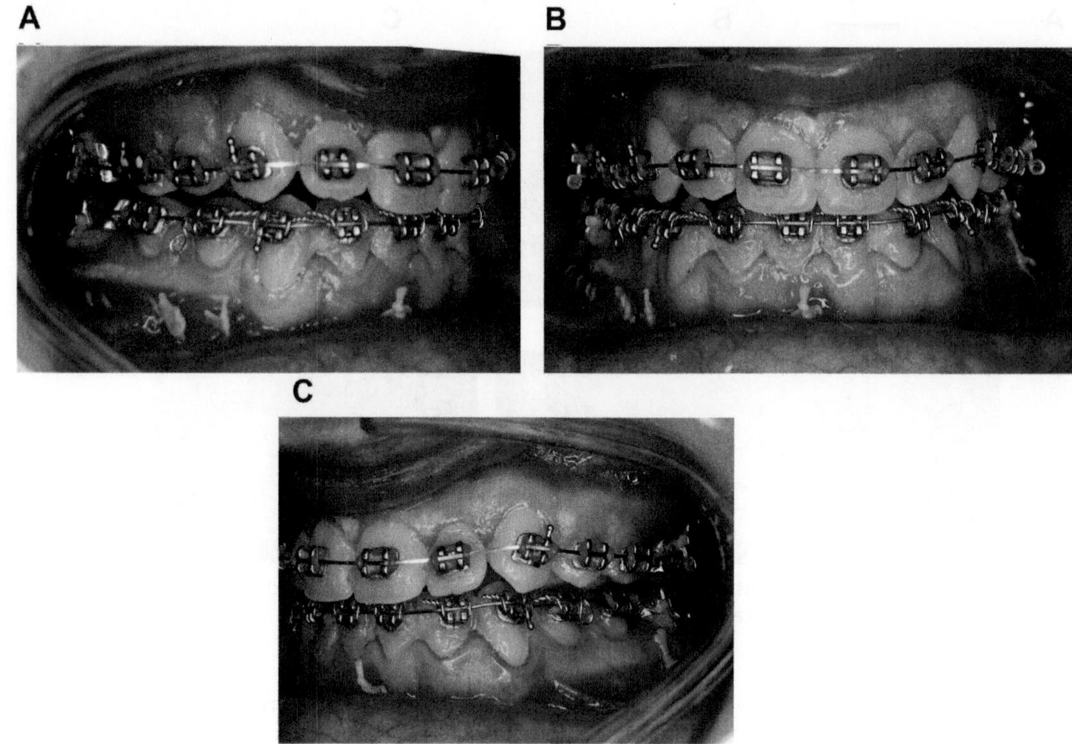

Fig. 6. Postsurgical occlusal result. (*A*) Right buccal occlusion. (*B*) Frontal occlusion. (*C*) Left buccal occlusion.

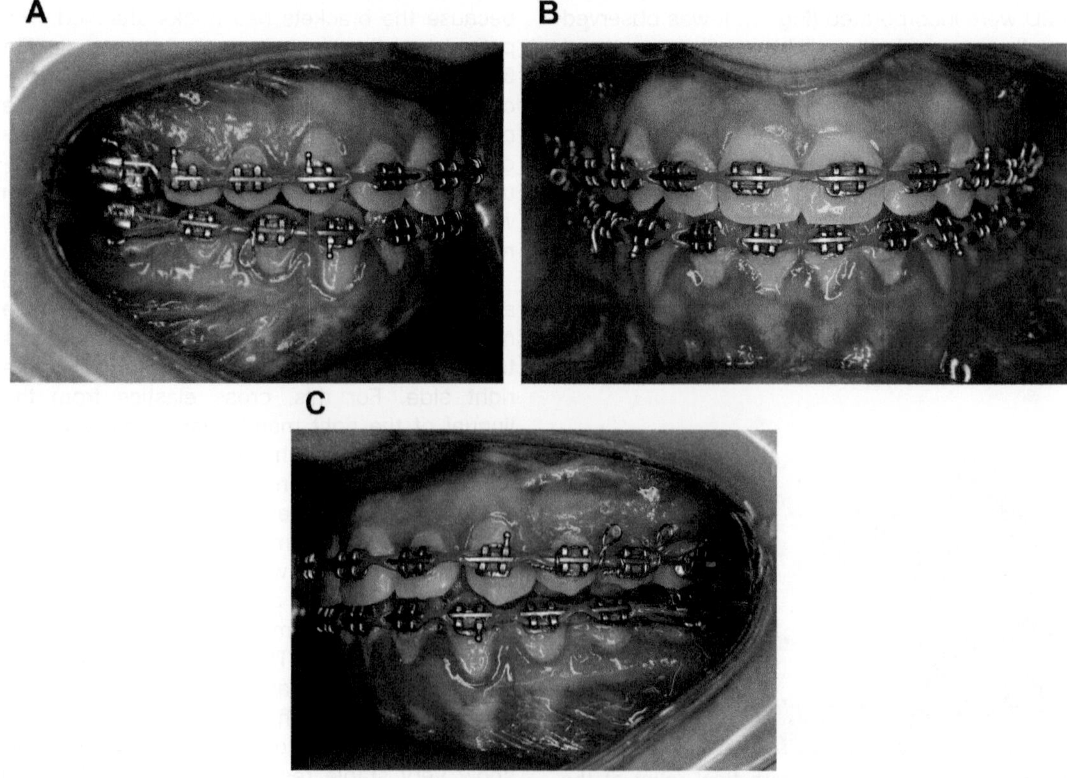

Fig. 7. Occlusion 2 months after surgery. (*A*) Right buccal occlusion. (*B*) Frontal occlusion. (*C*) Left buccal occlusion.

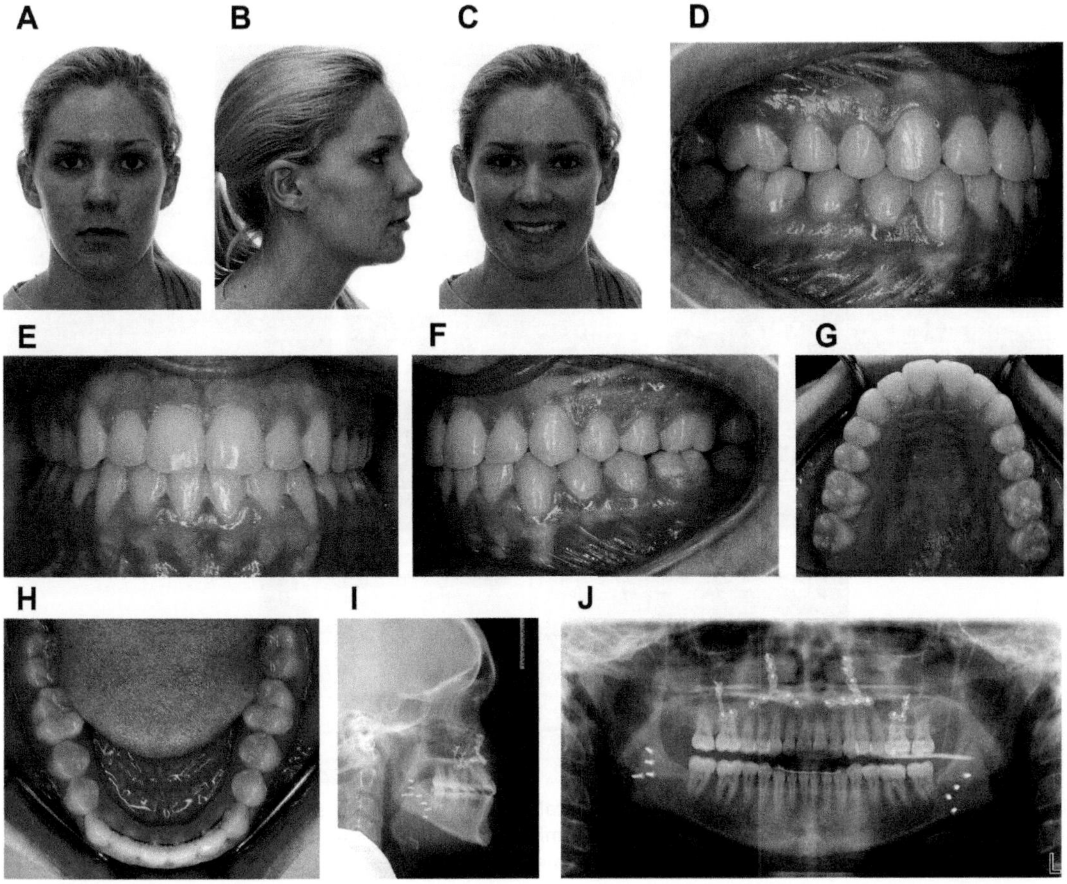

Fig. 8. Posttreatment records of patient 1. (*A*) Frontal, (*B*) profile, and (*C*) smile photographs. (*D*) Right buccal occlusion. (*E*) Frontal occlusion. (*F*) Left buccal occlusion. (*G*) Maxillary occlusal arch. (*H*) Mandibular occlusal arch. (*I*) Lateral cephalogram. (*J*) Panoramic radiograph.

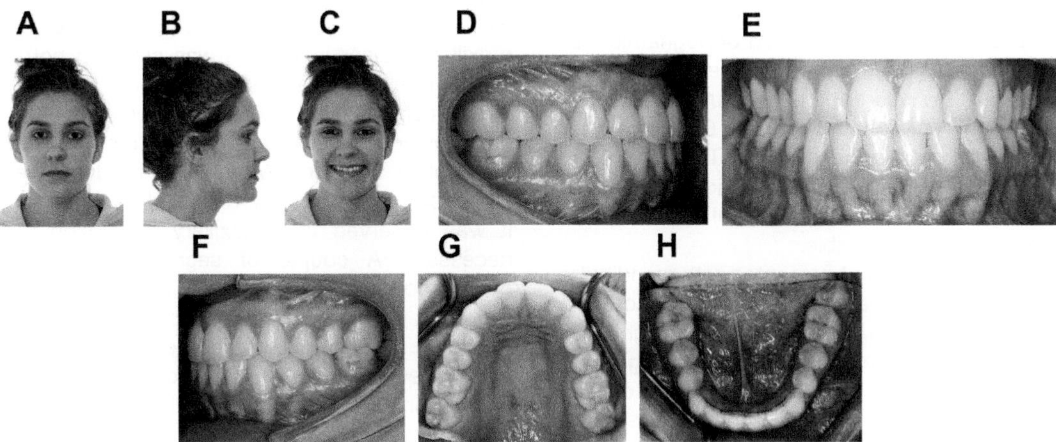

Fig. 9. Five-year retention records. (*A*) Frontal, (*B*) profile, and (*C*) smile photographs. (*D*) Right buccal occlusion. (*E*) Frontal occlusion. (*F*) Left buccal occlusion. (*G*) Maxillary occlusal arch. (*H*) Mandibular occlusal arch.

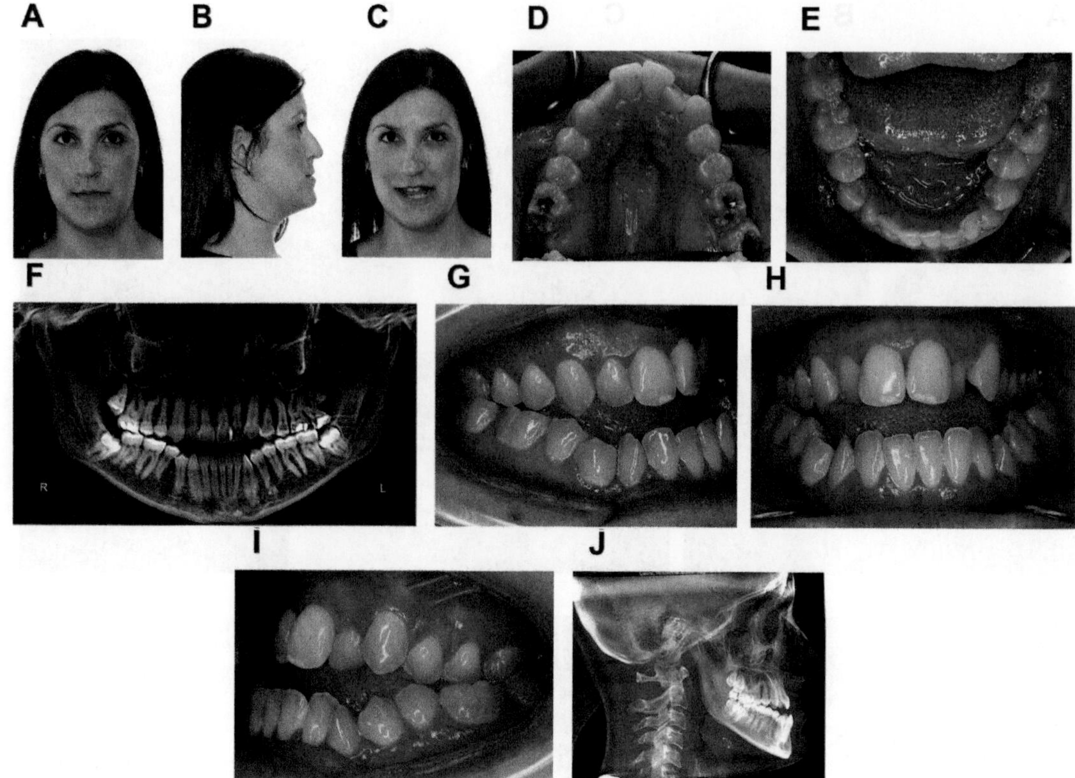

Fig. 10. Pretreatment records of patient 2. (*A*) Frontal, (*B*) profile, and (*C*) smile photographs. (*D*) Maxillary occlusal arch. (*E*) Mandibular occlusal arch. (*F*) Panoramic radiograph. (*G*) Right buccal occlusion. (*H*) Frontal occlusion. (*I*) Left buccal occlusion. (*J*) Lateral cephalogram.

Patient 2

A more complex patient was treated with the surgery-first approach, which included maxillary segmentation and the use of temporary anchorage devices for specific tooth movements. A 28-year-old female patient presented with chief complaint of an open bite and narrow maxilla. The patient had been told that she needed orthognathic surgery to address her dentofacial deformity, which required a 2-phase approach including a SARPE followed by orthognathic surgery 6 months after the surgical maxillary expansion. The patient did not want to have 2 separate surgical procedures and wanted to address her facial esthetic concerns as soon as possible.

Clinically, the patient presented with mandibular prognathism, maxillary deficiency, specifically in the perinasal region, long lower facial height, and mandibular asymmetry to the left side (**Fig. 10**A–C). The patient had slightly reduced incisor display at rest and on smile. The maxilla was constricted (**Fig. 10**D) with wide buccal corridors. The smile arch was reversed due to an anterior open bite. Dentally, the patient had an extra mandibular incisor (**Fig. 10**E), was missing the maxillary right second M, and had impacted third molars (**Fig. 10**F). The malocclusion included a significant anterior open bite with bilateral crossbite and lower midline deviated 2 mm to the left (**Fig. 10**G–I). A Class III molar and canine occlusion with a negative overjet also was observed. The maxillary incisor inclination was close to normal with retroclined mandibular incisors (**Fig. 10**J). The patient had mild to moderate maxillary and mandibular crowding accounting for the extra mandibular incisor. When the models were occluded to approximate a Class I malocclusion, it was observed that maxillary expansion was necessary. A couple of segmented maxillary dental models were prepared to analyze if a 2-piece or a 3-piece maxilla would result in an adequate occlusion anteroposteriorly and vertically. Because both types of segmentation resulted in similar occlusal relationships, the patient opted for a 2-piece maxillary surgery (**Fig. 11**). This option would give the patient a transitory diastema after surgery. Once the

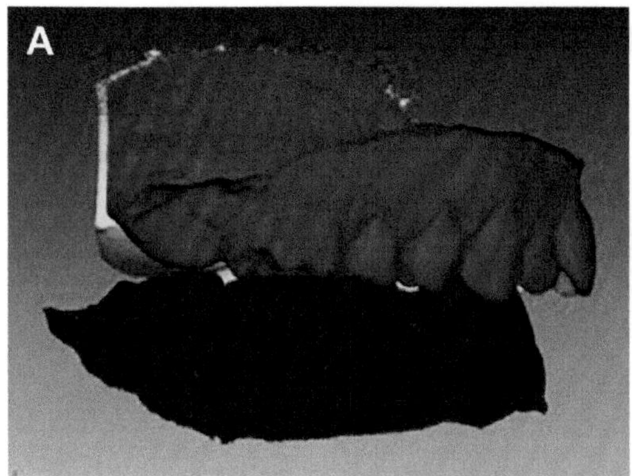

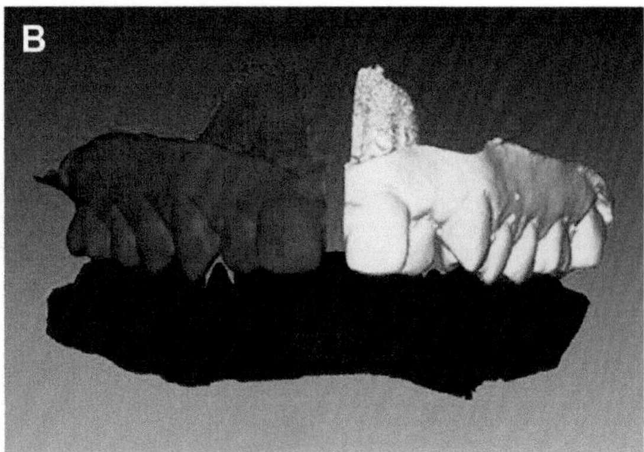

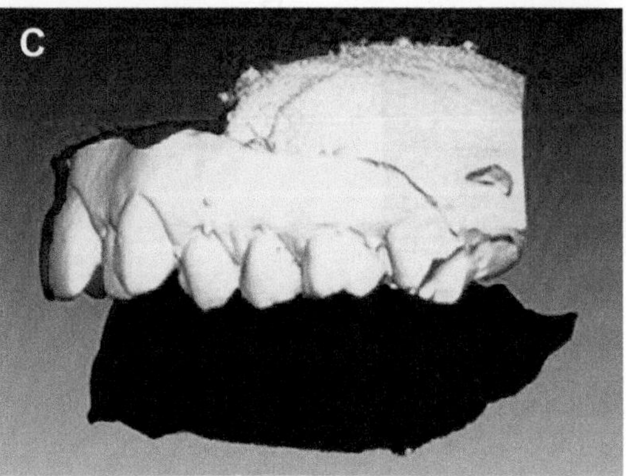

Fig. 11. Virtual maxillary segmentation and planned occlusion. (*A*) Right buccal view. (*B*) Frontal view. (*C*) Left buccal view.

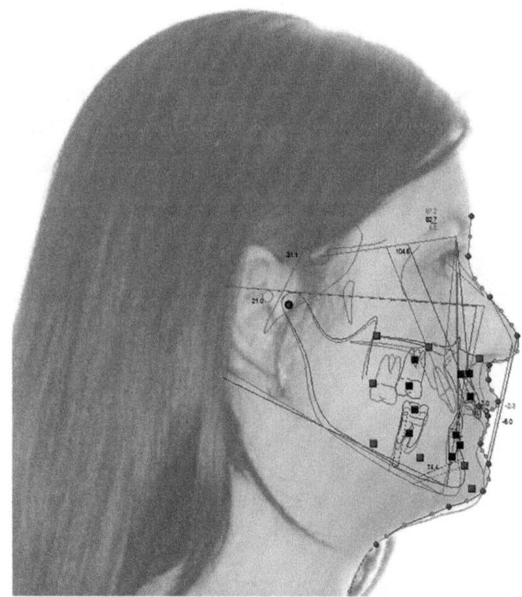

Fig. 12. Two-dimensional surgically planned movements.

appropriate occlusion was determined, the 2D skeletal changes were determined (**Fig. 12**). In this patient, the best esthetic prediction was obtained with 6 mm maxillary advancement measured at the central incisor edge while maintaining the mandible in the same anteroposterior position. Vertically the maxilla was to be impacted posteriorly approximately 2.5 mm bilaterally. The maxillary incisor was planned to be brought down vertically approximately 2 mm for better incisor show. The mandible autorotated with Menton moving up 5 mm. A bilateral setback with a jaw movement was planned to address the mandibular asymmetry. This specific movements were incorporated to the 3D plan for better visualization of the corrections in all planes (**Fig. 13**). Finally, the patient was also overcorrected to an edge-to-edge Class II molar relationship.

The day before surgery, 0.016 x 0.022-inch stainless steel braided wires were bent passively in both the maxillary and mandibular arches (**Fig. 14**). The mandibular left lateral incisor was not bonded, as it was to be extracted during surgery. Maxillary miniplates were placed to control the orthodontic movement after surgery for some maxillary distalization of the buccal segments and extrusion of the right third

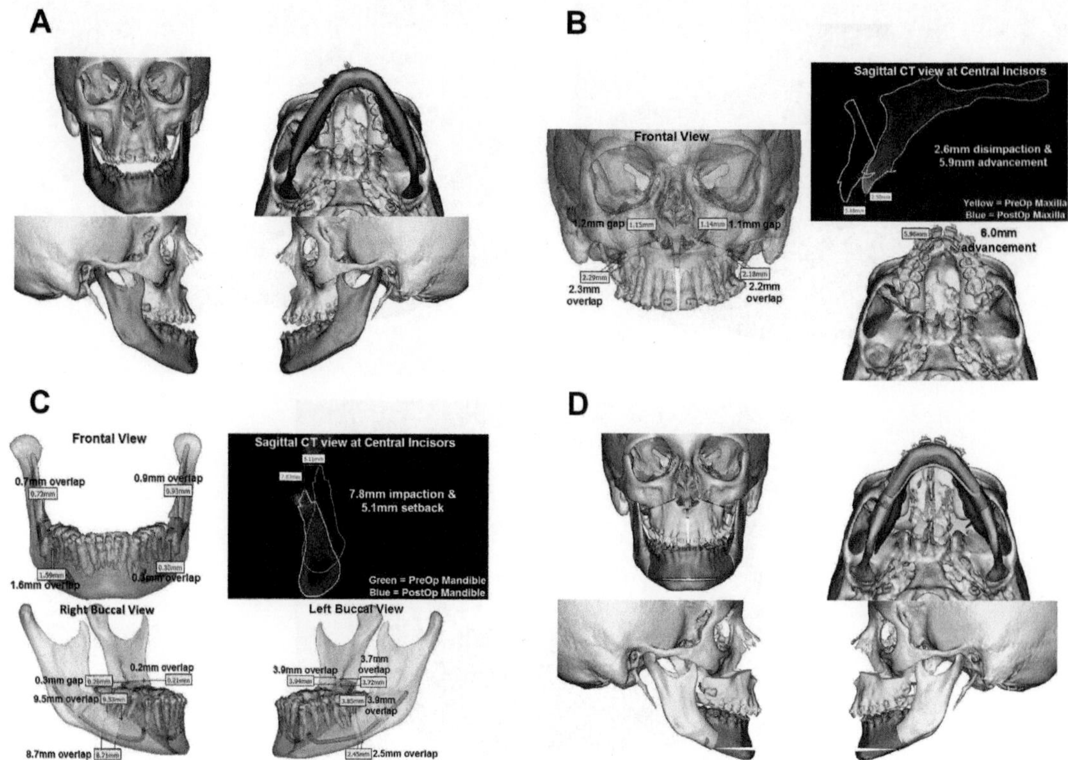

Fig. 13. Three-dimensional surgically planned movements. (*A*) Pretreatment CBCT. (*B*) Maxillary surgical movements. (*C*) Mandibular surgical movements. (*D*) Final predicted outcomes with all osteotomies.

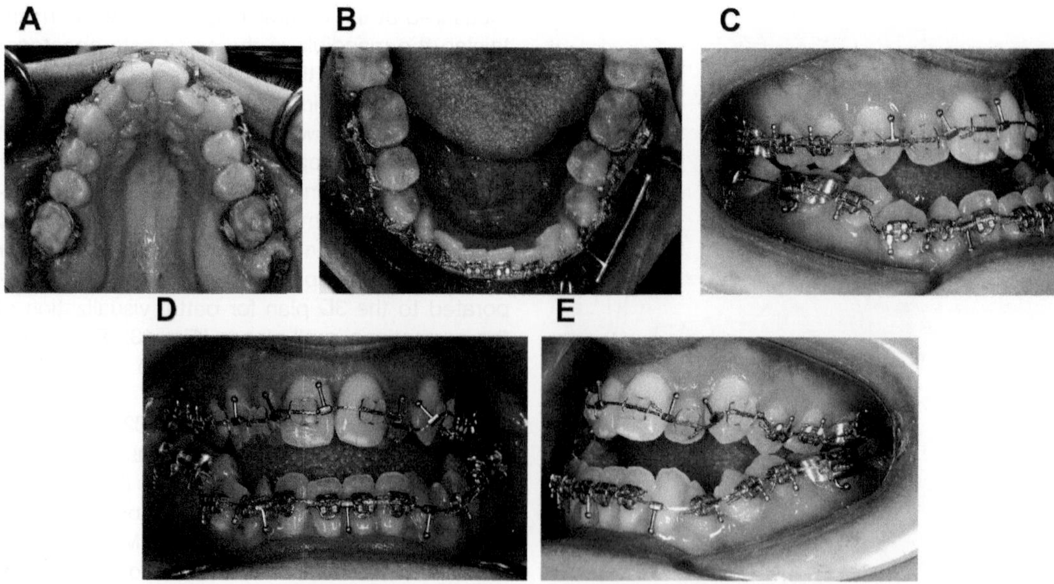

Fig. 14. Presurgical orthodontic wires. (*A*) Maxillary occlusal view. (*B*) Mandibular occlusal view. (*C*). Right buccal view. (*D*) Frontal view. (*E*) Left buccal view.

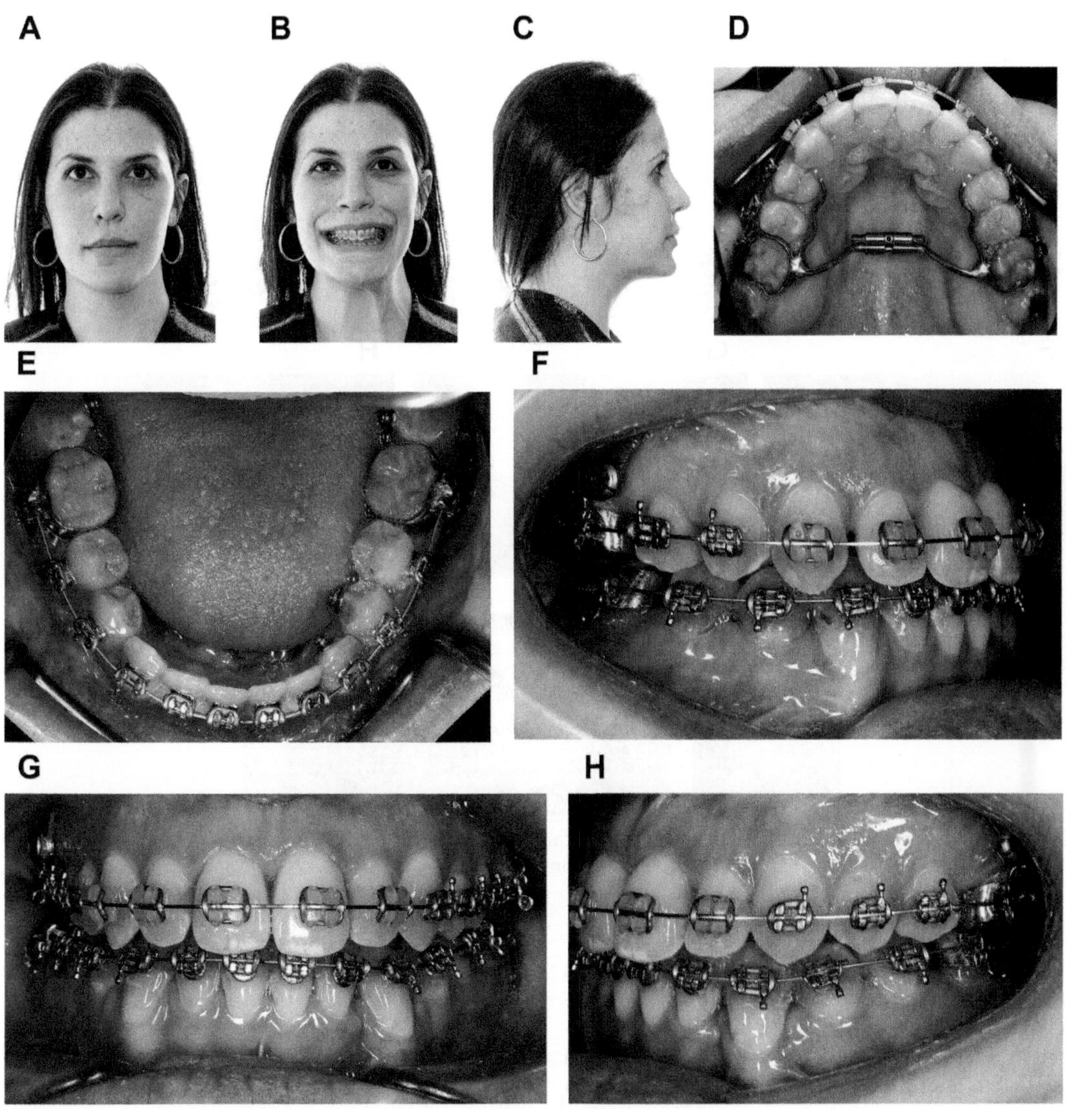

Fig. 15. Six-month facial esthetics and occlusal progress. (*A*) Frontal, (*B*) profile, and (*C*) smile photographs. (*D*) Maxillary occlusal arch. (*E*) Mandibular occlusal arch. (*F*) Right buccal occlusion. (*G*) Frontal occlusion. (*H*) Left buccal occlusion.

molar into the arch. The other third molars were to be extracted during surgery.

The patient presented 5 weeks after surgery for splint removal and initiation of orthodontic tooth movement. Upper and lower 0.016-inch NiTi archwires were placed to align and level the arches. The patient had limited opening, which prevented delivery of a maxillary transpalatal arch. Only 6 months after surgery a rapid maxillary expander appliance was inserted. At this point, good facial esthetics (**Fig. 15**A–C) with the surgery and good occlusal relationship were noted (**Fig. 15**D–H). Alignment and leveling were continued and space closure of the extracted supernumerary incisor closed. A 0.017 x 0.025-inch Beta titanium segmental archwire was delivered from the right miniplate to extrude the right third molar into occlusion (**Fig. 16**).

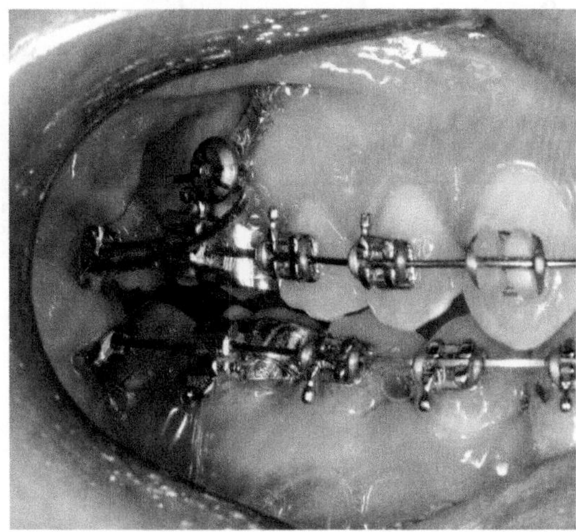

Fig. 16. Cantilever arm from miniplate to extrude impacted third molar into the missing second M site.

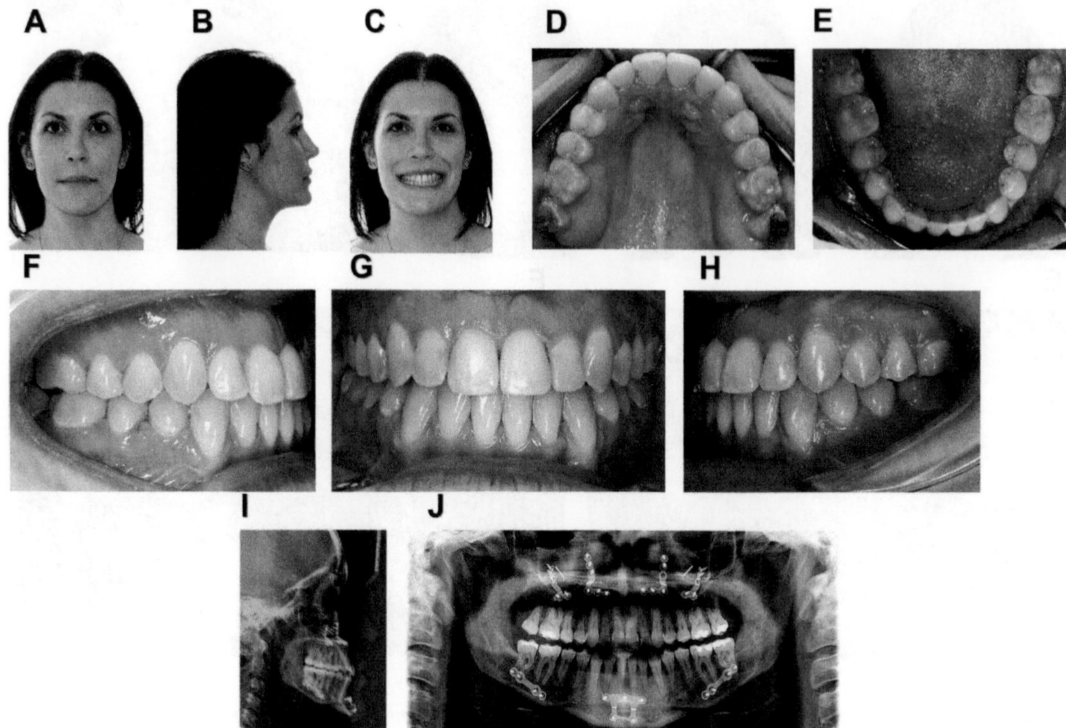

Fig. 17. Posttreatment records of patient 2. (*A*) Frontal, (*B*) profile, and (*C*) smile photographs. (*D*) Right buccal occlusion. (*E*) Frontal occlusion. (*F*) Left buccal occlusion. (*G*) Maxillary occlusal arch. (*H*) Mandibular occlusal arch. (*I*) Lateral cephalogram. (*J*) Panoramic radiograph.

Sixteen months after surgery, the patient was finished. Excellent facial esthetic and occlusal results were achieved as observed in **Fig. 17**. Thermoplastic Essix retainers were given to maintain the occlusal results. Long-term stability can be observed in **Fig. 18**. Two years after surgery, the facial esthetics and occlusal results have been adequately maintained. The patient is extremely satisfied with the results and the relatively short duration of treatment.

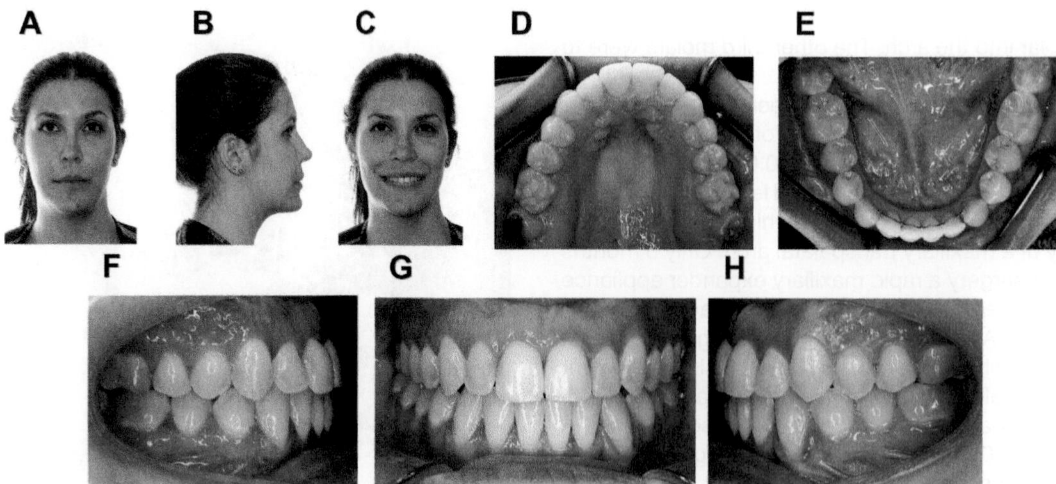

Fig. 18. Two-year retention records. (*A*) Frontal, (*B*) profile, and (*C*) smile photographs. (*D*) Right buccal occlusion. (*E*) Frontal occlusion. (*F*) Left buccal occlusion. (*G*) Maxillary occlusal arch. (*H*) Mandibular occlusal arch.

SUMMARY

Surgery-first is a paradigm shift in orthognathic surgery. Its approach is justified from a patient-centered treatment strategy. Treatment duration may be reduced in certain patients in whom no significant orthodontic movements are required. Skeletal anchorage with this approach offers a mechanical advantage that allows implementation of this technique to most dentofacial deformities. Future directions are the implementation of this approach with clear aligner therapy for an adult population opting for facial and occlusal changes without visible orthodontic appliances.

ACKNOWLEDGMENTS

The authors acknowledge Drs Greg Ross and Jonathan Dzingle who contributed to the orthodontic treatment of the patients reported in this article. Also, we acknowledge Drs David Shafer and Derek Steinbacher for performing the orthognathic surgeries on these patients.

REFERENCES

1. Pelo S, Gasparini G, Garagiola U, et al. Surgery-first orthognathic approach vs traditional orthognathic approach: oral health-related quality of life assessed with 2 questionnaires. Am J Orthod Dentofacial Orthop 2017;152(2):250–4.
2. Zingler S, Hakim E, Finke D, et al. Surgery-first approach in orthognathic surgery: Psychological and biological aspects—a prospective cohort study. J Craniomaxillofac Surg 2017;45(8):1293–301.
3. Behrman SJ, Behrman DA. Oral surgeons' considerations in surgical orthodontic treatment. Dent Clin North Am 1988;32(3):481–507.
4. Nagasaka H, Sugawara J, Kawamura H, et al. "Surgery first" skeletal Class III correction using the Skeletal Anchorage System. J Clin Orthod 2009;43(2):97–105.
5. Hernandez-Alfaro F, Guijarro-Martinez R, Peiro-Guijarro MA. Surgery first in orthognathic surgery: what have we learned? A comprehensive workflow based on 45 consecutive cases. J Oral Maxillofac Surg 2014;72(2):376–90.
6. Jeong WS, Choi JW, Kim DY, et al. Can a surgery-first orthognathic approach reduce the total treatment time? Int J Oral Maxillofac Surg 2017;46(4):473–82.
7. Peiro-Guijarro MA, Guijarro-Martinez R, Hernandez-Alfaro F. Surgery first in orthognathic surgery: a systematic review of the literature. Am J Orthod Dentofacial Orthop 2016;149(4):448–62.
8. Uribe F, Adabi S, Janakiraman N, et al. Treatment duration and factors associated with the surgery-first approach: a two-center study. Prog Orthod 2015;16:29.
9. Diaz PM, Garcia RG, Gias LN, et al. Time used for orthodontic surgical treatment of dentofacial deformities in white patients. J Oral Maxillofac Surg 2010;68(1):88–92.
10. O'Brien K, Wright J, Conboy F, et al. Prospective, multi-center study of the effectiveness of orthodontic/orthognathic surgery care in the United Kingdom. Am J Orthod Dentofacial Orthop 2009;135(6):709–14.
11. Slavnic S, Marcusson A. Duration of orthodontic treatment in conjunction with orthognathic surgery. Swed Dent J 2010;34(3):159–66.
12. Yang L, Xiao YD, Liang YJ, et al. Does the surgery-first approach produce better outcomes in orthognathic surgery? A systematic review and meta-analysis. J Oral Maxillofac Surg 2017;75(11):2422–9.
13. Nurminen L, Pietila T, Vinkka-Puhakka H. Motivation for and satisfaction with orthodontic-surgical treatment: a retrospective study of 28 patients. Eur J Orthod 1999;21(1):79–87.
14. Choi SH, Shi KK, Cha JY, et al. Nonsurgical miniscrew-assisted rapid maxillary expansion results in acceptable stability in young adults. Angle Orthod 2016;86(5):713–20.
15. Villegas C, Janakiraman N, Uribe F, et al. Rotation of the maxillomandibular complex to enhance esthetics using a "surgery first" approach. J Clin Orthod 2012;46(2):85–91 [quiz: 123].

Idiopathic Condylar Resorption
What Should We Do?

Louis G. Mercuri, DDS, MS[a,b,*], Chester S. Handelman, DMD[c,1]

KEYWORDS

• Idiopathic condylar resorption (ICR) • Progressive condylar resorption (PCR)
• Temporomandibular joint replacement (TMJR)

KEY POINTS

- Idiopathic condylar resorption (ICR), alternatively called progressive condylar resorption, is an uncommon aggressive form of degenerative disease of the temporomandibular joint (TMJ) seen mostly in adolescent and young women.
- The orthodontist is likely to have contact with patients afflicted with ICR in the following 2 contexts. The first include patients who spontaneously manifest ICR independent of surgical intervention and second, those who develop ICR during orthodontic treatment or in retention.
- TMJ intraarticular pathologic disorders, such as ICR, must be considered as pathologic entities in dental circles the same way our orthopedic colleagues discuss all other joint pathology. Failure to do this only exacerbates the problems associated with TMJ disorders in general for patients, clinicians, insurance companies.

INTRODUCTION

Idiopathic condylar resorption (ICR), alternatively called progressive condylar resorption (PCR), is an uncommon, aggressive form of degenerative disease of the temporomandibular joint (TMJ) seen mostly in adolescent and young women.[1–3] This disorder is very rarely seen in men. Constitutional risk factors include hormonal imbalance (↓estrogen, ↓17β-estradiol) and nutritional status (↓ Vitamin D, ↓ dietary Omega-3 fatty acids).[4,5] Bruxism, third molar extractions, orthodontics, and orthognathic surgery have been hypothetically implicated as resulting in compressive TMJ overloading and are thought to be possible causes of ICR.[6] In patients with ICR the intrinsic adaptive capacity of their joints to withstand mechanical loads is exceeded by functional demands; essentially they are a vulnerable subset of the population.[7] The rarity of this disease is shown in a survey of 59 orthodontists; only 56 cases of ICR were reported out of the thousands of patients seen in their practices.[1]

PATHOPHYSIOLOGY

ICR is best described as a localized pathologic disorder of the TMJ characterized by lysis and repair of the articular fibrocartilage and underlying subchondral bone.[3] This condition leads to loss of condylar bone mass, decrease of mandibular ramal height, steep mandibular and occlusal plane angles, and apertognathia. Most of the pathologic process is localized to the mandibular condyles.

Disclosure Statement: Dr L.G. Mercuri is a compensated clinical consultant for TMJ Concepts and holds stock in TMJ Concepts. Dr C.S. Handelman has nothing to disclose.
[a] Department of Orthopaedic Surgery, Rush University Medical Center, 1611 West Harrison Street, Chicago, IL 60612, USA; [b] TMJ Concepts, 6059 King Drive, Ventura, Ca 93003, USA; [c] Department of Orthodontics, College of Dentistry University of Illinois, 801 South Paulina, Chicago, IL 60612, USA
[1] Present address: 1044 Judson Avenue, Evanston, IL 60202.
* Corresponding author. 604 Bonnie Brae Place, River Forest, IL 60305.
E-mail address: lgm@tmjconcepts.com

Oral Maxillofacial Surg Clin N Am 32 (2020) 105–116
https://doi.org/10.1016/j.coms.2019.09.001
1042-3699/20/

The active phase of ICR often is associated with limited jaw opening and TMJ pain, followed by condylar head flattening. This alteration may eventually develop a compatible articulation with a remodeled posterior articular eminence slope permitting redistribution of functional loads and restoring mandibular mobility.[3]

ICR occurring before the completion of growth results in a shorter mandibular condyloid process, ramus and body, compensatory growth at the gonial angle (causing an antigonial notch deformity), and an increase in anterior facial vertical dimension. As ramus height decreases, there is compensatory increase in the coronoid process length and anterior open bite development. A tendency for a reduction in airway size secondary to decreased mandibular growth in the immature skeleton, as well as in the patient who has completed growth, leads to progressive mandibular retrusion and the risk of developing sleep apnea.[3]

HISTORY

A careful history can reveal the probable diagnosis of ICR. A report of a sudden change in occlusion is nearly pathognomonic of ICR. Unfortunately, this change may occur during orthodontic treatment, when it easily can be misinterpreted as being due to unfavorable growth, tongue thrust, or it might be regarded as an adverse response to treatment mechanics.

A history of autoimmune and collagen diseases should be part of the historical questioning. A history of TMJ discomfort and disc displacement may be a factor, because several patients with ICR report pain or other TMJ disorder symptoms and have displaced discs on imaging.[8] It should be remembered that disc displacement occurs in a significant number of asymptomatic individuals and disc displacement may not lead to TMJ pathology.[9–11] In a survey of a group of orthodontists only one-half of the ICR cases reported TMJ discomfort.[1] A history of facial trauma, especially when the TMJ is involved, is important as a possible cause of condylar resorption.[1,6] Fortunately, only rarely does a trauma case evolve into ICR.

IMAGING

The orthopantomogram (OPG) is the least expensive imaging modality for gross evaluation of the mandibular condyle. Pathognomonic imaging signs such as loss of condylar bone mass, flattening of the anterior or superior aspect of the condyle, as well as a distal inclination of the condylar neck can be easily observed on an OPG.[12]

A cephalogram will exhibit a decreased posterior facial height, increased anterior facial height, increased overjet, and anterior open bite. Serial cephalograms taken during the active stages of ICR using the suggested superimposition on basion along the basion-nasion plane will show a more mesial position of articulare[1] (**Fig. 1**). Serial cephalometric tracings of a case of ICR superimposed as discussed earlier show the typical skeletal changes as well as the anterior movement of articulare relative to basion (**Fig. 2**).

Cone beam computed tomography (CBCT) is definitive as it permits a 3-dimensional evaluation of the condyle and condylar degeneration, for example, subchondral Ely cyst formation, erosion, flattening and loss of the dense cortical layer, as well as subcortical bone loss[3] (see **Fig. 2**).

MRI is the preferred technique for investigation of the soft tissues of the TMJ, disk derangement, and inflammation. The T1-weighted MRI is helpful to identify disc position, the presence of alteration in bone, and soft tissue anatomy, whereas the T2-weighted MRI is helpful to identify any inflammatory response as well as mandibular condyle bone marrow edema.[2,3]

Bone scintigraphy, using technecium-99, can be used to assess whether there are any active bony

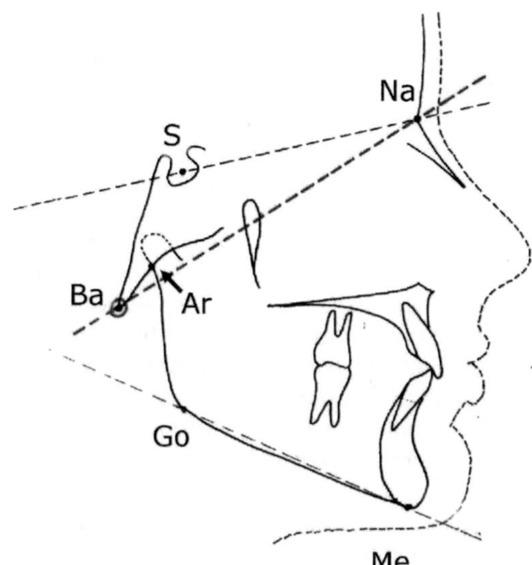

Fig. 1. Cephalometric tracing using nasion (Na) to basion (Ba) plane with the recommended superimposition point at basion. With active ICR, superimposed tracings will often show articulare (Ar) moving in an anterior direction.[1] Articulare is the point where the posterior of the ramus crosses the Na-Ba plane. It represents the movement of the condyle, which is often difficult to trace especially in advanced ICR cases.[1]

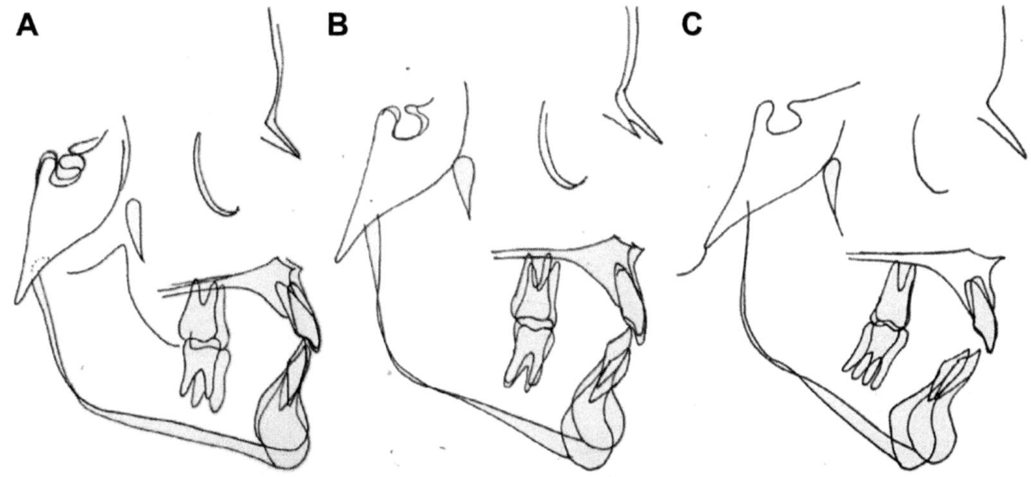

Fig. 2. Cephalometric tracings of progressing stages of ICR superimposed on the nasion-basion plane at basion. (*A*) Preorthodontic treatment at age 10 years, 3 months, traced in black. Occlusion class I deep bite with no signs of ICR. Postorthodontic treatment at age 13 years, 4 months, traced in red. Early stages of ICR as articulare advanced anteriorly relative to basion. Growth masked this early stage of ICR. (*B*) Tracing at 13 years, 4 months in red and at 14 years, 3 months in blue. Mandibular rotation results in anterior open bite. Condylar resorption is demonstrated by advancement of articulare. (*C*) Tracing at 14 years, 3 months in blue and age 15 years, 10 months in black. The mandible has shortened and has continued clockwise rotation resulting in severe Class II open bite. (*From* Handelman CS, Greene CS. Progressive/idiopathic condylar resorption: an orthodontic perspective. Sem Ortho. 2013;19:60; with permission.)

changes; but its specificity has been reported as not sufficient to assess state of stability/remission of those changes.[3]

PRELIMINARY DIAGNOSIS

Early diagnosis of ICR should include a careful examination of the mandibular condyle and condyloid process on the screening OPG. Signs of bony condylar changes or condyloid process shortening may be present despite absence of clinical symptoms. The suspicion and recognition of these imaging changes, plus awareness of any clinical sign and symptoms, may be an indication for the need for more sophisticated imaging (CBCT, MRI, bone scintigraphy), blood testing, and consultation. Blood testing to rule out high inflammatory arthritic diseases include erythrocyte sedimentation rate, C-reactive protein, antinuclear antibody, rheumatoid factor, and anticyclic citrullinated peptide. Vitamin D and 17β-estradiol levels should also be examined.[4–6,13] CBCT is pathognomic for normal, early degenerative change, advanced changes, and repair once active ICR goes into remission[3] (**Fig. 3**).

ORTHODONTIC MANAGEMENT

The orthodontist is likely to have contact with patients afflicted with ICR in the following 2 contexts. The first include patients who spontaneously manifest ICR independent of surgical intervention. The most troubling are those who develop ICR during orthodontic treatment or in retention. These patients are almost always young adolescent women, whereas others are afflicted in their late teens or early twenties. Their clinical history shows that their occlusion was acceptable in the past, but within a relatively brief time period they have deteriorated. The second group includes patients who have undergone orthognathic surgery for correction of any one or more of the following conditions: anterior open bite, mandibular retrognathia, or long anterior face height. Following surgery, the intermaxillary correction seems to be successful, but by the third to sixth month afterward the correction starts to fail to a variable extent. The extent of the relapse varies from minimal to almost return to the presurgical state.

Do these 2 groups of patients have different problems, either clinically or pathophysiologically? Or are they the same, only manifested at somewhat different ages and under different circumstances? In both cases, most of these patients share similarities in sex, age, malocclusion, skeletal pattern, and condylar pathology. With the exception of subjects with known medical or traumatic causality,[13] these patients are described as having an "idiopathic" problem (ie, ICR).

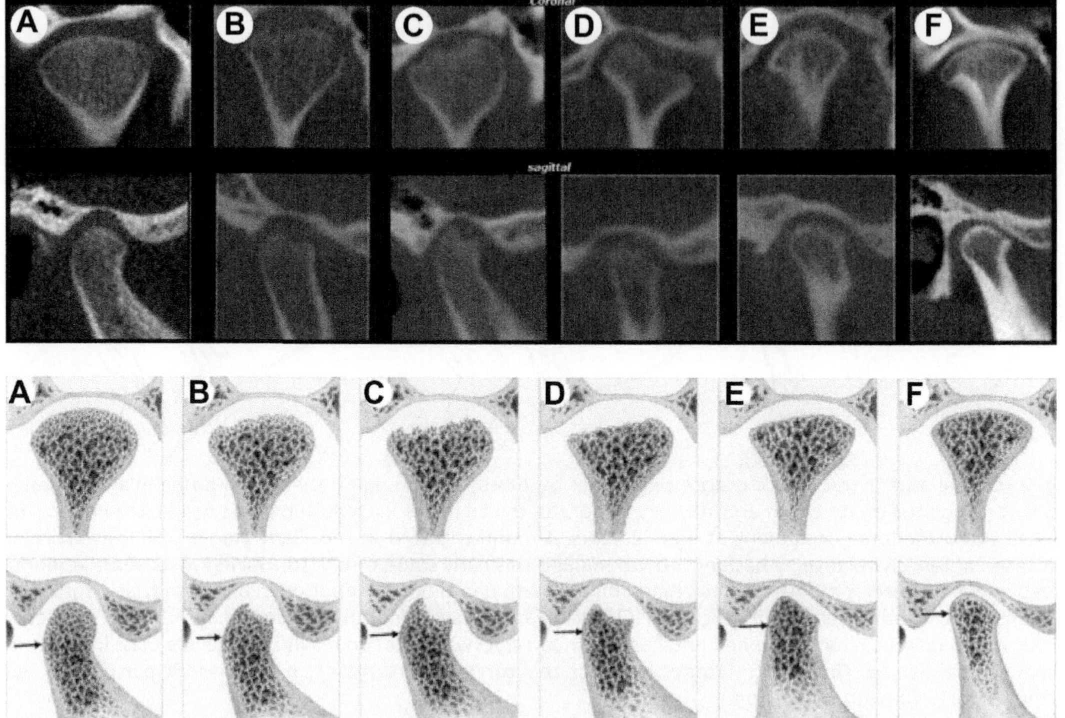

Fig. 3. Imaging stages of ICR. CBCT TMJ images (*top*) and anatomic images (*bottom*) displayed in paracoronal and parasagittal plane. (*A*) Normal, (*B*) beginning of active destructive stage, (*C*) continuing destructive stage, (*D*) beginning of repair stage, (*E*) advanced repair stage, (*F*) stable stage. Arrows pointing to the mandibular condyle. (*From* Hatcher DC. Progressive condylar resorption: pathologic processes and imaging considerations. Sem Ortho. 2013;19:104; with permission.)

Sex and Age

ICR is a disease of young women in their preteens or early twenties. Many diseases have a higher incidence in either men or women. It is unusual for a disease to be clustered almost completely within one gender when the sexual organs are not directly involved. Arnett and colleagues[4–6] have made a case for low serum 17 β-estradiol as a major factor in progressive condylar resorption. They state that the use of oral contraceptives and abnormal menstrual cycles are often seen in women with severe condylar resorption.

But why should there be a preponderance of adolescent and young women in the ICR population? The premenstrual woman may have insufficient circulating estrogen to initiate condylar pathology, but then there is the onset of menses. The age of expression of ICR is in adolescent and young women up to the late twenties. Interestingly, there seems to be an unexplained "burnout" of the resorption process in afflicted individuals sometime in the mid-twenties. However, the involved joints will always be subject to reactivation of the destructive phase when exposed to excessive functional demands even into adulthood.[3] It is best to consider the involved joints as in "remission" rather than healed.

Can the preadolescent facial type and occlusion predict later ICR? Not necessarily. **Fig. 2** illustrates a subject who during adolescence developed ICR/PCR, but as young girl had a Class I malocclusion without a hint of her future disease.

Mechanical Loads

The healthy TMJ that undergoes natural remodeling can withstand and adapt to heavy mechanical loads that are frequently experienced, including parafunctional habits such as nocturnal bruxism, orthodontic procedures such as wearing elastics, and orthopedic appliances such as Herbst or chin cup. However, a certain subset of adolescent and young adult women seem to be susceptible to developing degenerative joint disease that progresses to condylar resorption when their TMJs are exposed to excessive mechanical loading.[6] Orthodontic treatment and third molar extractions have been indicted as possible causes of ICR/PCR.[6] Statistics indicate that this is a very rare disease[1] and a large percentage of the young have had orthodontic treatment and/or third molar removal. Therefore, it is problematic to assign cause of a rare disease to a common experience. However, in those rare subjects whose condyles are undergoing an early, often undetected, stage of ICR/PCR, orthodontic treatment and/or third molar extractions may overwhelm the adaptive capacity of their vulnerable condyles. Even healthy joints cannot withstand extreme mechanical loads that exceed their adaptive capacity, for example, severe trauma.

ORTHOGNATHIC SURGERY AS A RISK FACTOR

Orthognathic surgery for the correction of the Class II open bite malocclusion usually involves maxillary impaction via a LeFort I osteotomy to induce mandibular closing rotation, combined with mandibular advancement via bilateral sagittal split osteotomies (BSSO). Both surgeries will cause a sudden repositioning of the condyles in the fossae and thereby alter both the direction and the magnitude of the mechanical load in the TMJs.[6,12] In most patients following surgery the joints will remodel and adapt to this change; but in some patients the remodeling capacity of their TMJs is exceeded by the functional demands of these sudden anatomic changes, and their condyles resorb.[6]

Arnett and colleagues[6] have demonstrated that the use of bicortical screws to fixate the mesial and distal segments during BSSO can rotate the condylar segments either laterally or medially in the glenoid fossa. This torquing of the condyle could initiate condylar resorption. To minimize torquing they suggest using titanium bone plates adapted to the outer cortical surfaces of the 2 segments with unicortical screw fixation to minimize this problem. They also point out that overseating the condyle in the fossa during BSSO can cause compression resulting in dysfunctional remodeling of the joint.[6]

In a study by Peacock and colleagues,[14] the incidence for condylar resorption following maxillary surgery for correction of Class II open bite malocclusions was less than after surgeries involving both jaws (9% compared with 23%). However, most severe Class II open bite patients will benefit from having bimaxillary surgery as well as advancement genioplasty in order to maximize facial aesthetics. Hoppenreijs and colleagues[12] also demonstrated that the initial correction can relapse due to condylar resorption by the sixth month, and this resorption can continue for up to 3 years.

DIAGNOSIS OF THE PATIENT WITH IDIOPATHIC CONDYLAR RESORPTION

Occlusal Appliances: Diagnostic Aspects

Occlusal appliances used only at night time are suggested as a joint stabilizing modality in ICR cases when there is joint pain and dysfunction as well as before orthognathic surgery.[6] An often-overlooked use is its potential as a diagnostic tool for determining cessation of the resorptive process. Patients suspected of having ICR should be fitted with a maxillary occlusal appliance with contact registered on all the mandibular teeth. If the lower incisors no longer register contact at a future evaluation, this indicates further joint degeneration and active disease.[1] An occlusal appliance should routinely be placed following orthognathic surgery and orthodontic treatment of patients with ICR at the time of retention both to reduce the forces on the TMJ and to evaluate stability of the correction.[1]

Idiopathic Condylar Resorption Treatment Options: What to Do

The following is a listing of treatment options that depend on severity, activity stage of ICR, and patient wishes.

No treatment: this is a possible option when ICR no longer is active, especially when the disfigurement of the facial soft tissue is moderate and acceptable for the patient. Usually the occlusion is only on the most distal molars with a variable anterior open bite. A full coverage occlusal appliance should be used at night to manage pain and avoid excessive forces on the TMJ.

Maintenance during active ICR: no active orthodontic or surgical treatment should be performed as this could accelerate condylar resorption. A full coverage occlusal appliance is used to manage the forces on the TMJ and for diagnosis of active disease. Follow-up at 6-month intervals with serial cephalometric radiographs (superimpose on the nasion-basion plane at basion). CBCT scans are taken annually to observe condylar anatomy to determine if the head of the condyle is in the active, destructive phase, varying stages of repair or the healed stable stage (see **Fig. 3**). It is best to wait 6 months to 1 year before treatment is initiated after the stable stage is achieved.

Orthodontic treatment: this is contraindicated during the active phase of ICR. First, it could accelerate condylar resorption and second it would expose the orthodontist to litigation if the

ICR progresses. Once the ICR is in remission, orthodontic treatment without follow-up jaw surgery is feasible in only a few patients with ICR—those with moderate skeletal and occlusal discrepancies. Their condylar resorption usually started after growth completion and their condition may better be described as "degenerative joint disease."

Most patients with ICR present with considerable condylar destruction with resulting soft tissue disfigurement and extreme Class II open bite malocclusions and require comprehensive orthognathic surgical procedures. In all cases before surgery orthodontic treatment is required to align the teeth in both jaws for maximum occlusion following repositioning of one or both jaws.

Orthognathic surgery: surgery places an enormous functional demand on the compromised adaptive capacity of even the healed condyle. One approach is to delay surgery until the patient is in the mid-twenties when the so-called burn out stage has occurred. Variable postsurgical relapse may still occur. Patients with the usual disfiguring malformation associated with ICR often wish correction before the college years when the disease may still be active. There are several papers that indicate that 30% of women following orthognathic surgery for Class II open bite develop postsurgical relapse of variable amounts of the correction.[15–20]

Medical management with orthognathic surgery: Arnette and Gunson have proposed pharmacologic and physiologic control of the resorptive process for a period of time both before and after orthognathic reconstruction. They recommend antiinflammatory medication such as the nonsteroidal antiinflammatory drugs (Naproxen, Celebrex, Feldene), vitamin D and calcium supplementation (both of which are known to increase bone density), and an antioxidant diet. When pursuing the medical management route proposed by Arnett and Gunson,[4–7] it is essential that a colleague rheumatologist with an understanding of this pathology prescribe and monitor any biological medication such as methotrexate or etanercept used as part of this regimen.[18,19] Gunson and Arnette have reported success in individual cases using these procedures.[5] The advantage of medical management of TMJ surgery is lifetime maintenance of the patient's own TMJ.

Surgical management of ICR using total alloplastic temporomandibular joint replacement (TMJR): the presence of an adverse mechanical and biological environment promoting osteoclastic pathologic activity over osteoblastic activity as found with ICR compromises the surgical options of autogenous reconstruction with a costochondral graft,[14] orthognathic surgery,[15–19] and/or distraction osteogenesis.[21]

Wolford and Gonçalves reported a protocol using salvageable intraarticular discs. The protocol includes removing the tissue pathology from the joint, repositioning and stabilizing the disc to the condyle with a Mitek anchor (Mitek Surgical Products, Westwood, MA), bimaxillary surgery with counterclockwise rotation of the maxillomandibular complex, and other adjunctive procedures such as turbinectomy and genioplasty. However, these investigators stated that the results using this protocol are best when it is used within 4 years of ICR signs and symptoms and most importantly, when the articular disc is intact. After 4 years, discs in this disease may become significantly deformed or fragmented and are unsalvageable. In such cases, the investigators recommend alloplastic TMJ replacement.[2,22]

It seems that an ICR surgical management option that does not depend on the compromised mechanical and biological adaptive capacity of the TMJ and surrounding tissues should be considered. Total alloplastic TMJ replacement, because it is a biomechanical rather than biological solution to the management of anatomically distorted dysfunctional joints resulting from pathology or end-stage disease, provides such an option. Individually customized patient-fitted TMJR fossa and ramus (condyle) components are designed and manufactured from a stereolithic model generated from the patient's protocol computed tomographic scan data to mimic the anatomic contours of the structures they are intended to replace (**Fig. 4**).

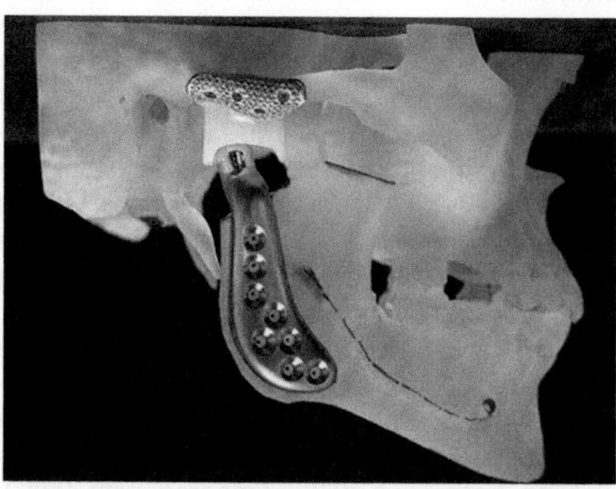

Fig. 4. Image of custom TMJR on stereolithic model. Fossa component is ultrahigh molecular weight polyethylene bearing surface backed by a commercially pure titanium mesh. Ramus component is titanium alloy with a cobalt chrome molybdenum condylar head. Screws are titanium alloy (TMJ Concepts, Ventura, CA).

Table 1
Patients with ICR managed surgically between 2001 and 2010

Patient	Diagnosis	Treatment	Result	Treatment	Result	Management	Status
DT	Cl II	Ortho BSSO	ICR	CCG	PCR	BTMJR	LTFU
CP	Cl II	Ortho BSSO	ICR	Refused Tx			LTFU
LS	Cl II	Ortho BSSO	ICR	CCG	PCR	BTMJR	Stable
PP	ICR			OA		Ortho BTMJR	Stable
TD	Cl II	Ortho BSSO	ICR	OA	PCR	Ortho BTMJR	Stable
YF	ICR			OA		OA	PCR
SC	ICR					BTMJR	Stable
JL	ICR					BTMJR	Stable
TM	ICR					BTMJR	Stable
JF	ICR					BTMJR	Stable
EF	ICR	Ortho		Refused Tx			LTFU
KP	ICR	Le Fort I BSSO	PCR			BTMJR Genio	Stable
MS	ICR					Ortho BTMJR	Stable
NC	ICR					LeFort I BTMJR	Stable
AI	Cl II	Ortho BSSO	PCR			LeFort I BTMJR	Stable

All bilateral alloplastic temporomandibular joint replacement cases remain stable without revision to date.
Abbreviations: BTMJR, bilateral alloplastic TMJ replacement; CCG, costochondral (rib) graft; Genio, genioplasty; LTFU, lost to follow-up; OA, occlusal appliance; Ortho, orthodontics; Tx, treatment.

At implantation, these TMJR components are adapted and fixed in a stable and close fashion to the bony surfaces of the temporal bone and mandibular ramus.[23–26]

There is always a component of counterclockwise mandibular rotation in the surgical management of ICR. Expecting an avascular autogenous rib graft or an ICR-compromised condyloid process

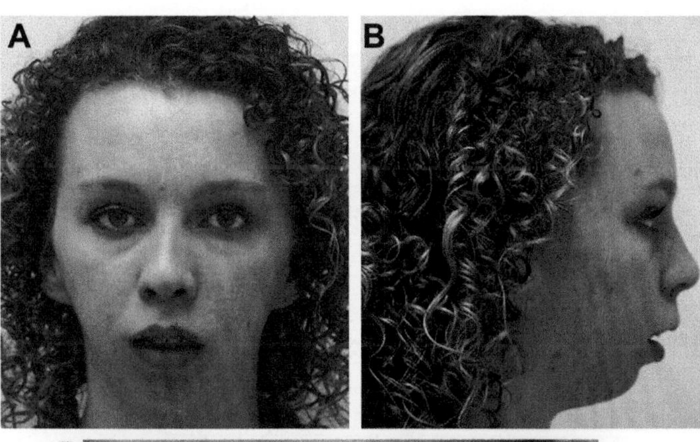

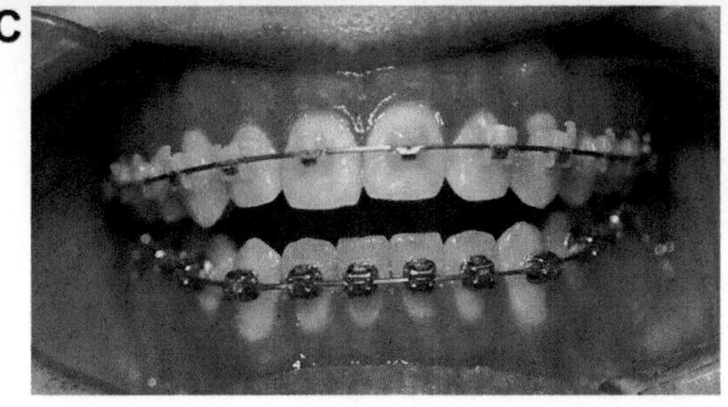

Fig. 5. This is a 15-year-old who presented from her orthodontist with a chief complaint of increasing bilateral temporomandibular joint pain and increasing anterior open bite. Her past medical history was unremarkable except for dysmenorrhea managed with birth control medication. Rheumatoid work-up was negative.

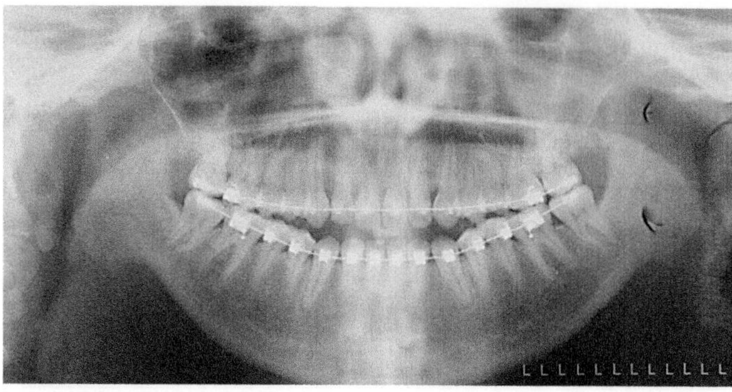

Fig. 6. Orthopantomogram demonstrated bilateral condylar resorption.

remnant after orthognathic surgery or distraction to withstand the muscle and other soft tissue forces generated by such movements under functional loading short or long term seems fraught with the potential for relapse if one considers the effects of muscle forces on bone.[27] The long-term stability using TMJR in the management of ICR cases is well documented (**Table 1**).[24,28–30]

The relative disadvantages of TMJR include (1) cost of the device; (2) material wear and failure; (3) uncertainty about long-term stability; and (4) the fact that alloplastic implants will not follow a patient's growth.[31]

Considering the demographics of ICR/PCR, longevity of any TMJR must be an important consideration. Because this is a biomechanical rather than a biological solution, future planning must be made for revision surgery to remove scar tissue from the articulating components of the implant. Eventually replacement of the implant

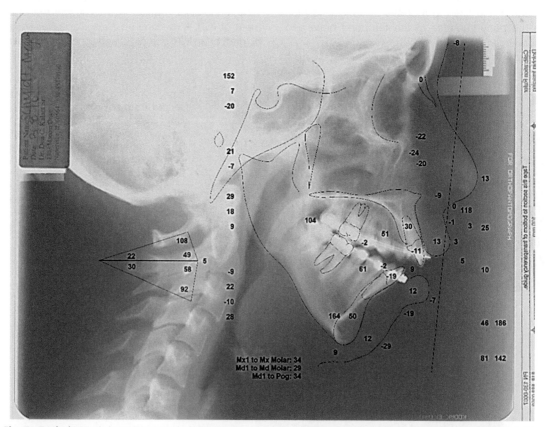

Fig. 7. Cephalometric imaging revealed steep mandibular and occlusal plane angles, anterior open bite and chin deficiency.

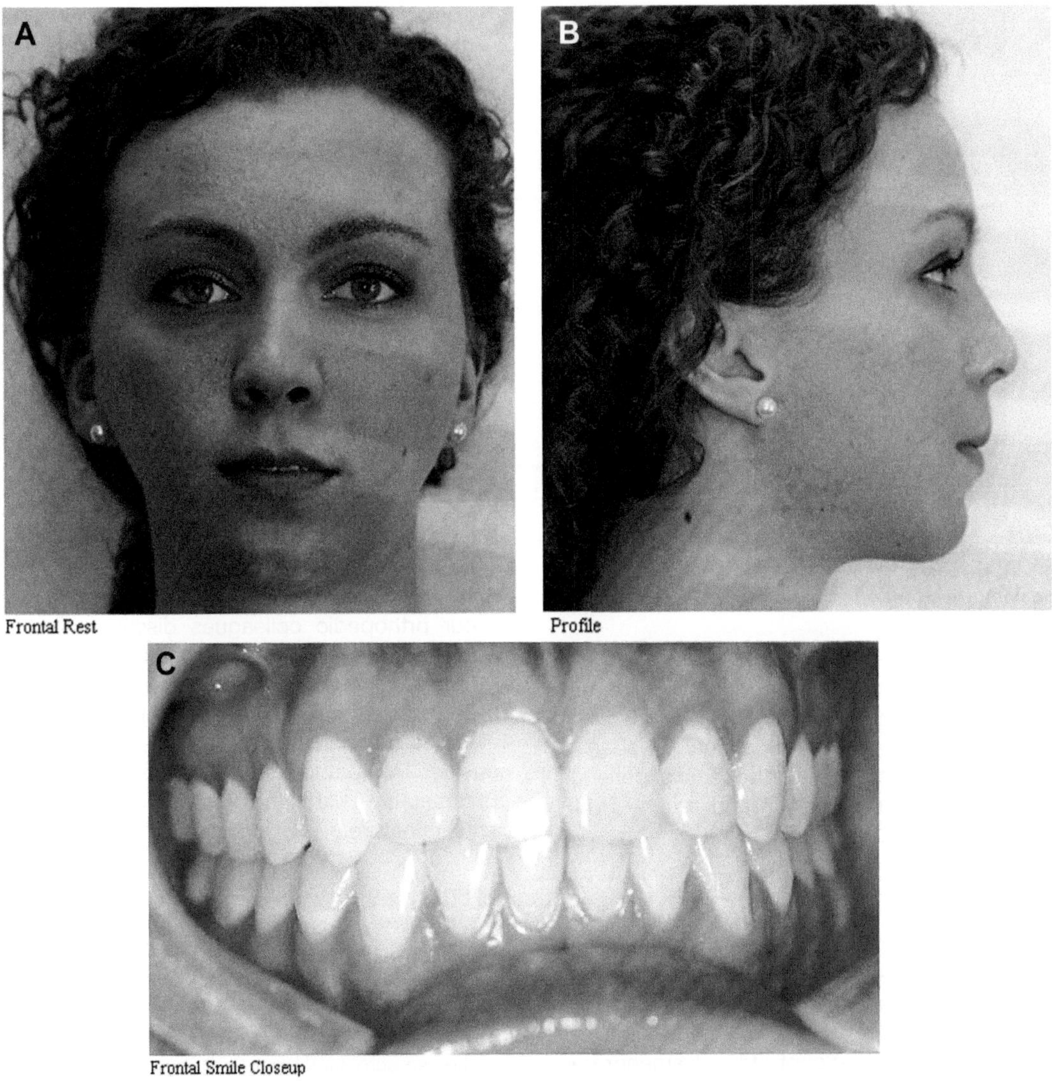

Frontal Rest

Profile

Frontal Smile Closeup

Fig. 8. A diagnosis of progressive condylar (PCR) resorption was made and a management plan was designed to include bilateral temporomandibular joint replacements with patient-fitted alloplastic prostheses (TMJ Concepts, Ventura, CA) as well as an advancement genioplasty. 6 years post-operatively, she has good mandibular function, facial form, stable and repeatable occlusion and no complaints of joint pain.

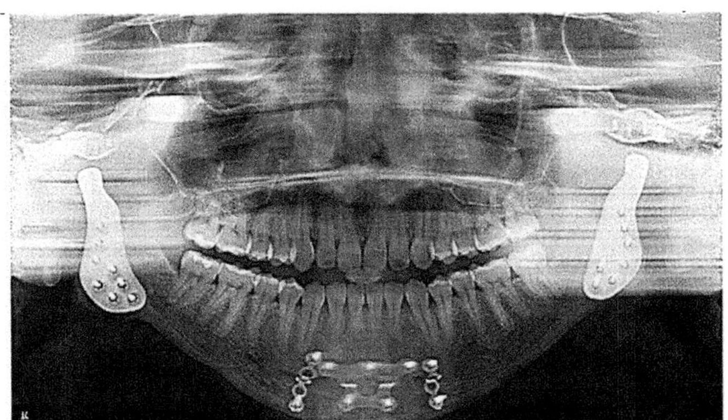

Fig. 9. 6-year post-operative orthopantomographic images.

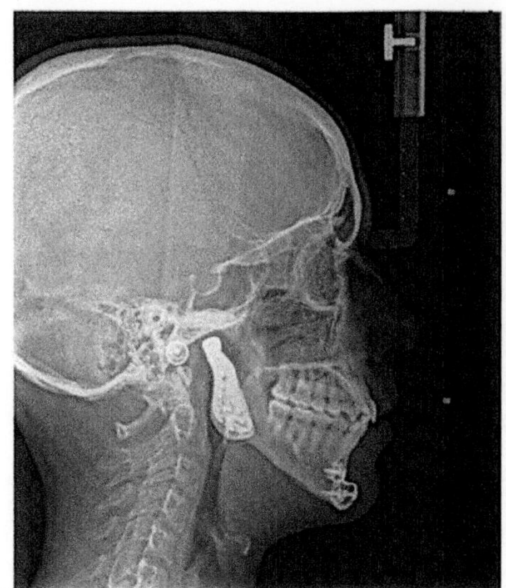

Fig. 10. 6-year post-operative cephalometric image reveal improved maxillomandibular relationships.

over time due to material wear and/or failure may be required. At present, patients are advised that these devices may have a functional life span of 10 to 15 years based on the orthopedic experience in total joint arthroplasty[32,33] and recent TMJR long-term outcomes results.[25–28,34–46]

CASE EXAMPLE

A 15-year-old girl presented from her orthodontist with a chief complaint of progressive bilateral TMJ pain and increasing anterior open bite over the past 2 years (**Fig. 5**). Her past medical history was unremarkable except for dysmenorrhea managed with β-estradiol medication. Rheumatoid workup was negative.

Physical examination revealed decreased maximal interincisal opening (MIO), mandibular retrognathia, anterior open bite, steep mandibular and occlusal planes, and bilateral TMJ and masticatory muscle pain to palpation. Orthopantomogram demonstrated loss of condylar bone stock bilaterally (**Fig. 6**). Cephalometric imaging confirmed the clinical findings (**Fig. 7**).

A diagnosis of progressive condylar resorption was made and a management plan was designed to include bilateral TMJ replacements with patient-fitted alloplastic prostheses (TMJ Concepts, Ventura, CA) as well as an advancement genioplasty.

Six years postoperatively, she has good mandibular function, facial form, stable and repeatable occlusion, and no complaints of joint pain (**Fig. 8**). Orthopantomogram (**Fig. 9**) and cephalometric imaging demonstrate good positioning of the TMJ replacement components, good facial form, as well as stable skeletal and occlusal relationships (**Fig. 10**).

SUMMARY

Long-term successful outcomes of both nonsurgical and surgical ICR management ultimately rely on the stability and strength of pathologically affected local TMJ articular and soft tissue elements.[24] However, Mehra and colleagues[29] and Alsabban and colleagues[47] recently have stated that ICR management is controversial and that there are to date no published randomized clinical trials to compare the outcomes of the various nonsurgical and surgical ICR treatment options.

Finally, it should be emphasized that TMJ intraarticular pathologic disorders, such as ICR, must be considered as pathologic entities among dentists and specialists the same way our orthopedic colleagues discuss all other joint pathologies. Failure to do this only exacerbates the problems associated with TMJ disorders in general for patients, clinicians, insurance companies, etc., because they do not consider TMJ pathology or orthopedic pathology, but rather that TMJ pathologic disorders are purely dental in nature.

REFERENCES

1. Handelman CS, Greene CS. Progressive/idiopathic condylar resorption: an orthodontic perspective. Semin Orthod 2013;19:55–70.
2. Wolford LM, Goncalves JR. Condylar resorption of the temporomandibular joint: how do we treat it? Oral Maxillofac Surg Clin North Am 2015;27:47–67.
3. Hatcher DC. Progressive condylar resorption: pathologic processes and imaging considerations. Semin Orthod 2013;19:97–105.
4. Gunson MJ, Arnett GW, Formby B, et al. Oral contraceptive pill use and abnormal menstrual cycles in women with severe condylar resorption: a case for low serum 17 beta-estradiol as a major factor in progressive condylar resorption. Am J Orthod Dentofacial Orthop 2009;136:772–9.
5. Gunson MJ, Arnett GW, Milam SB. Pathophysiology and pharmacologic control of osseous mandibular condylar resorption. J Oral Maxillofac Surg 2012;70:1918–34.
6. Arnett GW, Gunson MJ. Risk factors in the initiation of condylar resorption. Semin Orthod 2013;19:81–8.
7. Haskin CL, Milam SB, Cameron IL. Pathogeneis of degenerative joint disease in the human temperomandibular joint. Crit Rev Oral Biol Med 1995;6:248–77.

8. Link JJ, Nickerson JW. Temperomandibular joint internal deragnements in orthognathic surgery population. Int J Adult Orthodon Orthognath Surg 1992; 7:161–9.
9. Dolwick MF. Intra-articular disc displacement, Part I: its questionable role in temporomandibular joint pathology. J Oral Maxillofac Surg 1995;53:1069–72.
10. Manfredini D, Perinetti G, Guarda-Nardini L. Dental malocclusion is not related to temporomandibular joint clicking: a logistic regression analysis in a patient population. Angle Orthod 2014;84:310–5.
11. Manfredini D, Lombardo L, Siciliani G. Temporomandibular disorders and dental occlusion. A systematic review of association studies: end of an era? J Oral Rehabil 2017;44:908–23.
12. Hoppenreijs TJM, Freihofer HPM, Stoelinga PJW, et al. Condylar remodeling after LeFort I and bimaxillary osteotomies in patients with anterior open bite. A clinical and radiological study. Int J Oral Maxillofac Surg 1998;27:81–91.
13. Sarver D, Janyavula S. Condylar degeneration and diseases - local and systemic etiologies. Semin Orthod 2013;19:89–96.
14. Peacock ZS, Lee CCY, Troulis MJ, et al. Long-term stability of condylectomy and costochondral graft reconstruction for treatment of idiopathic condylar resorption. J Oral Maxillofac Surg 2019;77(4): 792–802.
15. Kerstens HC, Turnizing DB, Golding RP, et al. Condylar atrophy and osteoarthrosis after bimaxillary surgery. Oral Surg Oral Med Oral Pathol 1990; 69:274–80.
16. Moore KE, Gooris PJ, Stoelinga PJ. The contributing role of condylar resorption to skeletal relapse following mandibular advancement surgery: report of five cases. J Oral Maxillofac Surg 1991;49:448–60.
17. Bouwman JP, Kerstens HC, Tanzing DB. Condylar resorption in orthognathic surgery. The role of intermaxillary fixation. Oral Surg Oral Med Oral Pathol 1994;78:138–41.
18. Merkx MAW, Van Damme PA. Condylar resorption after orthognathic surgery. Evaluation of treatment in 8 patients. J Craniomaxillofac Surg 1994;22:53–8.
19. Ince DO, Ince A, Moore TL. Effect of methotrexate on the temporomandibular joint and facial morphology in juvenile rheumatoid arthritis patients. Am J Orthod Dentofacial Orthop 2000;118:75–83.
20. Carrasco R. Juvenile idiopathic arthritis overview and involvement of the temporomandibular joint: prevalence, systemic therapy. Oral Maxillofac Surg Clin North Am 2015;27:1–10.
21. Schendel SA, Tulashe JF, Link DW III. Idiopathic condylar resorption and micrognathia: the case for distraction osteogenesis. J Oral Maxillofac Surg 2007;65:1610–6.
22. Mercuri LG, Abramowicz S. Temporomandibular joint arthritic disease. In: Farah C, Balasubramaniam R, McCullough M, editors. Contemporary oral medicine. New York: Springer International Publishing; 2018. p. 1919–54.
23. Mercuri LG. A rationale for total alloplastic temporomandibular joint reconstruction in the management of idiopathic/progressive condylar resorption. J Oral Maxillofac Surg 2007;65:1600–9.
24. Mercuri LG. Alloplastic total joint replacement: a management option in emporomandibular joint condylar resorption. Semin Orthod 2013;19:116–26.
25. Coleta KE, Wolford LM, Gonçalves JR, et al. Maxillo-mandibular counter-clockwise rotation and mandibular advancement with TMJ Concepts total joint prostheses: part II–airway changes and stability. Int J Oral Maxillofac Surg 2009;38:228–35.
26. Coleta KE, Wolford LM, Gonçalves JR, et al. Maxillo-mandibular counter-clockwise rotation and mandibular advancement with TMJ Concepts total joint prostheses: part IV–soft tissue response. Int J Oral Maxillofac Surg 2009;38:637–46.
27. Burr DB. Muscle strength, bone mass, and age related bone loss. J Bone Miner Res 1997;12: 1547–51.
28. Pinto LP, Wolford LM, Buschang PH, et al. Maxillo-mandibular counter-clockwise rotation and mandibular advancement with TMJ Concepts total joint prostheses: part III–pain and dysfunction outcomes. Int J Oral Maxillofac Surg 2009;38:326–31.
29. Mehra P, Nadershah M, Chigurupati R. Is alloplastic temporomandibular joint reconstruction a viable option in the surgical management of adult patients with idiopathic condylar resorption? J Oral Maxillofac Surg 2016;74:2044–54.
30. Chigurupati R, Mehra P. Surgical management of idiopathic condylar resorption: orthognathic surgery versus temporomandibular total joint replacement. Oral Maxillofac Surg Clin North Am 2018;30: 355–67.
31. Mercuri LG, Swift JQ. Considerations for the use of alloplastic temporomandibular joint replacement in the growing patient. J Oral Maxillofac Surg 2009; 67:1979–90.
32. Salvati E, Wilson P, Jolley MA. A ten-year follow-up study of our first one hundred consecutive Charnley total hip replacements. J Bone Joint Surg Am 1981; 63A:753–76.
33. Schulte KR, Callaghan JJ, Kelley SS, et al. The outcome of Charnley total hip arthroplasty with cement after a minimum of twenty-year follow-up. The results of one surgeon. J Bone Joint Surg Am 1993;75A:961–75.
34. Mercuri LG. The use of alloplastic prostheses for temporomandibular joint reconstruction. J Oral Maxillofac Surg 2000;58:70–5.
35. Mercuri LG. End-stage TMD and TMJ reconstruction [Chapter: 52]. In: Miloro M, Ghali G, Larsen P, et al, editors. Peterson's principles of oral & maxillofacial

surgery. 3rd edition. Shelton, (CT): PMPH, USA Ltd; 2012. p. 1173–86.

36. Mercuri LG. Alloplastic TMJ replacement. Rationale for custom devices. Int J Oral Maxillofac Surg 2012;41:1033–40.
37. Mercuri LG. The role of patient-fitted devices in total temporomandibular joint replacement. Revista Española de Cirugía Oral y Maxilofacial 2013;35:1–10.
38. Wolford LM, Cottrell DA, Henry CH. Temporomandibular joint reconstruction of the complex patient with the Techmedica custom-made total joint prosthesis. J Oral Maxillofac Surg 1994;52:2–10.
39. Mercuri LG, Wolford LM, Sanders B, et al. Custom CAD/CAM total temporomandibular joint reconstruction system: preliminary multicenter report. J Oral Maxillofac Surg 1995;53:106–15.
40. Mercuri LG. Considering total alloplastic temporomandibular joint replacement. Cranio 1999;17:44–8.
41. Mercuri LG. Subjective and objective outcomes in patients reconstructed with a custom-fitted alloplastic temporomandibular joint prosthesis. J Oral Maxillofac Surg 1999;57:1427–30.
42. Oral Maxillofac Surg Clin N Amer. In: Donlon WC, editor. Total temporomandibular joint reconstruction, vol. 12. Philadelphia: Saunders; 2000.
43. Mercuri LG, Wolford LM, Sanders B, et al. Long-term follow-up of the CAD/CAM patient fitted alloplastic total temporomandibular joint reconstruction prosthesis. J Oral Maxillofac Surg 2002;60:1440–8.
44. Wolford LM, Dingworth DJ, Talwar RM, et al. Comparison of 2 temporomandibular joint prosthesis systems. J Oral Maxillofac Surg 2003;61:685–90.
45. Mercuri LG, Giobbe-Hurder A. Long-term outcomes after total alloplastic temporomandibular joint reconstruction following exposure to failed materials. J Oral Maxillofac Surg 2004;62:1088–96.
46. Wolford LM, Mercuri LG, Schneiderman ED, et al. Twenty-year follow-up study on a patient-fitted temporomandibular joint prosthesis: the techmedica/TMJ concepts device. J Oral Maxillofac Surg 2015;73:952–60.
47. Alsabban L, Amarista FJ, Mercuri LG, et al. Idiopathic condylar resorption: a survey and review of the literature. J Oral Maxillofac Surg 2018;76(11): 2316.e1–13.

Interdisciplinary Management of Dentofacial Deformity in Juvenile Idiopathic Arthritis

Peter Stoustrup, DDS, PhD[a], Thomas Klit Pedersen, DDS, PhD[a,b], Sven Erik Nørholt, DDS, PhD[b,c], Cory M. Resnick, DMD, MD[d,e], Shelly Abramowicz, DMD, MPH[f,*]

KEYWORDS

- Juvenile idiopathic arthritis • Temporomandibular joint • Dentofacial deformity

KEY POINTS

- Temporomandibular joint (TMJ) arthritis impacts mandibular growth and development.
- This can result in skeletal deformity, such as facial asymmetry and malocclusion asymmetry.
- This article reviews the unique properties of TMJ and dentofacial growth and development in the setting of juvenile idiopathic arthritis.
- Specific orthopedic/orthodontic and surgical management of children with TMJ arthritis is discussed.
- The importance of interdisciplinary collaboration is highlighted.

Juvenile idiopathic arthritis (JIA) was previously known as juvenile chronic arthritis in Europe and as juvenile rheumatoid arthritis in North America. The International League of Associations for rheumatology unified the terminology in 1995 with a revision in 2004.[1,2] Today, JIA is categorized into 7 subtypes (systemic arthritis, oligoarthritis, rheuma-factor positive polyarthritis, rheuma-factor negative polyarthritis, psoriatic arthritis, enthesitis-related arthritis, undifferentiated arthritis). JIA is a diagnosis of exclusion in children 16 years or younger who have a history of joint pain, swelling, limited range of motion, and calor (heat) for at least 6 weeks.[1,2]

JIA can affect any joint; the temporomandibular joint (TMJ) is one of the joints most frequently involved[3–6] and can be the only joint involved.[7] The orofacial consequences of TMJ arthritis range from a mild asymptomatic presentation only visible on MRI to orofacial pain, dysfunction, and/or dentofacial deformity, with an impact on quality of life.[3,4,8–13] Orofacial manifestations of TMJ arthritis can appear early in the disease course and may persist into adulthood.[14,15]

All authors contributed equally to the content of the article.
Disclosure Information: The authors have nothing to disclose.

[a] Section of Orthodontics, Aarhus University, Vennelyst Boulevard 9-11, 8000 Aarhus C, Denmark; [b] Department of Oral and Maxillofacial Surgery, Aarhus University Hospital, Aarhus, Palle Juul-Jensens Boulevard 165, 8200 Aarhus N, Denmark; [c] Section of Oral Maxillofacial Surgery, Aarhus University, Vennelyst Boulevard 9-11, 8000 Aarhus, Denmark; [d] Department of Plastic and Oral Surgery, Boston Children's Hospital, 300 longwood Avenue, Boston, MA 02115, USA; [e] Oral and Maxillofacial Surgery, Harvard School of Dental Medicine, Harvard Medical School, Boston, MA, USA; [f] Department of Surgery, Division of Oral and Maxillofacial Surgery, Emory University School of Medicine, Children's Healthcare of Atlanta, Emory University, 1365 Clifton Road, Building B, Suite 2300, Atlanta, GA 30322, USA
* Corresponding author.
E-mail address: sabram5@emory.edu

Oral Maxillofacial Surg Clin N Am 32 (2020) 117–134
https://doi.org/10.1016/j.coms.2019.09.002

An algorithm for management of the dentofacial deformity from JIA has recently been published.[16] This algorithm presents a combination of surgical and nonsurgical orthodontic strategies (eg, orthopedic appliance) that emphasizes the importance of interdisciplinary collaborative efforts. The aim of the present article is to review orthodontic and surgical management of patients with TMJ arthritis and resulting dentofacial deformity. The article reviews the unique properties of the TMJ and dentofacial growth and development while focusing on TMJ involvement from JIA.

TERMINOLOGY

The present article adheres to TMJaw consensus-based standardized terminology[17] (**Table 1**). "TMJ arthritis" indicates the presence of active TMJ inflammation. In contrast, "TMJ involvement" is a less restrictive term embracing all abnormalities presumed to be a consequence of TMJ arthritis. The presence of active inflammation ("TMJ arthritis") is not a prerequisite for the use of the term "TMJ involvement." However, "TMJ arthritis" assumes "TMJ involvement." The terms "TMJ deformity" and "dentofacial deformity" refer to arthritis-induced osseous changes.[17]

Table 1
Consensus-based, interdisciplinary, standardized operational terminology

Term	Definition
TMJ arthritis	Active inflammation in the TMJ
TMJ involvement	Abnormalities presumed to be the result of TMJ arthritis
TMJ arthritis management	Diagnosis, treatment, and monitoring of TMJ arthritis and involvement
Dentofacial deformity	Abnormality in growth, development, structure, and/or alignment of the facial bones and dentition
TMJ deformity	Abnormality in growth, development, or structure of the osseous and/or soft tissue components of the TMJ
TMJ symptoms	Patient or parent-reported conditions related to TMJ arthritis or involvement
TMJ dysfunction	Physician-reported functional examination abnormalities related to TMJ arthritis or involvement

Abbreviation: TMJ, temporomandibular joint.

Data from Stoustrup P, Resnick CM, Pedersen TK, et al. Standardizing terminology and assessment for orofacial conditions in juvenile idiopathic arthritis: international, multidisciplinary consensus-based recommendations. J Rheumatol. 2019;46(5):518-22.

TEMPOROMANDIBULAR JOINT: A UNIQUE JOINT

The TMJ is a complex joint composed of the condylar head and the temporal bone with an interposed disc. Condylar cartilage on the mandibular condyle is an important intra-articular mandibular growth site, and is considered a secondary cartilage due to its embryonic origin.[18–20] Condylar cartilage serves as functional cartilage and as a site of bone formation where environmental and genetic factors contribute to mandibular growth and development.[20,21] Unique structural features make the TMJ and growing mandible particularly vulnerable to TMJ inflammation and mechanical loading. This vulnerability originates from the unique developmental, anatomic, and histologic properties of the TMJ compared with other synovial joints: the intra-articular location of the condylar growth site, the condylar cartilage type (fibrocartilage), the ossification process (endochondral), the cellular organization of the condylar cartilage, the matrix composition, the multidirectional condylar growth capacity, the unique cartilage response to altered TMJ function, and the late cartilage maturation.[18–21]

TEMPOROMANDIBULAR JOINT ARTHRITIS

The pathologic mechanism of arthritis-induced dentofacial deformity is still not fully understood. However, during the past decade, there has been a fundamental shift in the conceptual framework of the relationship between TMJ arthritis and dentofacial deformity. The traditional view has been challenged; dentofacial deformity is no longer considered the outcome of a degenerative process alone.[22] Development of arthritis-induced dentofacial deformity is now understood to be a complex, multifactorial condition mediated by growth retardation, degeneration, deformity, mechanical overloading, dysfunction, and dentofacial compensation.[23]

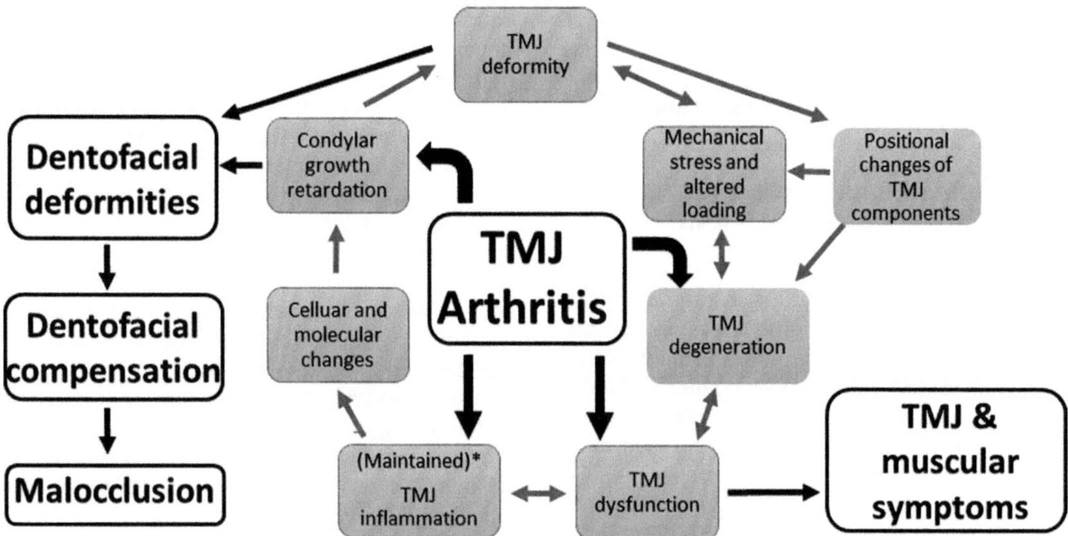

Fig. 1. From TMJ arthritis to malocclusion. Model for arthritis-initiated processes causing malocclusion and orofacial symptoms in skeletally immature subjects. TMJ arthritis can directly impact condylar cartilage homeostasis causing mandibular growth retardation/TMJ degeneration and TMJ dysfunction (*thick black arrows*). In turn, this may alter TMJ function (mechanical stress and loading) initiating a progressive inflammatory cycle promoting further mandibular growth retardation and degeneration (*blue boxes*). The net result is dentofacial deformity followed by dentofacial compensation and malocclusion (*thin black arrows*). TMJ dysfunction also may initiate TMJ and orofacial muscular symptoms. [a] Suboptimal joint function may induce continuous progression of dentofacial deformity through the low-grade inflammatory cycle (*blue boxes*) despite successful anti-inflammatory treatment.

Fig. 1 shows a model explaining arthritis-initiated processes causing malocclusion, dentofacial deformity, and orofacial symptoms. TMJ arthritis can have a direct impact on condylar cartilage causing mandibular growth retardation and degeneration. These changes induce TMJ deformity and dysfunction and may lead to increased joint friction, mechanical stress, and excessive joint loading. These pathologic mechanisms exceed the adaptive capacity of the articular structures and perpetuate the cycle of deformity and dysfunction.[24] Metabolic changes in the articular structures and underlying bone then impair condylar growth and alter dentofacial development, and maintain low-grade inflammation that further perpetuates mandibular growth retardation and breakdown (see **Fig. 1**). Suboptimal joint function may induce continuous progression of dentofacial deformity. The chronic low-grade inflammation induced by TMJ dysfunction may continue to exacerbate the TMJ destruction even after the arthritis-induced inflammation has resolved or been medically controlled (see **Fig. 1**). This emphasizes the importance of optimal TMJ function: dynamic mechanical loading is an important stimulus for condylar growth and development and for TMJ cartilage homeostasis.[25] Importantly, TMJ involvement does not arrest condylar growth; mandibular growth and development is still seen in skeletally immature patients with TMJ arthritis. However, TMJ arthritis retards and alters the condylar growth potential with impact on the general mandibular growth and development.[26,27]

In vitro studies have found evidence that functional cyclic tensile strain is protective of inflammation by reducing the catabolic effects of tumor necrosis factor (TNF)-α on chondrocytes.[25,28,29] Tabeian and colleagues[29] suggest that functional loading with oral physiotherapy or orthodontic splints may reduce the catabolic effect of TNF-α in the TMJ. The beneficial effects of functional joint loading on inflammation and condylar growth at a histologic level has previously been demonstrated in an experimental model by von Bremen and colleagues,[30] who showed that TMJ loading with mandibular advancement splints had beneficial histologic effects on inflammation and condylar growth.

In growing patients, the intra-articular location of mandibular growth cartilage make the joint specifically vulnerable to inflammation, degeneration, and functional overloading. In contrast, the intra-articular cartilage location is also believed to play a crucial role in the regenerative capacity of the mandibular condyle in subjects with low disease activity.[31,32]

TEMPOROMANDIBULAR JOINT ARTHRITIS AND DENTOFACIAL GROWTH AND DEVELOPMENT

In healthy, skeletally immature children, condylar vertical growth and development is a key component for normal mandibular morphologic development. The normal mandible elongates vertically; simultaneously, bone apposition at the posterior border of the ramus and compensatory resorption at the anterior ramus occur. Posterior vertical growth causes the mandible to rotate in an anterior direction, leading to elongation. The space created between the maxilla and the mandible provides space for tooth eruption and dentoalveolar vertical development.[18,19,21,25]

TEMPOROMANDIBULAR JOINT INVOLVEMENT IN GROWING PATIENTS

In JIA, TMJ involvement can disturb mandibular growth and development (**Fig. 2**). The timing of TMJ arthritis onset and growth disruption influences the subsequent consequence on dentofacial growth and development (**Fig. 3**), and, as such, is important with respect to the choice of management.

In skeletally immature patients, TMJ arthritis impairs condylar growth, thereby decreasing mandibular *posterior* vertical development and secondarily reducing *posterior* vertical maxillary development.[26] Reduced posterior height inhibits normal mandibular anterior rotation. When both joints are involved, this creates mandibular retrognathism (see **Fig. 2**). Decreased posterior vertical mandibular development leads to compensatory growth and development of the mandibular body and dentoalveolar structures, decreasing vertical space for dental eruption posteriorly. As a result, the occlusal plane becomes steep. Reduced vertical mandibular posterior height facilitates only limited mandibular anterior rotation, and the mandible becomes retrognathic.

Long-term bilateral TMJ involvement can lead to dentofacial deformity as depicted in **Fig. 3**A: reduced vertical posterior ramus height, and a retrognathic, posteriorly rotated, mandible with significant dentoalveolar compensations. A longitudinal cephalometric study has shown that this characteristic abnormal morphology is mostly established between the ages of 9 and 12 years, coinciding with the mandibular growth spurt.[26]

Unilateral TMJ involvement creates mandibular asymmetry with asymmetric condyle-ramus unit and a cant of the mandibular occlusal plane. The severity of both types of deformities depends on the time of JIA onset and the degree of growth retardation and TMJ degeneration. The growing maxilla adapts to the asymmetric mandible, resulting in a maxillary occlusal cant and yaw/roll deformity. TMJ arthritis may start on one side and later

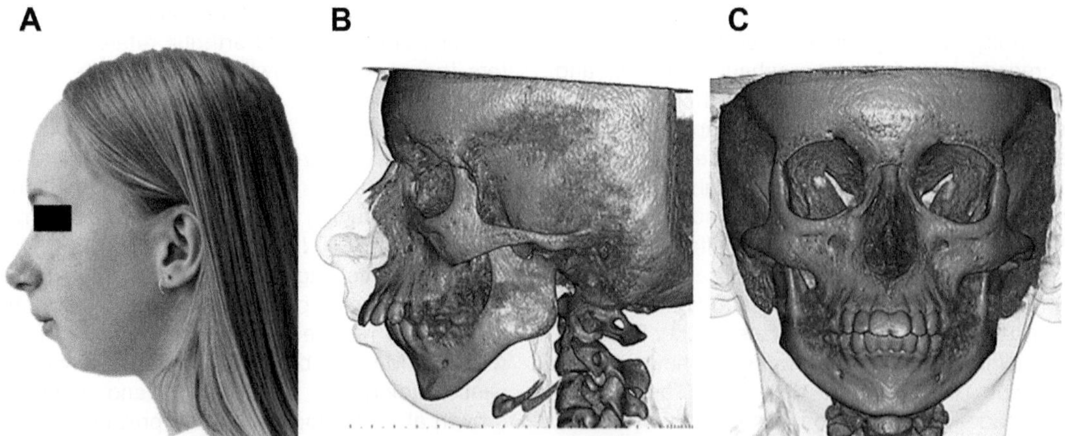

Fig. 2. Long-term bilateral TMJ arthritis. Thirteen-year-old girl with JIA (extended oligoarticular subtype) and long-term bilateral TMJ involvement. (*A*) Profile photo: Moderate facial convexity due to mandibular retrusion. (*B*) CBCT shows reduced vertical ramus height has led to a posterior mandibular rotation and a retrognathic mandible with significant mandibular dentoalveolar compensations. (*C*) CBCT shows mostly symmetric mandible despite of bilateral TMJ involvement.

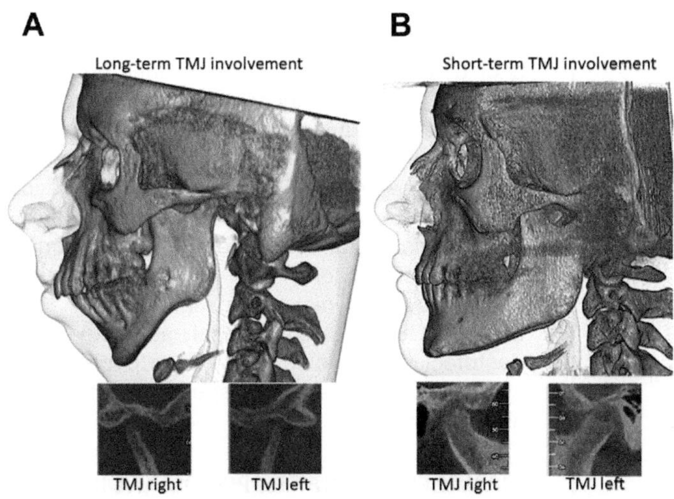

Fig. 3. Early versus late onset of TMJ arthritis. (*A*) Early onset of TMJ arthritis in skeletally immature patient: 17-year-old boy with JIA (oligoarticular subtype) and long-term bilateral TMJ involvement (>7 years) with onset before the dentofacial growth spurt. CBCT shows significant degree of dentofacial deformity: reduced mandibular height, mandibular posterior rotation. The dentofacial deformity has led to significant abnormal mandibular dentoalveolar compensation (increased mandibular dentoalveolar height and proclined lower incisors). Cross-sectional cuts show abnormal condylar morphology. (*B*) Late onset of TMJ arthritis in skeletally mature patient: 16-year-old boy with JIA (oligoarticular extended subtype) and onset of bilateral TMJ arthritis after the dentofacial growth spurt. CBCT shows normal dentofacial development and no significant dentoalveolar compensations. Cross-sectional cuts show significant degree of bilateral condylar deformity. Also notice difference in airway volume.

progress to the contralateral side; the degree of asymmetry and retrognathism depends on the timing of involvement with relation to growth trajectory.

Prediction of the dentofacial deformity resulting from TMJ arthritis is complicated by a nonlinear association between the severity of TMJ deformity (condylar flattening or erosion) and the degree of dentofacial deformity.[22] This complicates clinical decision making as, for example, imaging may find only a minor TMJ deformity in a patient with severe dentofacial deformity and, conversely, advanced TMJ deformity does not always denote a significant facial abnormality (see **Fig. 3**). It is important to notice additional effect from the underlying genetic influence of dentofacial development; patients with JIA with a genetically determined retrognathism and mandibular posterior growth pattern might have a worse deformity.

TEMPOROMANDIBULAR JOINT INVOLVEMENT IN NONGROWING PATIENTS

TMJ arthritis in skeletally mature individuals leads to a different dentofacial deformity. TMJ arthritis may promote degeneration and deformity of the TMJ components (eg, condyle, fossa, and disc) leading to loss of condylar height and an unstable occlusion. In turn, the mandibular condyle shifts to a more anterior position in the glenoid fossa, causing the mandible to rotate in a posterior direction. Together with the loss of condylar height, this manifests as an open bite and enlarged overjet due to mandibular posterior rotation.[23] In contrast to the skeletally immature patient, TMJ arthritis after skeletal maturation affects only condylar/ramus height, mandibular position, occlusion, and TMJ function, but does not induce the extensive morphologic abnormalities seen in growing patients (see **Fig. 3**B).

TEMPOROMANDIBULAR JOINT SYMPTOMS AND DYSFUNCTION

Orofacial signs and symptoms are common in patients with TMJ involvement from JIA, but children may be asymptomatic in early stages of the disease.[13–15] In contrast, signs and symptoms can also occur relatively early in the disease course and persist into adulthood.[14,15] TMJ symptoms and dysfunction may be present without the presence of TMJ inflammation.[10,13] The most common findings are presented in **Box 1**. Constant orofacial symptoms are rare; most patients report moderate, transient pain during function.[11,12] Symptoms may be directly attributed to TMJ arthritis and/or may be due to the TMJ dysfunction that results from TMJ deformation and chronic low-grade inflammation **Fig. 1**.

Internal joint derangement and crepitation may develop during the teenage years in patients with long-term TMJ involvement. This, in turn, leads to additional loading of the TMJ and associated structures causing muscle hyperactivity and further dysfunction and symptoms.

Box 1
Most common orofacial symptoms and dysfunctions associated with JIA

Symptoms

Fluctuating symptoms mainly from the TMJ and the masseter muscle regions

Orofacial symptoms during mandibular function

TMJ symptoms during mastication (eg, fatigue)

Complaints of reduced mouth opening capacity

TMJ morning stiffness

Impact of orofacial symptoms on general quality of life

Dysfunctions

Reduced mouth opening capacity

Mandibular deviation at maximal mouth opening position

TMJ pain on palpation

Masticatory muscle pain on palpation

Abbreviations: JIA, juvenile idiopathic arthritis; TMJ, temporomandibular joint.

Symptoms are a poor predictor of TMJ arthritis[33,34]; orofacial symptoms and dysfunction are common in patients without JIA and, even when present in a patient with JIA, may not be directly caused by autoimmune-induced inflammation.

DIFFERENTIAL DIAGNOSIS

TMJ arthritis is a condition meeting the diagnostic criteria of temporomandibular disorders (TMDs): the orofacial dysfunction and symptoms caused by TMJ arthritis/involvement are comparable to those encountered in other TMD subsets.[35,36] Differential TMD diagnoses are important clinical considerations in patients with JIA who present orofacial signs and symptoms. Conditions like idiopathic condylar resorption and symptomatic disc displacement without reduction may present orofacial signs and symptoms comparable to JIA-associated orofacial conditions.[37,38]

DIAGNOSIS OF TEMPOROMANDIBULAR JOINT ARTHRITIS

Although clinical examination has been shown to be a poor predictor of TMJ arthritis,[9,10,33,34,39] when conducted in a standardized fashion, it provides important information regarding the orofacial health of subjects with JIA. Detection of TMJ dysfunction and/or dentofacial deformity should prompt referral for further examinations.[40,41] Contrast-enhanced MRI of the TMJs is the gold standard for diagnosis of TMJ arthritis.[33,34] Computerized tomography (CT) and cone-beam CT (CBCT) provide information regarding morphology of the TMJ and the dentofacial deformity, and are helpful in planning operative correction.[16,17] Consensus-based standards for clinical examination, TMJ MRI, and CT/CBCT 3-dimensional assessment of dentofacial morphology have been published to standardize these aspects of JIA assessment.[41–43]

MANAGEMENT OF TEMPOROMANDIBULAR JOINT INVOLVEMENT IN JUVENILE IDIOPATHIC ARTHRITIS

The objectives of TMJ arthritis management are to provide timely diagnosis, reduce TMJ inflammation, alleviate orofacial symptoms, optimize orofacial function, normalize dentofacial growth, and correct dentofacial deformity. Diverse manifestations of TMJ arthritis highlight the importance of a collaborative, interdisciplinary management approach involving pediatric rheumatologists, radiologists, oral and maxillofacial surgeons, and orthodontists.

Management of Temporomandibular Joint Arthritis (Inflammation)

Control of systemic arthritis is paramount to optimal TMJ management. Although limited evidence exists of the effect of systemic anti-inflammatory treatment on TMJ arthritis in JIA, aggressive systemic medication is considered an important aspect of management.[32,44] Traditionally, intra-articular TMJ corticosteroid injections (IACIs) were used to decrease inflammation.[45,46] However, emerging evidence from animal and human studies has shown only transient effects outweighed by risk of mandibular growth retardation and intra-articular calcifications in growing patients following IACI.[46–48] Routine and repetitive use of TMJ IACIs in growing subjects is no longer encouraged,[49] although limited application can be indicated in case of sustained pain and/or limited function caused by refractory inflammation.

Management of Orofacial Symptoms and Dysfunction

Several modalities can be applied for the management of orofacial symptoms and dysfunction. It is beyond the scope of this article to review these modalities, but they are listed in **Box 2**. In general, their use is based mainly on evidence derived from other TMD conditions.

Management of Dentofacial Deformity

Management of a complicated dentofacial growth abnormality and associated malocclusion demands comprehensive understanding of etiologic processes related to arthritis-induced dentofacial deformity. Before choice of management, the following issues must be addressed: (1) general disease activity, (2) inflammatory status and stability of the TMJs, (3) progression of dentofacial deformity during the past 12 months, (4) level of skeletal maturity and continued mandibular growth potential, and (5) severity of the dentofacial deformity.[16]

Management of dentofacial deformities involves options: (1) Interceptive, growth-adaptive initiatives in skeletally immature subjects with a dentofacial deformity (ie, nonsurgical orthopedic appliance treatment). A combination of orthopedic appliance and distraction osteogenesis (DO) can be considered in severe cases. (2) Corrective surgical interventions for an existing advanced dentofacial deformity in skeletally mature patients or TMJ replacement. Early application of interceptive, growth-adaptive initiatives does not preclude future corrective surgical management. The combination of these 2 modalities has been recommended in the recent management algorithm of dentofacial deformity in JIA.[16]

Box 2
Management of orofacial symptoms and dysfunction associated with JIA

Management strategies

Patient information

Pain-coping strategies (avoidance of pain triggers)

Change/adjustment to general medication

Oral splint (stabilization splint)

Orofacial physiotherapy and home exercises

Intra-articular TMJ steroid injection[a]

Intra-articular lavage/arthrocentesis

[a] Intra-articular steroid injections may be used cautiously in patients with refractory TMJ arthritis and orofacial symptoms. However, intra-articular steroid is not recommended in routine treatment of TMJ arthritis due to unwanted side effects (ie, growth retardation and intra-articular calcification).

REMOVABLE ORTHOPEDIC APPLIANCE TREATMENT IN SKELETALLY IMMATURE PATIENTS

The purpose of an orthopedic appliance is to improve or normalize mandibular growth and development: posterior vertical mandibular dimension, mandibular length, and mandibular symmetry. Observational studies have described the effects of orthopedic appliance treatment in JIA.[27,50–54] Orthopedic treatment will avoid the need for later surgical treatment in some patients.[16] Barriers to routine use include full-time use, the year-long use of the splint from early signs of dentofacial deformity to end of growth, need for substantial patient compliance, need for orthodontic visits every 6 to 8 weeks, lack of reimbursement in the North American insurance system, need for a knowledgeable practitioner, and the risk of caries and/or periodontal disease adjacent to the splint. Despite these challenges, orthopedic appliance treatment is used by several European centers and is part of the contemporary treatment algorithm for minor to moderate dentofacial deformities.

Initiation of orthopedic treatment early in the development of the dentofacial deformity is crucial to a successful outcome with this management modality. Correction of minor to moderate dentofacial asymmetry can be achieved with orthopedic appliances.[27,53] Just like with non-JIA patients treated with orthopedic appliances, "good" and "poor" responders are found within the JIA group.[55] In case progression of the dentofacial deformity occurs despite orthopedic treatment, distraction osteogenesis can be considered. Two types of removable orthopedic appliances have been proposed for management of deformities in skeletally immature patients with JIA: the activator and the distraction splint (**Fig. 4**).

THE DISTRACTION SPLINT

In 1995, Pedersen and colleagues[56] proposed the use of the distraction splint for management of JIA-induced dentofacial deformities (see **Fig. 4**C, D). This is an acrylic splint covering the occlusal surfaces of the mandibular canines, premolars, and molars. The splint is periodically adjusted so that it gradually "unloads" the TMJs and positions the mandible in the midline. The splint (1) allows for mandibular vertical

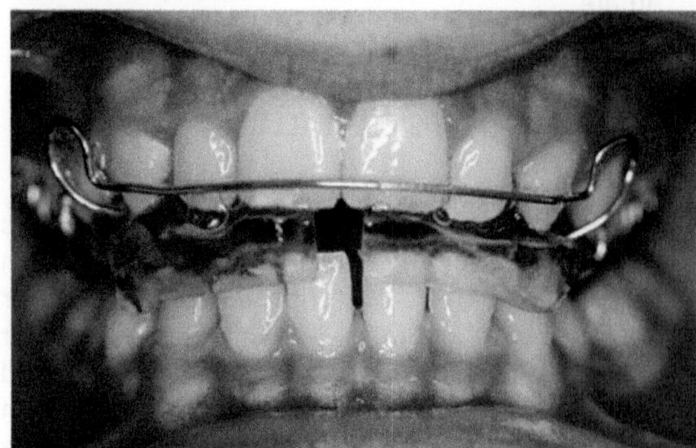

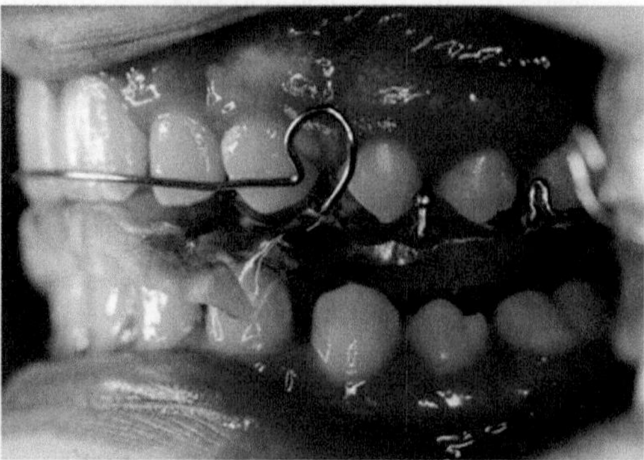

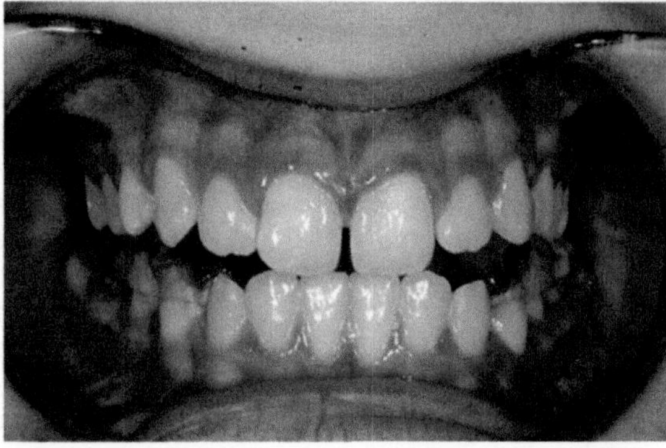

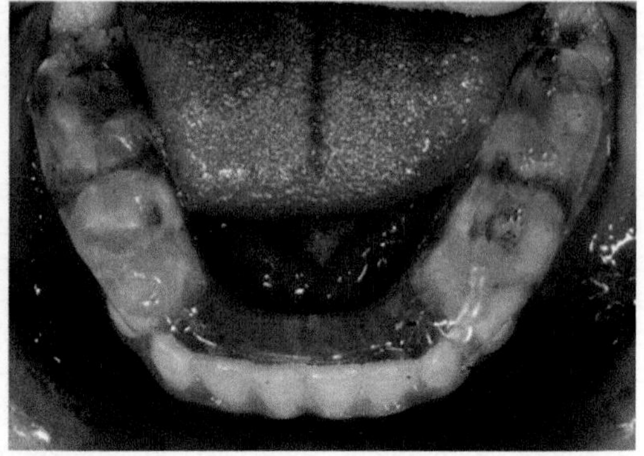

Fig. 4. Orthopedic appliances. Two types of removable orthopedic appliances for management of dentofacial deformities in growing subjects with JIA and TMJ involvement. (*A*) *The activator* is an acrylic monoblock that promotes mandibular advancement. The activator is worn almost full-time for 6 to 12 months during the dentofacial growth spurt. (*B*) The posterior extension of the activator. Selective grinding of the posterior acrylic cover allows for control of tooth eruption useful for management of occlusal canting. (*C*) *The distraction splint* is an acrylic splint covering the posterior mandibular dentition. (*D*) The posterior extension of the distraction splint.

growth and development, (2) guides the mandible to a symmetric position, (3) promotes anterior mandibular advancement, (4) enables control of tooth eruption and relative intrusion of teeth in specific regions, and (5) limits unbeneficial dentoalveolar compensation.[56] **Fig. 5** demonstrates the principles of the distraction splint. The appliance is worn full-time, including during eating, from diagnosis of the dentofacial deformity until limited mandibular growth exists (see **Fig. 4**). "Distraction" is achieved by gradual increase in the height of the splint on the side(s) of TMJ involvement: approximately 0.25 to 0.5 mm of acrylic is added to the splint every eighth week.[56] In subjects with unilateral TMJ involvement, the splint is adjusted mainly on the affected side to allow for mandibular repositioning as illustrated in **Fig. 6**. Lack of occlusal incisal coverage allows for normalized dentoalveolar development in the incisal region. The distraction splint is adjusted to prevent overeruption of the first and second mandibular molars (**Fig. 7**). In patients with bilateral TMJ involvement, the bilateral posterior open bite allows for anterior mandibular rotation, which corrects intermaxillary sagittal discrepancy and decreases anterior facial height. The posterior open bite may be corrected by selective grinding of the distraction splint (see **Fig. 7**) or by transition to an activator appliance that may produce further mandibular advancement.[55]

In patients with unilateral TMJ involvement, the full-time wear of the splint will create a large posterior open bite in the affected side and a minor open bite in the nonaffected side (**Figs. 8** and **9**). The posterior open bite allows for correction of occlusal canting. Use of the distraction splint leads to comparable vertical growth between the affected and unaffected sides in patients with unilateral TMJ involvement[27,53] (see **Figs. 8** and **9**).

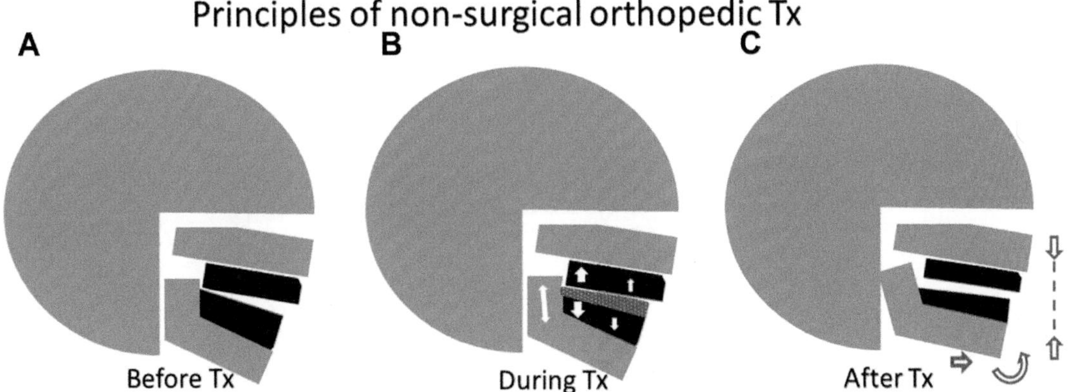

Fig. 5. Orthopedic treatment of bilateral TMJ involvement in skeletally immature subjects. (*A*) Before treatment: Mandibular deformity caused by long-term TMJ involvement consists of retrognathic, posteriorly rotated mandible and intermaxillary sagittal discrepancy. (*B*) During distraction splint treatment, the splint is worn full-time. The splint height is gradually increased every sixth to eighth week, which promotes increased mandibular vertical growth and encourages dentoalveolar development by relative intrusion of the posterior teeth. Long-term splint use creates a posterior open bite allowing for mandibular anterior rotation when the splint is no longer used. (*C*) After treatment: Normalized skeletal and dentoalveolar development allows for mandibular anterior rotation with correction of the intermaxillary sagittal discrepancy and a reduced anterior facial height. Vertical dentoalveolar development (eruption of teeth from the posterior maxilla) can be initiated. Tx, treatment.

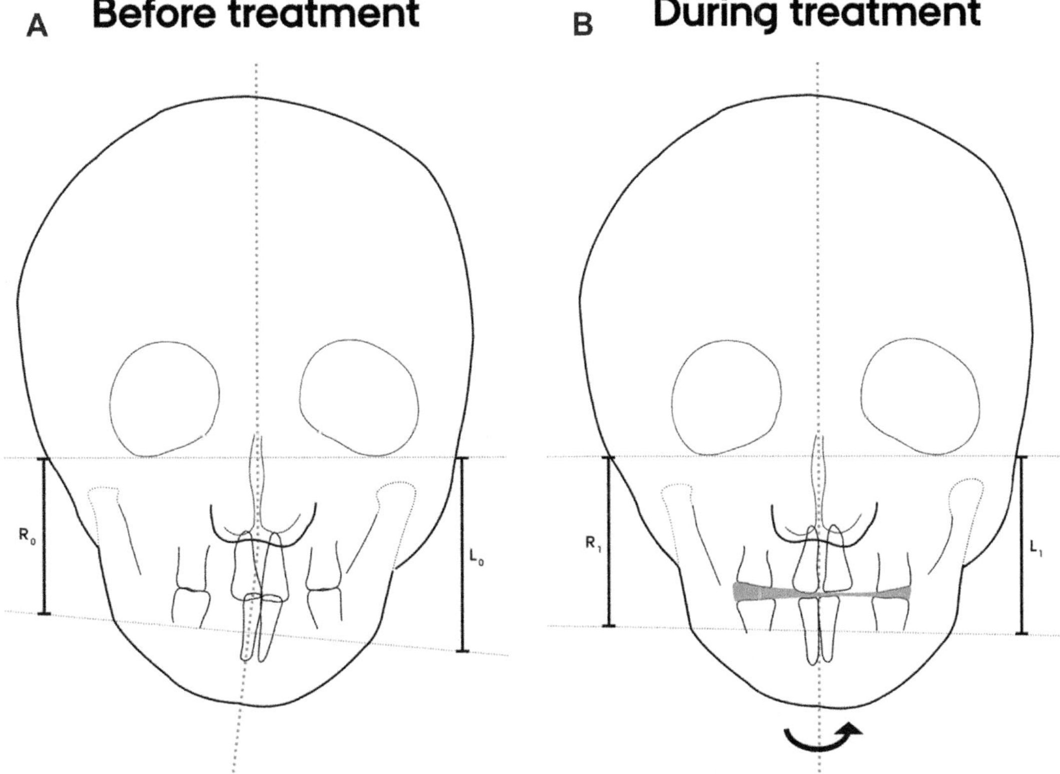

Fig. 6. Orthopedic treatment of unilateral TMJ involvement in skeletally immature subjects. (*A*) Before distraction splint treatment. Unilateral TMJ involvement (*right side*) has led to reduced vertical right-sided mandibular development, dentofacial asymmetry, and a canted occlusal plan. Dentofacial asymmetry is illustrated by the reference lines R_0 and L_0. (*B*) During distraction splint treatment, the height of the splint is gradually increased on the right side. This distraction of the normalized mandibular skeletal and dentofacial development on the right side and repositions the mandible in a more symmetric position. Long-term treatment will reduce dentofacial asymmetry, as illustrated by the reference lines R_1 and L_1.

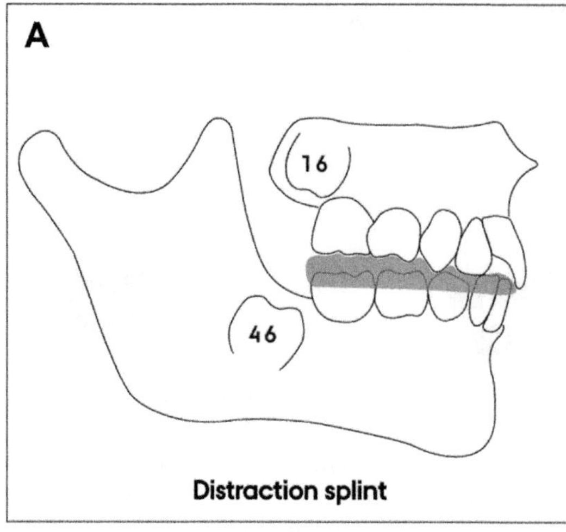

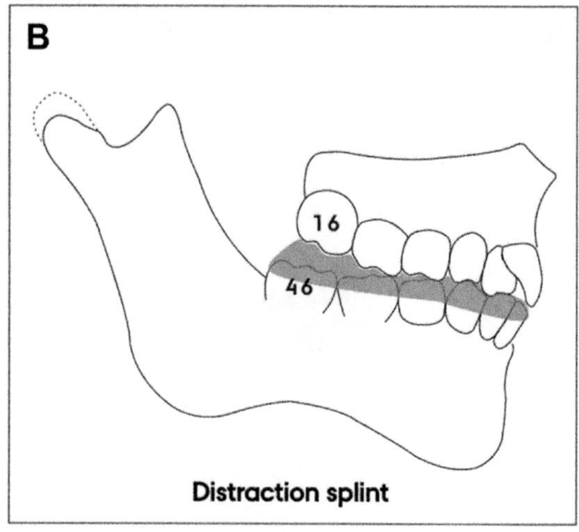

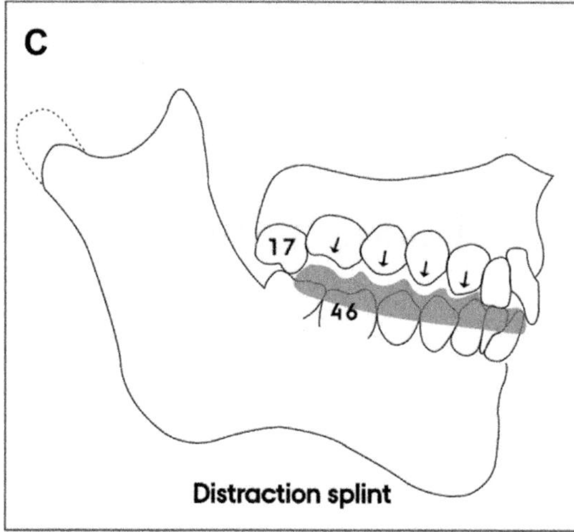

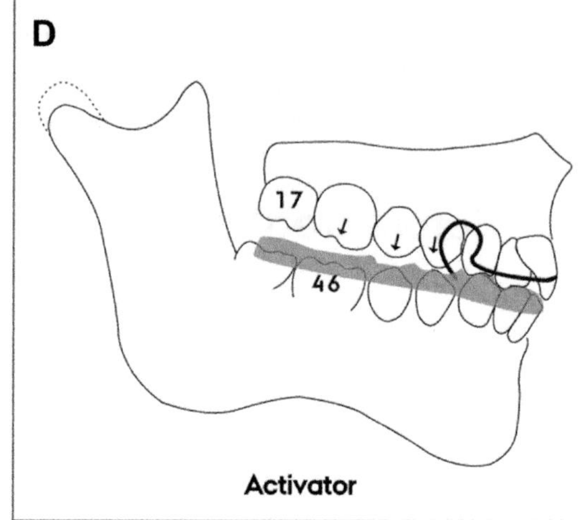

Fig. 7. Orthopedic treatment and tooth eruption. (*A*) Distraction splint treatment in the primary dentition. (*B*) Distraction splint in the mixed dentition after eruption of first upper[16] and lower molars.[46] Eruption of the permanent molars is prevented and creates a posterior open bite that allows for mandibular anterior rotation when the splint is no longer used, as illustrated in **Fig. 5**C. (*C*) After mandibular growth spurt, the open bite correction consists of guided tooth eruption. Selective grinding of the distraction splint allows for guided eruption of the upper posterior dentition (indicated with *black arrows*) beneficial for correction of occlusal canting. (*D*) After mandibular growth spurt, transition into an activator appliance treatment is an alternative to the option presented in Fig. 7C. This allows for guided tooth eruption combined with management of intermaxillary sagittal discrepancy. Arrows indicate tooth eruption after selective grinding of the activator.

THE ACTIVATOR

The activator is another type of orthopedic removable appliance proposed for management of JIA-induced dentofacial deformities from bilateral TMJ involvement.[50,52,55] The activator is an acrylic splint (monoblock) covering upper and lower dentition (see **Fig. 4**A, B). The appliance is used "full-time" to "16 hours per day." The activator promotes anterior mandibular advancement to correct the sagittal intermaxillary discrepancy and enables control of tooth eruption. In contrast to the distraction splint, the activator does not need periodic adjustment because encouraging vertical growth is not its main purpose. It is most often used only during the years of dentofacial growth.[50–52,55] Patient compliance is an issue to this modality because of the considerable size of the appliance.

Subsequent use of the activator, after treatment with distraction splint, enables effective correction of occlusal canting by selective grinding of the activator, which guides dental eruption[55] (see **Fig. 7**).

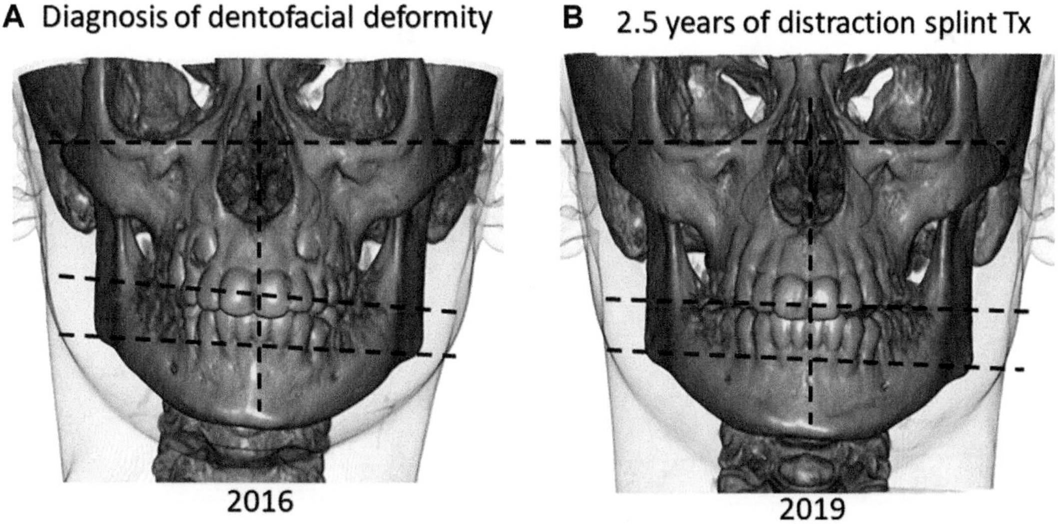

A Diagnosis of dentofacial deformity

B 2.5 years of distraction splint Tx

2016

2019

Fig. 8. Skeletal effect of orthopedic appliance treatment. Thirteen-year-old girl with JIA (oligoarticular subtype) and right-sided unilateral TMJ involvement. (*A*) Dentofacial deformity (at age 10) before distraction splint treatment was initiated. (*B*) Dentofacial deformity after 2.5 years of orthopedic appliance treatment. Notice normalized mandibular development on the right side, reduced occlusal canting, and reduced mandibular asymmetry. Tx, treatment.

FIXED ORTHODONTIC APPLIANCES

Little is known about the effects of a fixed orthodontic appliances in the management of JIA-induced dentofacial deformities; evidence is based mainly on empirical observations. There is a general lack of knowledge of how the underlying autoimmune systemic disease and the systemic treatment modalities applied (methotrexate, nonsteroidal anti-inflammatory drugs, and biologic drugs) influence aspects of orthodontic treatment like tooth movement rate, bone remodeling, and the risk of root resorption.

In general, fixed orthodontic treatment is considered a modality to establish the occlusion after treatment with a removable orthopedic appliance; a final settling of the occlusion to compensate for minor dental discrepancies. Caution should be taken before applying orthodontic principles from the non-JIA population as the sole treatment principle of moderate/large dentofacial deformities caused by JIA (eg, skeletal discrepancies, distal occlusion, increased horizontal overjet), as normal growth, essential for optimal orthodontic treatment in healthy patients, may be impaired. Persistent orthodontic efforts to correct sagittal discrepancies may cause unwanted dentoalveolar compensation and root resorption. Vertical control of dentoalveolar growth and development is a key aspect of the management of JIA-induced dentofacial deformities.[55] However, this may be compromised in the efforts to advance a retrognathic mandible. In the non-JIA population, 2 recognized orthodontic principles are applied in the treatment of distal occlusion and sagittal discrepancies: (1) the "bite-jumping" device: a protrusive appliance mounted at the upper molars to the lower canines (eg, Herbst appliance); and (2) "class II elastics": intermaxillary elastics from the anterior upper dentition to the posterior lower jaw (**Fig. 10**). These principles are not contraindicated in JIA; however, they should be cautiously used, as uncritical use of these biomechanical principles may further aggravate arthritis-induced dentofacial deformities such as posterior mandibular rotation, steepening of the occlusal plane, excessive lower incisor proclination, and increased anterior face height (see **Fig. 10**). Although proclination of the lower incisors may reduce the horizontal overjet, these dentoalveolar compensations complicate any future treatment involving combined efforts of orthognathic surgery and orthodontics.

The commercialization of the orthodontic temporary anchorage device (TAD), small titanium implants, has introduced new treatment modalities to the orthodontic tool box (**Fig. 11**). In skeletally mature subjects, TAD-assisted intrusion of upper and lower molars may affect a correction of an anterior open bite and facilitate mandibular anterior rotation. The biomechanical principles are somewhat comparable to the

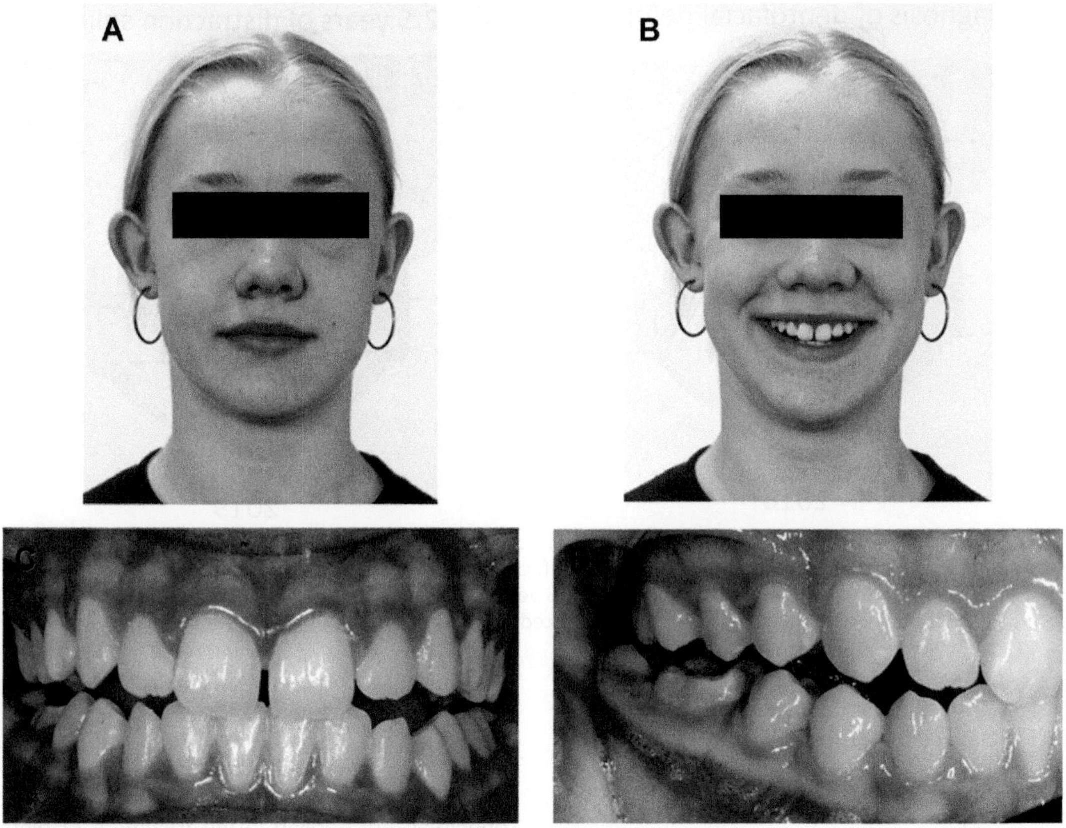

Fig. 9. Dentoalveolar effects of orthopedic appliance treatment (continuation from **Fig. 8**). Facial and dentoalveolar effect after 2.5 years of distraction splint treatment. Thirteen-year-old girl with JIA (oligoarticular subtype) and right-sided unilateral TMJ involvement. (*A*, *B*) After 2.5 years of distraction splint treatment, only minor dentofacial deformity remains with (*C*, *D*) minimal dentoalveolar effects. A bilateral posterior open bite is created; most pronounced in the affected right side. Minor posterior open bite is created on the left side because of full-time wear of the splint. Notice the normal development of the incisal area. Guided tooth eruption will be used to correct the posterior open bite (eruption from posterior maxilla left side and from posterior mandible right side) and minimize occlusal canting (principles described in **Fig. 7**C, D).

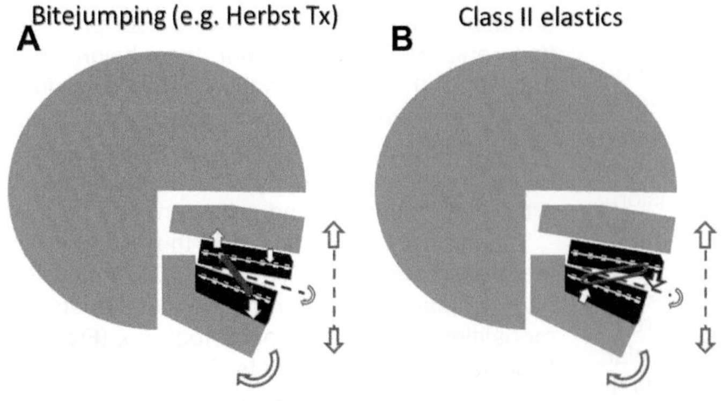

Fig. 10. Effects of orthodontic treatment principles. Orthodontic biomechanical principles from the non-JIA population should be cautiously used in the management of JIA-induced dentofacial deformity due to risk of unwanted side effects. (*A*) Treatment with bite-jumping device: This protrusive appliance has the potential to intrude upper posterior dentition and the dentition in the lower front. In turn, this may lead to a steeping of the occlusal plane, a mandibular posterior rotation, and an increased anterior face height. (*B*) Treatment with intermaxillary class II elastics has the potential to extrude upper front teeth and lower posterior teeth. In turn, this may also create unwanted effects with a steeping of the occlusal plane, a mandibular posterior rotation and an increased anterior face height.

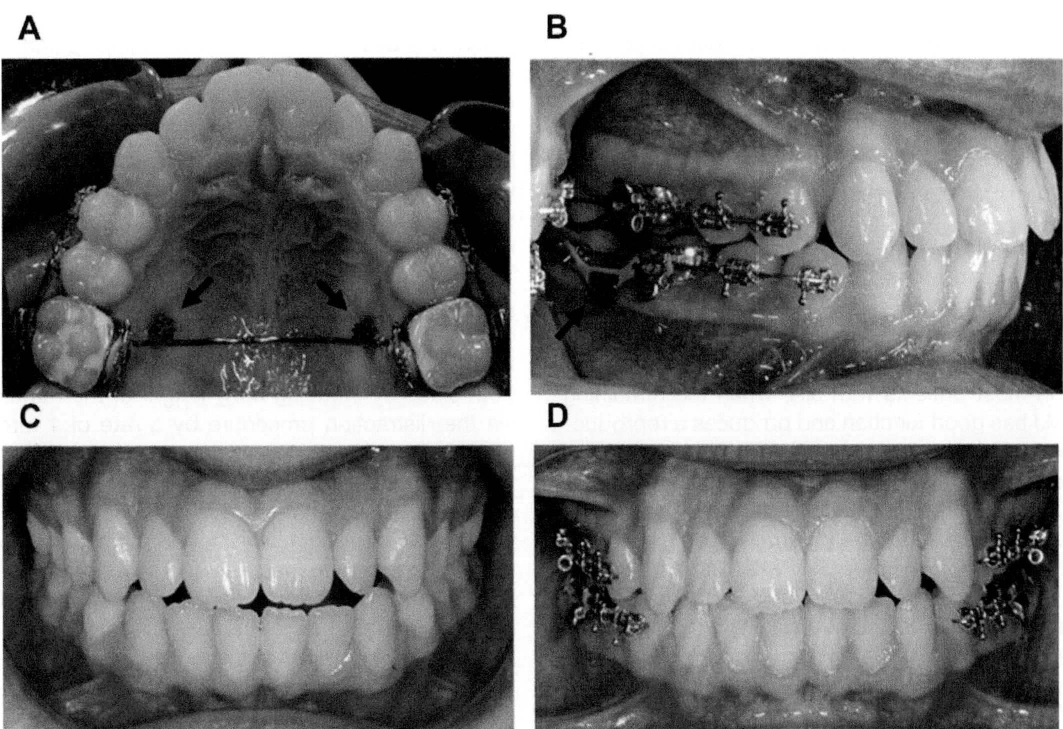

Fig. 11. Orthodontic treatment with TAD. Orthodontic correction of anterior open bite by TAD-assisted intrusion of posterior dentition. (*A*, *B*) TADs have been inserted (*black arrows*). Elastics from TADs to orthodontic appliance and intrusion of the posterior dentition. (*C*) Pre-orthodontic occlusion with anterior open bite. (*D*) Occlusion after intrusion of posterior dentition with correction of the anterior open bite.

approach exploited during distraction splint treatment in growing subjects regarding the dentoalveolar effect (see **Fig. 5**).

TRANSITION TO SURGICAL MANAGEMENT

Orthognathic surgery should be considered if orthopedic appliance treatment is insufficient to normalize the dentofacial deformity to an acceptable level.[16] DO can be used both during and after growth.[57,58] If DO is conducted in growing individuals, the orthodontist must manage the postsurgical residual growth and dentoalveolar development by means of orthopedic and/or orthodontic appliances. Combined orthognathic surgery and orthodontic treatment should be postponed until skeletal maturity. Decision making depends on close collaboration between the orthodontist and oral maxillofacial surgeon.

SURGICAL CORRECTION OF DENTOFACIAL DEFORMITY

Before initiation of surgical treatment, specific information is necessary regarding (1) general disease activity and TMJ stability, (2) progressing deformity of the facial skeleton over the past 12 months, (3) the age and skeletal maturity of the patient, and (4) the severity of the skeletal deformity.[16] The activity of the arthritis is assessed in collaboration with a pediatric rheumatologist; and in case of surgical treatment, any adjustments in medication are planned, such as drug holidays to promote wound healing. Dentofacial development is usually monitored by the orthodontist, who detects changes in morphology and occlusion before surgery. A developing deformity usually warrants a prolonged observation period before surgical correction is determined and initiated.

ANESTHESIA CONSIDERATIONS

Patients with JIA may pose a challenge for the anesthesiologist, as several factors negatively influence airway access. Typical findings include fusions in the cervical spine with diminished extension and flexion capacity, and a retrognathic mandible with reduced range of mouth opening. Consequently, the anesthesiologist may consider fiberoptic intubation.[59] Following surgery, any potential swelling in the floor of the mouth or pharyngeal region that can impact the airway may require prolonged intubation, as urgent reintubation may be difficult.

SURGICAL OPTIONS

Surgical management of arthritis-induced dentofacial deformities may involve orthognathic surgery (including DO), total alloplastic joint replacement (TJR), reconstruction with costochondral graft, or a combination.[58,60–63]

In most patients with JIA, when the remaining TMJ has good function and produces a reproducible stable position, the first choice of surgical treatment is a joint-preserving procedure. Orthognathic surgery is indicated in skeletally mature patients with moderate deformity and quiescent disease. The treatment plan is based on registrations similar to those required for routine orthognathic surgery patients, including clinical registrations of facial proportions and asymmetries, natural head position, and dental occlusion with the TMJ in an orthopedic stable relation. Virtual treatment planning is completed using a 3-dimensonal CBCT scan combined with an intraoral dental scan. The position of the condyles may be difficult to determine exactly, as some degree of joint deformity may already have occurred. The goal of surgical treatment is to anterior rotate, advance, and center the mandible as necessary to obtain a normal condylar/ramal position, improve the profile and airway space, correct the malocclusion, and eliminate asymmetry. Concomitant genioplasty is often indicated to achieve optimal esthetic results and to support lip function.[64] The advantage of orthognathic surgery is that it is based on well-known principles and is completed as a single surgical procedure using entirely intraoral access. Theoretic potential disadvantages are the risk of mechanical loading causing further progression of TMJ deformity leading to relapse and extensive stretching of soft tissues, which may increase the tendency for relapse.

DO is indicated in growing or skeletally mature patients with moderate to severe deformity and quiescent TMJ arthritis. The aim is to compensate for the lack of posterior vertical growth in one or both sides by inducing bony height of the ramus via the distraction procedure by a rate of 1 mm per day. Postoperatively, continued development of the jaw and dental occlusion in growing patients is supported by orthopedic/orthodontic appliance therapy. In approximately half of the cases, no further surgery is needed after DO; in others, finalizing orthognathic surgery is done after the end of growth. The last part of the surgical treatment is usually less extensive because of the effect obtained by DO (eg, a maxillary osteotomy for adjustment of the occlusion) (**Fig. 12**), compared with patients who await skeletal maturity before correction. Furthermore, DO is an option for treatment of severe mandibular retrognathia after the end of growth, provided that stable joint function is present. In such cases, the rationale is a gradual elongation of bone and soft tissue to reduce loading of the TMJs and minimize relapse caused by stretching the surrounding tissue.[58] If surgical correction of the maxillary position is indicated, this can be done at the time of removal of the distraction devices. Advantages of DO include the ability to provide skeletal correction during growth, and to

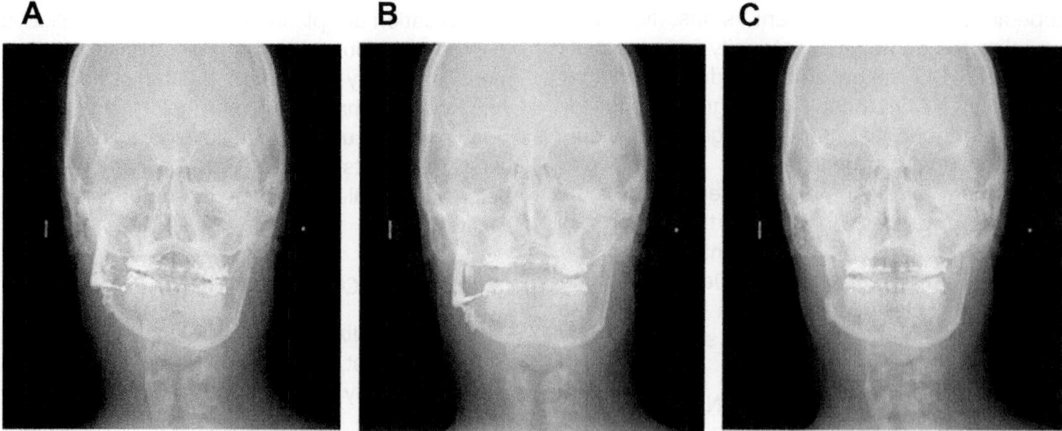

Fig. 12. DO: A 17-year-old girl with JIA and history of arthritis of right TMJ was treated with intraoral vertical DO of the ramus. (*A*) Frontal cephalogram of device inserted. (*B*) After 18-mm distraction. (*C*) At the time of removal of the device (3 months after insertion), a Le Fort I osteotomy was performed to level the maxilla.

achieve larger movements without bone grafts than by conventional orthognathic surgical procedures. Drawbacks are the need for at least 2 operations and the need for patients to activate the device during the treatment period.

A severe and prolonged course of TMJ arthritis can lead to extensive destruction, deformation, and impaired function that necessitates resection of either the condyle or the entire joint, including the fossa component. A joint-sparing reconstruction can be completed using an autologous graft; the most commonly used is the costochondral graft.[62] This method can be indicated in growing patients who need condylar replacement. However, because the autogenous graft is placed into an area of active synovitis, it has the same potential to resorb as the original mandibular condyle.

TJR may be the best reconstructive option if the active inflammation cannot be adequately medically controlled.[60] TJR is typically reserved for skeletally mature patients who present with a destroyed TMJ or uncontrollable TMJ disease,[65] although its use has been reported in growing patients.[66] Alloplastic TMJ replacement can be planned using 3-dimensional virtual planning with custom, patient-specific components. At surgery, the remaining condyle and disc are resected and both condylar and fossa components of the TJR are placed and fixated with titanium screws. An anterior rotation of the mandible can be incorporated in the prostheses, and, if indicated, a simultaneous Le Fort I osteotomy and genioplasty can be performed. The advantage of alloplastic TJR is that all pathology in the TMJ is eliminated and a stable position of the jaw is obtained. However, if placed in young individuals, the unknown longevity of the prosthesis and the risk of heterotopic bone formation should be taken into consideration.

SUMMARY

Patients with TMJ arthritis require specific expertise from an interdisciplinary team with members knowledgeable in JIA care. This article focuses on the unique properties of TMJ and dentofacial growth, and the effects of TMJ involvement from JIA. The importance of interdisciplinary collaboration among pediatric rheumatologists, maxillofacial surgeons, and orthodontists is illustrated, focusing on orthopedic/orthodontic treatment and surgical interventions.

ACKNOWLEDGMENT

The authors thank graphical designer Nikolai Lander, Aarhus University, for his help with illustrations.

REFERENCES

1. Petty RE, Southwood TR, Baum J, et al. Revision of the proposed classification criteria for juvenile idiopathic arthritis: Durban, 1997. J Rheumatol 1998;25(10):1991–4.
2. Petty RE, Southwood TR, Manners P, et al. International League of Associations for Rheumatology classification of juvenile idiopathic arthritis: second revision, Edmonton, 2001. J Rheumatol 2004;31(2):390–2.
3. Arvidsson LZ, Fjeld MG, Smith HJ, et al. Craniofacial growth disturbance is related to temporomandibular joint abnormality in patients with juvenile idiopathic arthritis, but normal facial profile was also found at the 27-year follow-up. Scand J Rheumatol 2010;39(5):373–9.
4. Cannizzaro E, Schroeder S, Muller LM, et al. Temporomandibular joint involvement in children with juvenile idiopathic arthritis. J Rheumatol 2011;38(3):510–5.
5. Kuseler A, Pedersen TK, Herlin T, et al. Contrast enhanced magnetic resonance imaging as a method to diagnose early inflammatory changes in the temporomandibular joint in children with juvenile chronic arthritis. J Rheumatol 1998;25(7):1406–12.
6. Stoll ML, Sharpe T, Beukelman T, et al. Risk factors for temporomandibular joint arthritis in children with juvenile idiopathic arthritis. J Rheumatol 2012;39(9):1880–7.
7. Hugle B, Spiegel L, Hotte J, et al. Isolated arthritis of the temporomandibular joint as the initial manifestation of juvenile idiopathic arthritis. J Rheumatol 2017;44(11):1632–5.
8. Frid P, Nordal E, Bovis F, et al. Temporomandibular joint involvement in association with quality of life, disability, and high disease activity in juvenile idiopathic arthritis. Arthritis Care Res 2017;69(5):677–86.
9. Koos B, Twilt M, Kyank U, et al. Reliability of clinical symptoms in diagnosing temporomandibular joint arthritis in juvenile idiopathic arthritis. J Rheumatol 2014;41(9):1871–7.
10. Muller L, Kellenberger CJ, Cannizzaro E, et al. Early diagnosis of temporomandibular joint involvement in juvenile idiopathic arthritis: a pilot study comparing clinical examination and ultrasound to magnetic resonance imaging. Rheumatology (Oxford) 2009;48(6):680–5.
11. Rahimi H, Twilt M, Herlin T, et al. Orofacial symptoms and oral health-related quality of life in juvenile idiopathic arthritis: a two-year prospective observational study. Pediatr Rheumatol Online J 2018;16(1):47.
12. Stoustrup P, Kristensen KD, Verna C, et al. Orofacial symptoms related to temporomandibular joint arthritis in juvenile idiopathic arthritis: smallest detectable difference in self-reported pain intensity. J Rheumatol 2012;39(12):2352–8.

13. Weiss PF, Arabshahi B, Johnson A, et al. High prevalence of temporomandibular joint arthritis at disease onset in children with juvenile idiopathic arthritis, as detected by magnetic resonance imaging but not by ultrasound. Arthritis Rheum 2008; 58(4):1189–96.
14. Resnick CM, Dang R, Henderson LA, et al. Frequency and morbidity of temporomandibular joint involvement in adult patients with a history of Juvenile Idiopathic Arthritis. J Oral Maxillofac Surg 2017;75(6):1191–200.
15. Stoustrup P, Glerup M, Bilgrau AE, et al. Cumulative incidence of orofacial manifestations in early juvenile idiopathic arthritis: a regional, three year cohort study. Arthritis Care Res (Hoboken) 2019. [Epub ahead of print].
16. Resnick CM, Frid P, Norholt SE, et al. An algorithm for management of dentofacial deformity resulting from juvenile idiopathic arthritis: results of a multinational consensus conference. J Oral Maxillofac Surg 2019;77(6):1152.e1-33.
17. Stoustrup P, Resnick CM, Pedersen TK, et al. Standardizing terminology and assessment for orofacial conditions in juvenile idiopathic arthritis: international, multidisciplinary consensus-based recommendations. J Rheumatol 2019;46(5): 518–22.
18. Enlow DH. Growth of the mandible. In: Enlow DH, Hans MG, editors. Essential of facial growth. Philadelphia: Saunders; 1996. p. 57–78.
19. Hinton RJ, Carlson DS. Regulation of growth in mandibular condylar cartilage. Semin Orthod 2005; 11:209–18.
20. Hinton RJ, Jing J, Feng JQ. Genetic influences on temporomandibular joint development and growth. Curr Top Dev Biol 2015;115:85–109.
21. Mao JJ, Nah HD. Growth and development: hereditary and mechanical modulations. Am J Orthod Dentofacial Orthop 2004;125(6):676–89.
22. Stoustrup PB, Ahlefeldt-Laurvig-Lehn N, Kristensen KD, et al. No association between types of unilateral mandibular condylar abnormalities and facial asymmetry in orthopedic-treated patients with juvenile idiopathic arthritis. Am J Orthod Dentofacial Orthop 2018;153(2):214–23.
23. Peltomäki T, Kreiborg S, Pedersen TK, et al. Craniofacial growth and dentoalveolar development in juvenile idiopathic arthritis patients. Semin Orthod 2015;21(2):84–93.
24. Tanaka E, Detamore MS, Mercuri LG. Degenerative disorders of the temporomandibular joint: etiology, diagnosis, and treatment. J Dent Res 2008;87(4): 296–307.
25. Betti BF, Everts V, Ket JCF, et al. Effect of mechanical loading on the metabolic activity of cells in the temporomandibular joint: a systematic review. Clin Oral Investig 2018;22(1):57–67.
26. Fjeld MG, Arvidsson LZ, Stabrun AE, et al. Average craniofacial development from 6 to 35 years of age in a mixed group of patients with juvenile idiopathic arthritis. Acta Odontol Scand 2009;67(3):153–60.
27. Gonzalez MF, Pedersen TK, Dalstra M, et al. 3D evaluation of mandibular skeletal changes in juvenile arthritis patients treated with a distraction splint: a retrospective follow-up. Angle Orthod 2016;86(5):846–53.
28. Agarwal S, Long P, Gassner R, et al. Cyclic tensile strain suppresses catabolic effects of interleukin-1beta in fibrochondrocytes from the temporomandibular joint. Arthritis Rheum 2001;44(3):608–17.
29. Tabeian H, Bakker AD, Betti BF, et al. Cyclic tensile strain reduces TNF-alpha induced expression of MMP-13 by condylar temporomandibular joint cells. J Cell Physiol 2017;232(6):1287–94.
30. von Bremen J, Kohler K, Siudak K, et al. Histologic effects of mandibular protrusion splints in antigen-induced TMJ arthritis in rabbits. Pediatr Rheumatol Online J 2017;15(1):27.
31. Arvidsson LZ, Flato B, Larheim TA. Radiographic TMJ abnormalities in patients with juvenile idiopathic arthritis followed for 27 years. Oral Surg Oral Med Oral Pathol Oral Radiol Endod 2009; 108(1):114–23.
32. Twilt M, Schulten AJ, Verschure F, et al. Long-term followup of temporomandibular joint involvement in juvenile idiopathic arthritis. Arthritis Rheum 2008; 59(4):546–52.
33. Kristensen KD, Stoustrup P, Kuseler A, et al. Clinical predictors of temporomandibular joint arthritis in juvenile idiopathic arthritis: a systematic literature review. Semin Arthritis Rheum 2016;45(6):717–32.
34. Rongo R, Alstergren P, Ammendola L, et al. Temporomandibular joint damage in juvenile idiopathic arthritis: diagnostic validity of diagnostic criteria for temporomandibular disorders. J Oral Rehabil 2019; 46(5):450–9.
35. Peck CC, Goulet JP, Lobbezoo F, et al. Expanding the taxonomy of the diagnostic criteria for temporomandibular disorders. J Oral Rehabil 2014;41(1):2–23.
36. Schiffman E, Ohrbach R, Truelove E, et al. Diagnostic criteria for temporomandibular disorders (DC/TMD) for Clinical and Research Applications: recommendations of the International RDC/TMD Consortium Network* and Orofacial Pain Special Interest Groupdagger. J Oral Facial Pain Headache 2014;28(1):6–27.
37. Kellenberger CJ, Bucheli J, Schroeder-Kohler S, et al. Temporomandibular joint magnetic resonance imaging findings in adolescents with anterior disk displacement compared to those with juvenile idiopathic arthritis. J Oral Rehabil 2019;46(1):14–22.
38. Naeije M, Te Veldhuis AH, Te Veldhuis EC, et al. Disc displacement within the human temporomandibular joint: a systematic review of a 'noisy annoyance. J Oral Rehabil 2013;40(2):139–58.

39. Abramowicz S, Susarla HK, Kim S, et al. Physical findings associated with active temporomandibular joint inflammation in children with juvenile idiopathic arthritis. J Oral Maxillofac Surg 2013;71(10):1683–7.
40. Stoustrup P, Koos B. Clinical craniofacial examination of patients with juvenile idiopathic arthritis. Semin Orthod 2015;21:7.
41. Stoustrup P, Twilt M, Spiegel L, et al. Clinical orofacial examination in juvenile idiopathic arthritis: international consensus-based recommendations for monitoring patients in clinical practice and research studies. J Rheumatol 2017;44(3):326–33.
42. Kellenberger CJ, Junhasavasdikul T, Tolend M, et al. Temporomandibular joint atlas for detection and grading of juvenile idiopathic arthritis involvement by magnetic resonance imaging. Pediatr Radiol 2018;48(3):411–26.
43. Stoustrup P, Iversen CK, Kristensen KD, et al. Assessment of dentofacial growth deviation in juvenile idiopathic arthritis: Reliability and validity of three-dimensional morphometric measures. PLoS One 2018;13(3):e0194177.
44. Ince DO, Ince A, Moore TL. Effect of methotrexate on the temporomandibular joint and facial morphology in juvenile rheumatoid arthritis patients. Am J Orthod Dentofacial Orthop 2000;118(1):75–83.
45. Stoll ML, Good J, Sharpe T, et al. Intra-articular corticosteroid injections to the temporomandibular joints are safe and appear to be effective therapy in children with juvenile idiopathic arthritis. J Oral Maxillofac Surg 2012;70(8):1802–7.
46. Stoustrup P, Kristensen KD, Verna C, et al. Intra-articular steroid injection for temporomandibular joint arthritis in juvenile idiopathic arthritis: a systematic review on efficacy and safety. Semin Arthritis Rheum 2013;(12):10.
47. Lochbuhler N, Saurenmann RK, Muller L, et al. Magnetic resonance imaging assessment of temporomandibular joint involvement and mandibular growth following corticosteroid injection in juvenile idiopathic arthritis. J Rheumatol 2015;42(8):1514–22.
48. Stoll ML, Amin D, Powell KK, et al. Risk factors for intraarticular heterotopic bone formation in the temporomandibular joint in juvenile idiopathic arthritis. J Rheumatol 2018;45(9):1301–7.
49. Resnick CM, Pedersen TK, Abramowicz S, et al. Time to reconsider management of the temporomandibular joint in juvenile idiopathic arthritis. J Oral Maxillofac Surg 2018;76(6):1145–6.
50. Farronato G, Carletti V, Maspero C, et al. Craniofacial growth in children affected by juvenile idiopathic arthritis involving the temporomandibular joint: functional therapy management. J Clin Pediatr Dent 2009;33(4):351–7.
51. Isola G, Ramaglia L, Cordasco G, et al. The effect of a functional appliance in the management of temporomandibular joint disorders in patients with juvenile idiopathic arthritis. Minerva Stomatol 2017;66(1):1–8.
52. Kjellberg H, Kiliaridis S, Thilander B. Dentofacial growth in orthodontically treated and untreated children with juvenile chronic arthritis (JCA). A comparison with Angle Class II division 1 subjects. Eur J Orthod 1995;17(5):357–73.
53. Stoustrup P, Kuseler A, Kristensen KD, et al. Orthopaedic splint treatment can reduce mandibular asymmetry caused by unilateral temporomandibular involvement in juvenile idiopathic arthritis. Eur J Orthod 2013;35(2):191–8.
54. von Bremen J, Ruf S. Orthodontic and dentofacial orthopedic management of juvenile idiopathic arthritis: a systematic review of the literature. Orthod Craniofac Res 2011;14(3):107–15.
55. Pedersen TK, Verna C. Functional and orthopedic treatment in developing dentofacial growth deviation in juvenile idiopathic arthritis. Semin Orthod 2015;21(2):134–9.
56. Pedersen TK, Gronhoj J, Melsen B, et al. Condylar condition and mandibular growth during early functional treatment of children with juvenile chronic arthritis. Eur J Orthod 1995;17(5):385–94.
57. Norholt SE, Jensen J, Schou S, et al. Complications after mandibular distraction osteogenesis: a retrospective study of 131 patients. Oral Surg Oral Med Oral Pathol Oral Radiol Endod 2011;111(4):420–7.
58. Norholt SE, Pedersen TK, Herlin T. Functional changes following distraction osteogenesis treatment of asymmetric mandibular growth deviation in unilateral juvenile idiopathic arthritis: a prospective study with long-term follow-up. Int J Oral Maxillofac Surg 2013;42(3):329–36.
59. Dravid RM, Popat M. Intubation during manual in-line stabilisation of the head and neck. Anaesthesia 2000;55(8):814–5.
60. Frid P, Resnick C, Abramowicz S, et al. Surgical correction of dentofacial deformities in juvenile idiopathic arthritis: a systematic literature review. Int J Oral Maxillofac Surg 2019;48(8):1032–42.
61. Leandro LF, Ono HY, Loureiro CC, et al. A ten-year experience and follow-up of three hundred patients fitted with the Biomet/Lorenz Microfixation TMJ replacement system. Int J Oral Maxillofac Surg 2013;42(8):1007–13.
62. Svensson B, Adell R. Costochondral grafts to replace mandibular condyles in juvenile chronic arthritis patients: long-term effects on facial growth. J Craniomaxillofac Surg 1998;26(5):275–85.
63. Svensson B, Feldmann G, Rindler A. Early surgical-orthodontic treatment of mandibular hypoplasia in

juvenile chronic arthritis. J Craniomaxillofac Surg 1993;21(2):67–75.
64. Precious DS, Delaire J. Correction of anterior mandibular vertical excess: the functional genioplasty. Oral Surg Oral Med Oral Pathol 1985;59(3):229–35.
65. Wolford LM, Mercuri LG, Schneiderman ED, et al. Twenty-year follow-up study on a patient-fitted temporomandibular joint prosthesis: the Techmedica/TMJ Concepts device. J Oral Maxillofac Surg 2015;73(5):952–60.
66. Mercuri LG, Swift JQ. Considerations for the use of alloplastic temporomandibular joint replacement in the growing patient. J Oral Maxillofac Surg 2009; 67(9):1979–90.

Comprehensive Post Orthognathic Surgery Orthodontics

Complications, Misconceptions, and Management

Larry M. Wolford, DMD[a,b,*]

KEYWORDS

• Palatal splint • Occlusal splint • Orthognathic surgery • Occlusal plane angle • Open bite • Maxillary osteotomies • Mandibular osteotomies • TMJ

KEY POINTS

- Know the postsurgery orthodontic mechanics to finalize dental, dentoalveolar, and skeletal relationships and identify those patients that may require aggressive orthodontic management to acquire a high-quality outcome.
- Use postsurgery orthodontic management techniques that are stable and predictable for specific dental and dentoalveolar factors and be aware of those orthodontic mechanics that have a negative impact on outcomes.
- Recognize immediate postsurgical short and long-term risks and complications of orthognathic surgery as well as the management to correct these challenging situations.
- Be aware of the temporomandibular joint conditions and pathologies that are common causes of long-term relapse.
- When temporomandibular joint problems develop after surgery, learn to identify the pathology and apply the indicated protocols, including possible surgical intervention.

INTRODUCTION

Postsurgical patient management is a critical factor for high-quality patient treatment and predictable outcomes in orthognathic surgery. However, a lack of understanding of proper patient management on the part of the surgeon and orthodontist can result in compromised or even disastrous results. Poor postsurgical orthodontic management after an initially great surgical result can produce a compromised or unacceptable outcome. Although often difficult, a compromised surgical result may be salvaged by aggressive postsurgical orthodontics. Surgeons and orthodontists must have the knowledge and ability to implement postsurgical management protocols and strategies to provide the best care and outcomes possible for their orthognathic surgery patients.

Disclosure: The author has nothing to disclose.

[a] Department of Oral and Maxillofacial Surgery, Texas A&M University College of Dentistry, Baylor University Medical Center – Private Practice, 3409 Worth Street, Suite #400, Dallas, TX 75246, USA; [b] Department of Orthodontics, Texas A&M University College of Dentistry, Baylor University Medical Center – Private Practice, 3409 Worth Street, Suite #400, Dallas, TX 75246, USA
* Department of Oral and Maxillofacial Surgery, Texas A&M University College of Dentistry, Baylor University Medical Center – Private Practice, 3409 Worth Street, Suite #400, Dallas, TX 75246.
E-mail address: Lwolford@drlarrywolford.com

Oral Maxillofacial Surg Clin N Am 32 (2020) 135–151
https://doi.org/10.1016/j.coms.2019.09.003
1042-3699/20/

Jaw deformities requiring orthognathic surgery often coexist with temporomandibular joint (TMJ) pathology. Unrecognized or untreated TMJ pathologies are one of the primary factors leading to postsurgical complications. TMJ surgery may be required in these coexisting situations. However, the TMJ surgery should be done before the orthognathic surgery in separate operations or perform the TMJ surgery followed by the orthognathic surgery at the same operation.[1,2] This article presents basic concepts, philosophies, treatment protocols, and other important information that can be helpful in postsurgical patient management.

SURGICAL FACTORS TO ENHANCE POSTSURGICAL ORTHODONTICS

The surgeon can simplify the postsurgical patient management and orthodontic requirements by the following methods: (1) Perform precise surgery; (2) segmentalize the maxilla when indicated to improve outcome stability; (3) use surgical stabilizing splints when indicated; (4) use rigid fixation; (5) graft maxillary bone defects with bone or synthetic bone[3–6]; (6) maximize occlusal interdigitation at surgery, and (7) Surgically correct preexisting TMJ pathology either at a separate surgical procedure before the orthognathic surgery or at the same operation as the orthognathic surgery. TMJ pathology is one of the most common factors that lead to relapse and failure of orthognathic surgical procedures.[7,8]

At the completion of surgery, a surgical stabilizing splint may be present and wired to the upper teeth. Light elastics (3.5 oz) are usually placed between the upper and lower arches in the cuspid and molar areas, and/or elsewhere if indicated, to (1) maximize the occlusal fit, (2) take stress off the muscles of mastication by providing extra vertical support to the jaws to improve patient comfort, and (3) reduce swelling in the TMJs, if TMJ surgery was simultaneously performed.

SPLINTS

Surgical stabilizing splints are indicated for providing the following: (1) Stability in multiple segmental surgery of the maxilla or mandible, (2) transverse stability when the maxilla and/or mandible have been expanded or narrowed, (3) occlusal support when key teeth are missing (ie, first, second, and third molars are missing in a quadrant), and (4) a means to interdigitate the occlusion if teeth are severely worn or missing. There are 2 basic types of maxillary splints for orthognathic surgery: the palatal splint (**Fig. 1**) and the occlusal splint (**Fig. 2**). If the maxilla and mandible are single pieces and the teeth can be appropriately interdigitated, then a final splint is usually not necessary in single or double jaw surgery.

Palatal Splint

This horseshoe-shaped splint (see **Fig. 1**) is preferred by the author because (1) it provides excellent stability, (2) the occlusal interrelationship of the dental arches can be maximized and observed (the teeth and occlusal relationships are not covered and hidden by the splint), (3) it is easier to keep the teeth and splint clean, (4) orthodontic treatment can be performed with the splint in place, including arch wire changes, (5) the splint can be left in place for extended time (2–3 months or longer if necessary), and (6) after removal, the splint can be modified to function as a retainer by adding clasps.

When fabricating the splint, the palatal tissues beneath the splint must have wax relief of about 1 to 2 mm on the dental model so the splint does not impinge on the soft tissues that could cause vascular compromise to the maxilla (see **Fig. 1**A, B). The palatal splint can be produced by virtual surgical planning technology (see **Fig. 1**C, D), designed to provide palatal soft tissue relief. The splint is stabilized to the maxilla with light, #28 gauge stainless steel wire placed through the splint and circumferentially around the first molars and first bicuspids (second bicuspids if the first bicuspids are missing) and wires twisted on the labial side of the teeth (see **Fig. 1**E, F). The interdigitation of the maxillary and mandibular arches can be seen because the splint does not interfere with the occlusion. The anterior teeth are not tied into the splint, but stabilized in position with the maxillary bone plates.

Occlusal Splint

The occlusal splint has the following advantages: (1) easy to construct, (2) provides transverse stability, and (3) it can lock-in the occlusion perhaps better than the palatal splint (see **Fig. 2**A). However, the occlusal splint presents the following possible complicating factors: (1) the clinician cannot see the occlusal inter-relationship of the teeth with the splint in place, (2) an occlusal interference caused by the splint could result in a malocclusion (see **Fig. 2**B), (3) postsurgical orthodontics could be much more difficult, (4) cannot change the arch wire or perform orthodontics with the splint in place, and (5) oral hygiene is

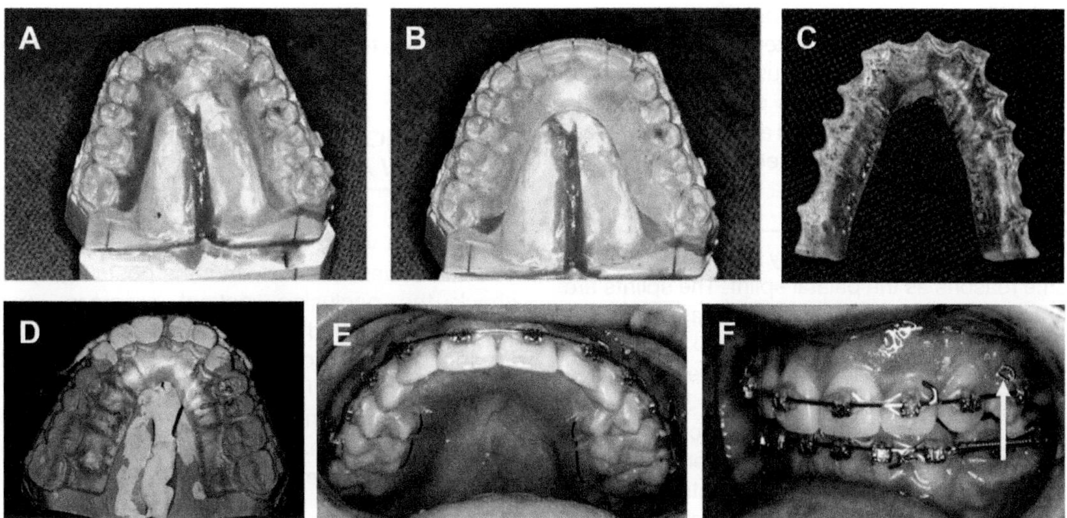

Fig. 1. (*A*) Traditional method of palatal splint construction requires waxing-out the palate to protect the soft tissues. (*B*) The splint has been constructed with holes placed between the teeth to accommodate circumferential wire placement around the first molar and first bicuspid. (*C*) A virtual surgical planning constructed splint using computer technology. (*D*) The splint is seen on the working model. (*E*) The splint is stabilized to the maxilla with 28-gauge stainless steel wire placed through the splint and circumferentially around the first molars and first bicuspids or second bicuspids. (*F*) The wires are twisted on the labial side of the teeth (*white arrows*).

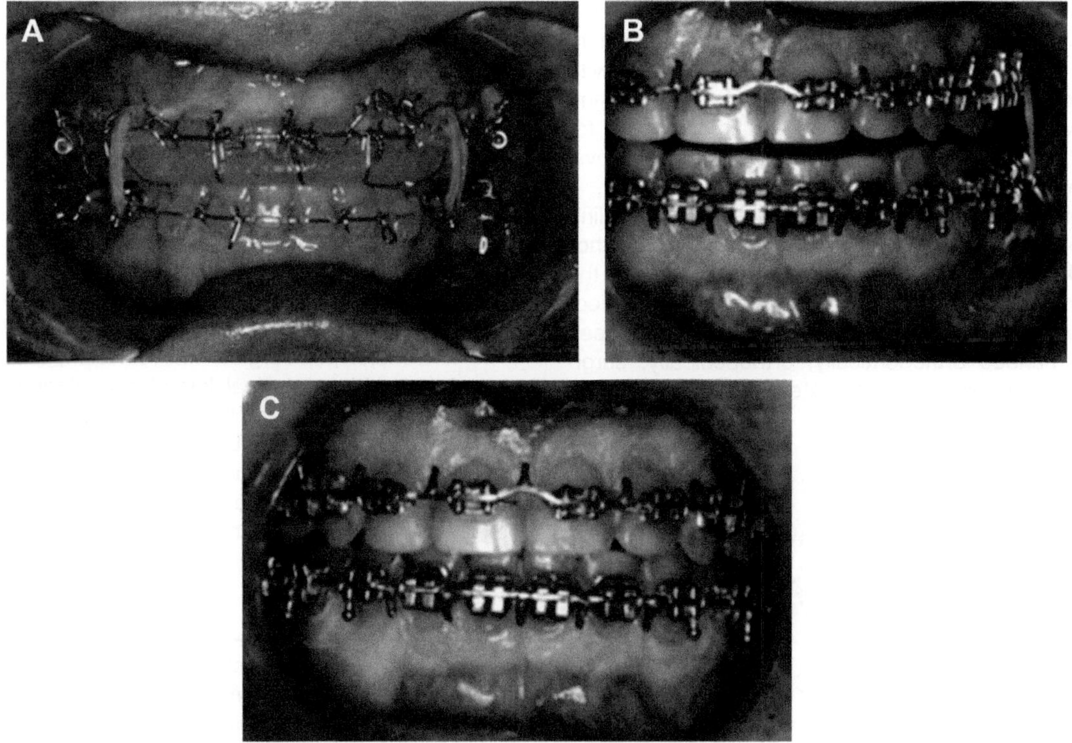

Fig. 2. (*A*) The occlusal splint is usually stabilized to the maxillary arch with wires placed through the buccal flange of the splint and around the adjacent orthodontic brackets on the teeth. The interdental relationship cannot be observed. (*B*) The occlusal splint has been removed and a malocclusion is present with premature contact of teeth created by the splint. (*C*) Placement of light to heavy elastics over a short or longer time may be required to get the occlusion into a good relationship.

more difficult and can cause discoloration, decalcification, and caries of the teeth where covered by the splint. The splint is usually stabilized to the maxillary arch with wires placed through the buccal flange of the splint and around the adjacent orthodontic brackets on the teeth.

Mandibular Splint

Mandibular splints (**Fig. 3**) may be indicated for the same reasons as the palatal splint. The splints are constructed to fit around the lingual aspect of the mandibular crowns, similar to the maxillary palatal splint. Therefore, these splints can be maintained in position for an extended time (2–3 months or longer) if required. The splint is secured to the mandibular arch by placing retention wires through the splint and circumferentially around the first molars and first bicuspids (second bicuspids if the first bicuspids are absent) (see **Fig. 3**). Using this splint design, orthodontic arch wire changes and mechanics can progress with the splint remaining in place.

Splint Removal

This process requires cutting and removing the retention wires and then removing the splint. For most cases with minimal palatal expansion, the palatal or occlusal splint can be removed at 1 to 2 months after surgery. An exception is with maxillary expansions greater than 3 to 4 mm, where the palatal splint can remain in position for 2 to 3 months or longer if required. After removal of the splint, particularly if removed early, a transpalatal arch bar, removable palatal splint, or heavy labial arch wire followed by postorthodontic retainers, can be used to maintain the maxillary expansions for an extended time period. Maxillary or mandibular arches that have been expanded orthodontically, orthopedically, surgically assisted, or by osteotomies will require long-term (1–2 years or longer) transverse stabilization after treatment to ensure a predictable outcome.

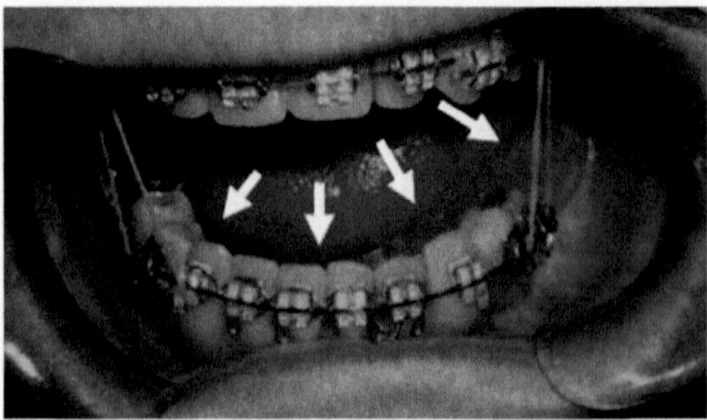

Fig. 3. A mandibular splint (*white arrows*) can be constructed similar to the palatal splint design and is stabilized to the mandibular teeth with wires placed through the splint and circumferentially around the adjacent teeth and twisted on the labial side.

POSTSURGICAL ORTHODONTICS

Postsurgical Appointments

The surgeon and/or orthodontist should see the patient on a weekly basis, or more often if indicated, for the first 1 to 2 months postsurgery to check the occlusion, patient progress, and make any indicated changes in the elastic or orthodontic mechanics to maximize the occlusal inter-relationship. If the occlusion fits properly, then elastics may not be necessary. As long as the occlusion remains stable, the time span between appointments can be increased.

Aggressive Postsurgical Orthodontics

If the occlusion is not perfect initially after surgery, then the surgeon and/or orthodontist must aggressively apply the appropriate elastic mechanics. Relatively light strength elastics (3.5 oz) will usually be adequate to correct the situation. However, occasionally heavier elastics may be necessary. Delays in addressing postsurgical occlusal imbalances results in much greater difficulties correcting the problem at a later time. If the occlusion was good at the completion of surgery, but a shift has occurred or open bite developed, this change is often due to occlusal interference. If light elastics do not reapproximate the occlusion, then placing heavy elastics in the appropriate direction for 30 minutes to 1 hour may settle the occlusion into position so that light elastics can then be used again (see **Fig. 2**B, C). Occasionally, equilibration of the teeth may be necessary to settle the occlusion into position. If there is a major postsurgical malocclusion, then assessment of postsurgical lateral cephalogram and TMJ tomograms may help to determine if it is a correctable problem orthodontically or if additional surgical intervention is required. If required, the sooner the surgical intervention is performed, usually the better situation for the patient and surgeon.

Elastics

Postsurgical interarch elastics are indicated for the following reasons: (1) maximize the occlusal fit, (2) provide orthodontic forces to correct postsurgical occlusal discrepancies, (3) take stress off the muscles of mastication to improve patient comfort immediately after surgery, (4) finalize the occlusion, and (5) minimize edema in the bilaminar tissues if simultaneous TMJ surgery was performed. Controlling the occlusion after surgery can generally be accomplished using elastics with one or more of the following vectors depending of the situation; that is, class II, class III, vertical, box, triangle, trapezoidal, rhomboidal, cross arch, anterior tangential, and so on. Usually only light force elastics of 3.5 oz with sizes of 1/8″, 3/16″, 1/4″, and 5/16″ are needed because teeth and bone segments can move faster after surgery. If the occlusion fits together very well, then elastics may not be necessary.

Vertical elastics

The use of anterior vertical elastics must be closely monitored. Although often necessary initially after surgery to maximize the occlusal fit, these elastics can also create unwanted dentoalveolar changes. Patients predisposed to these unwanted changes include (1) nasal airway obstruction that was not corrected at surgery, (2) habitually holding the jaws open, and (3) short roots. Holding the jaws apart for extended periods of time with anterior vertical elastics will extrude the anterior teeth and over time can increase the dentoalveolar bone height. With the arch wire engaging the molars, as the incisors are extruded, a reciprocal force tends to intrude the posterior teeth (**Fig. 4**). These changes may result in the development of posterior open bites, premature contact of the incisors, increased upper tooth-to-lip relationship, and increased mandibular and maxillary anterior vertical height (see **Fig. 4**). Avoiding these factors may include one or more of the following: (1) perform stable presurgical orthodontics and accurate surgery to decrease requirements for vertical elastics, (2) discontinue vertical elastics as soon as possible, (3) decrease daily time requirements for wearing elastics particularly during activities where the jaws will function in an open position, (4) use light vertical therapeutic clenching to minimize vertical forces, (5) correct nasal airway obstruction and sleep apnea issues by performing the appropriate surgical procedures so the patients can breathe through their noses instead of requiring mouth breathing, and (6) use Temporary anchoring devices (TADs) or similar devices with vertical elastics so that the stress is placed on the basal bone structures and not on the teeth.

If vertical elastics are necessary for an extended time, it may be important to maintain the palatal splint in place or have a heavy maxillary arch wire in position. The use of posterior vertical elastics will tend to narrow the transverse width of the maxillary arch tipping the posterior teeth palatally creating posterior cross-bite relationships.

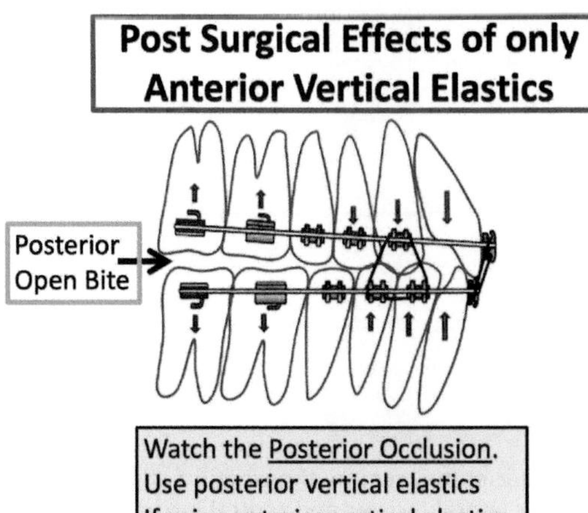

Fig. 4. Vertical elastics, if only used anteriorly, tend to extrude the anterior teeth and intrude the posterior teeth creating posterior open bites.

Power Chains

Avoid the use of power chains particularly in the upper arch after surgery. The use of power chains is a relatively common technique in the orthodontic finishing phase of treatment (**Fig. 5**A). However, postsurgical use of power chains and the forces created can extrude the anterior teeth, create increased torque on the incisors, tipping the incisor edges lingually and the root tips labially, as well as close space created to correct tooth size discrepancies. This can cause premature contact of the incisors with subsequent end-on incisor relationship and development of posterior open bites (**Fig. 5**B). When this problem is identified, the power chain should be immediately removed, and mechanics reversed to tip the incisor edges forward and the root tips posteriorly. Corrective treatment may involve reopening space between the lateral incisors and cuspids, intruding the incisors, and extruding the posterior teeth into occlusion. TADs could be required to intrude the incisors. Spacing created between the lateral incisors and cuspids can be eliminated post orthodontically with bonding, veneers, or crowns on the lateral incisors (**Fig. 6**).

Change Arch Wires

Segmental osteotomies in the maxilla or mandible commonly require the arch wire to be cut into sections. Generally, the arch wires can be changed at about 4 to 6 weeks after surgery. It is usually too uncomfortable for patients to tolerate the arch wire change before that time. If a palatal splint is in place, it can remain in place because it should not interfere with the arch wire change and the splint can continue to help with maxillary

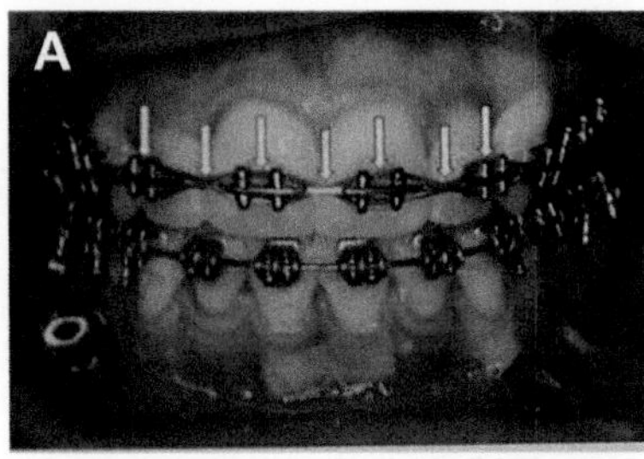

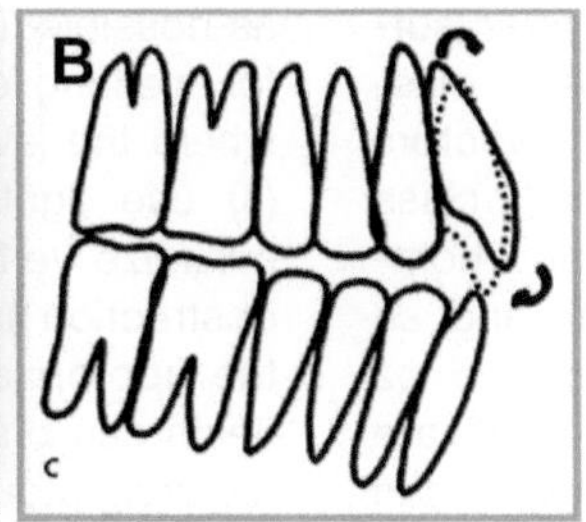

Fig. 5. (*A*) Postsurgical use of power chains and the forces created can extrude teeth and create increased torque on the incisors, tipping the incisor edges lingually and the root tips labially. (*B*) This can cause premature contact of the incisors with subsequent end-on incisor relationship and development of posterior open bites.

transverse stability. Occlusal coverage splints usually require removal before the arch wire can be changed.

Dental Arch Spacing

The correction of significant anterior tooth size discrepancies may require the creation of space in the upper arch between the lateral incisors and cuspids, and/or lateral incisors and central incisors to assure a good class I occlusal fit with proper over-jet/overbite relationship[9] (see **Fig. 6**A). It is very important in the postsurgical patient management phase that the space is maintained for subsequent bonding, veneers, or

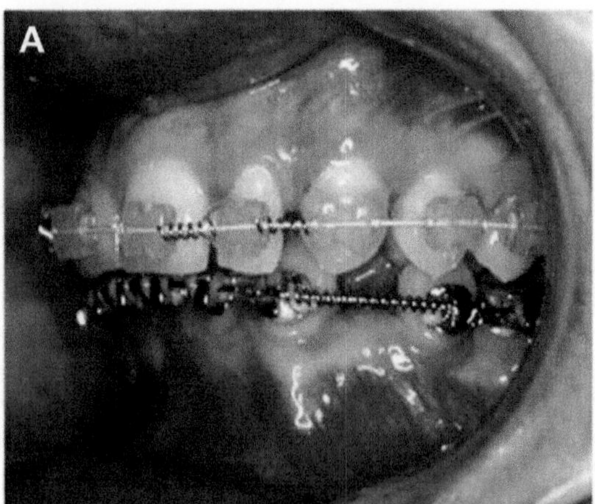

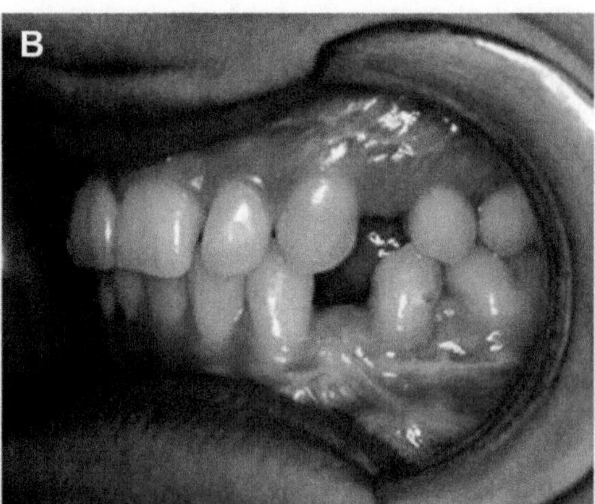

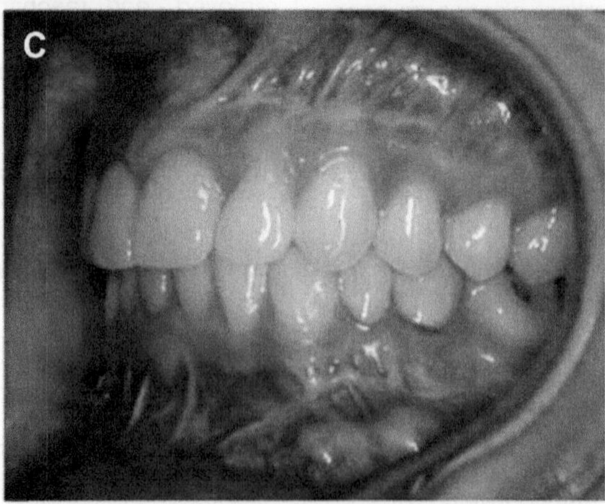

Fig. 6. (*A*) The correction of significant anterior tooth size discrepancies may require the creation of space in the upper arch usually between the lateral incisors and cuspids, and/or lateral incisors and central incisors (note the coil springs in position) to ensure a good class I occlusal fit with proper over-jet/overbite relationship. This case also opened bicuspid spaces as well. (*B*) It is very important that the spaces are maintained at the completion of orthodontics for (*C*) subsequent bonding, veneers, or crowns to correct for the tooth size discrepancy and to replace missing teeth.

crowns (see **Fig. 6**B, C). Do note close the space, because this can result in a significant malocclusion. A common postsurgery orthodontic practice is to close interdental spaces with a power chain (see **Fig. 5**). This can create major occlusal problems by downward and backward retraction of the maxillary incisors resulting in an end-on incisor relationship, posterior open bites, downward and backward rotation of the mandible, increased stress on the TMJs, and pain. If this situation occurs, the spaces need to be opened again with forward rotation of the incisors to improve the occlusal fit with subsequent restorative dentistry to eliminate the spaces with bonding, veneers, or crowns.

Tooth Movement

Teeth move more rapidly for about the first 6 months after surgery as compared with before the surgery. Relative to tooth movement, the orthodontist can usually accomplish in 1 to 2 weeks after surgery that took 3 to 4 weeks before surgery. This is because the bone metabolism and bone turnover increases substantially after surgery, allowing more rapid bone resorption and apposition in response to orthodontic forces, so the teeth move more quickly. In addition, with segmental maxillary surgery, the individual bone segments can also move some, providing increased flexibility of the teeth and bone units.

Finishing Orthodontics

It is important for the surgery patient to keep the orthodontic appliances on for a minimum of 4 to 6 months after orthognathic surgery, when appropriate rigid fixation techniques are used, to allow for initial bone healing as well as finish aligning, leveling, and stabilizing the occlusion. It usually takes 4 months to complete the initial postsurgical bone healing phase to where the maxilla and mandible should be skeletally stable, although the completion of bone healing will take about 1 year.[3,4] If inadequate rigid fixation was used or the maxillary bone was exceptionally thin, or uncontrolled clenching/bruxism is present, then orthodontic appliances may be required for a significantly extended time. The greater and more complex required surgical movements and presurgical orthodontic treatment mechanics, generally the longer the time requirements for the postsurgical orthodontic management. The orthodontist determines when the occlusion is maximized, stabilized, and the patient is ready for debanding and retainers.

Retainers

For patients who have undergone orthognathic surgery, with or without concomitant TMJ surgery, rigid retainers (Hawley or wraparound type) without occlusal coverage (**Fig. 7**) are recommended to provide transverse support to the width of the maxillary and mandibular dental arches, maintain the dental alignment, and allow for maximal interdigitation of the occlusion. Occlusal coverage retainers, such as Essex type (**Fig. 8**), should not be used because of vertical separation of the occlusion because this can create a malocclusion, usually with open bite situations anteriorly or posteriorly, unilaterally, or bilaterally. In addition, occlusal coverage retainers are usually flexible (see **Fig. 8**B) and do not provide adequate transverse stability resulting in transverse relapse in cases of surgical or orthodontic expansion or narrowing of the dental arches that can result in anterior open bite and posterior cross-bite relationships. Hawley or wraparound retainers are the devices of choice (see **Fig. 7**). For the mandibular arch where no expansion, narrowing, extrusion, intrusion, or other potential unstable orthodontics has occurred, a 3 $\times$ 3 or similar type of retainer may be adequate.

IDENTIFYING POSTSURGICAL PROBLEMS

This section discusses common problems that can be encountered after surgery and the management of those problems. If problems arise, early identification and appropriate management usually minimizes the subsequent adverse effects.

Infection

Although relatively uncommon, infections can occur after orthognathic surgery. Clinical signs of infection can include (1) elevated temperature, (2) usually unilateral swelling that gets progressively worse, (3) erythema (redness and hot feeling) over the area, (4) soft tissue induration (firmness) over area, (5) purulence (pus) coming out of incision areas or draining nasally or into the oropharyngeal area, (6) bad taste in mouth, (7) bad smell, (8) difficulties opening the jaws owing to associated muscle trismus, and (9) increased pain, particularly over the involved area. Sinus infections can also occur and generate clinical symptoms, such as (1) fullness and pressure in cheek and upper jaw, (2) increased sensitivity to maxillary teeth, (3) nasal and postnasal drainage of purulent material, (4) bad taste, (5) offensive

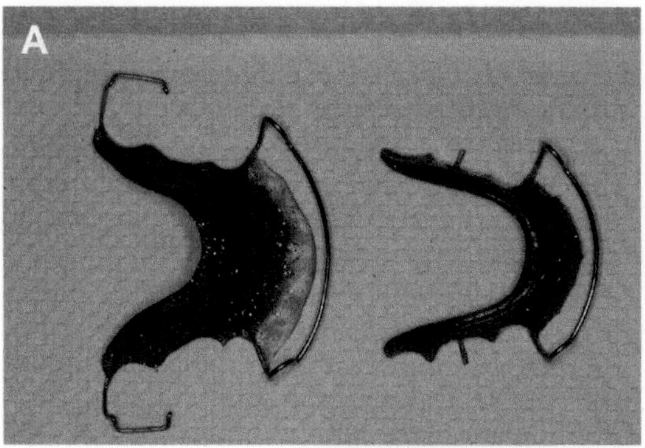

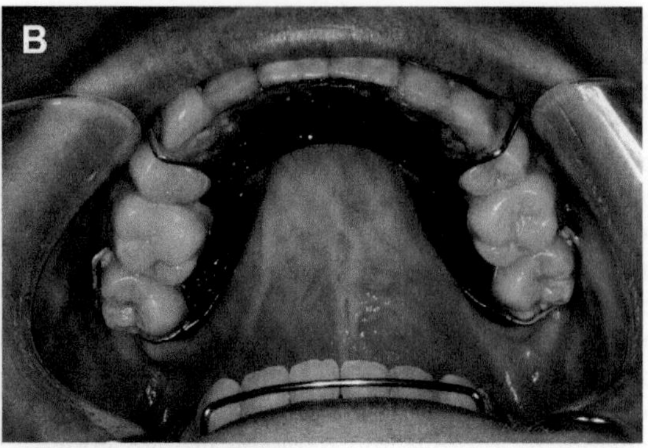

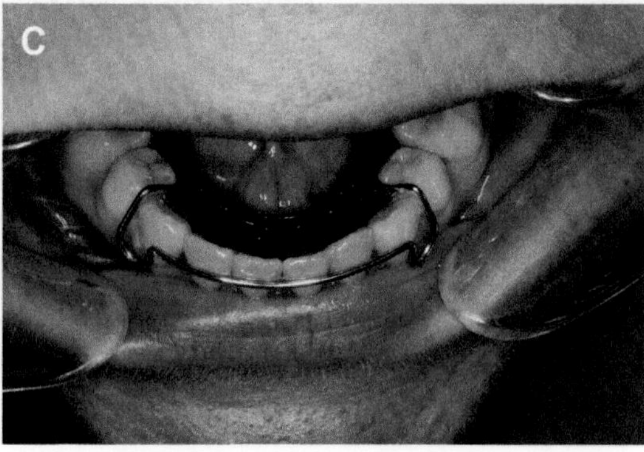

Fig. 7. (*A*) Rigid retainers (Hawley or wraparound types) without occlusal coverage are recommended to maintain dental alignment and provide transverse support to the maxillary (*B*) and mandibular (*C*) arches. (*C*) These retainers should allow maximal interdigitation of the occlusion.

smell, (6) pain, and (7) facial swelling. If any of these signs occur, the surgeon should be notified immediately so the etiology can be identified, cultures and sensitivities taken, drainage and irrigations performed if indicated, and the patient started on appropriate antibiotics. If an infection occurs and identified early, it is usually relatively easily managed. However, an infection could require additional management such as incision and drainage, irrigation protocol, antibiotics, debridement, scrubbing of devices such as bone plates, TMJ prostheses, and removal of infected bone grafts or hardware.

Tooth Discoloration

Although uncommon, a tooth may become discolored after orthognathic surgery. When this occurs, it is usually associated with a tooth adjacent to an interdental osteotomy, but not always. The discoloration is caused by disruption of the vessels to the pulp canal leading to hemorrhage or necrosis of the pulpal tissues. The viability of the tooth usually remains intact, but the vitality is lost. Treatment usually involves root canal therapy and bleaching, or if indicated, a veneer or crown.

Tooth Ankylosis

Tooth ankylosis can be present before surgery or develop as a result of the surgery. During surgery, ankylosis can develop as a result of cutting into the root of a tooth while an interdental osteotomy is being performed, or decreased vascularity to an alveolar segment that could cause loss of the periodontal ligament resulting in ankylosis. When ankylosis occurs, the affected tooth does not respond to orthodontic mechanics; rather, the tooth acts as an anchor and pulls the adjacent teeth toward the ankylosed tooth, which could create a malocclusion. Proper presurgery orthodontic preparation and careful surgery should prevent this problem from occurring. If an ankylosed tooth is identified after surgery and that tooth is out of occlusion, then the tooth should be disengaged from the arch wire and the rest of the teeth finalized and retained. The ankylosed tooth can be crowned, bonded, or a single tooth osteotomy can be performed to reposition it into the best occlusal fit.

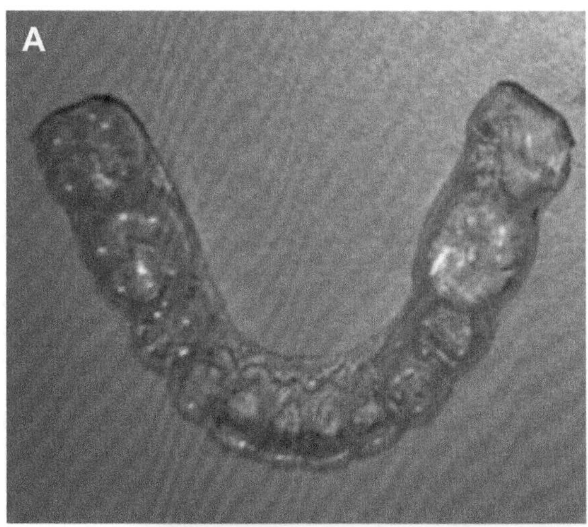

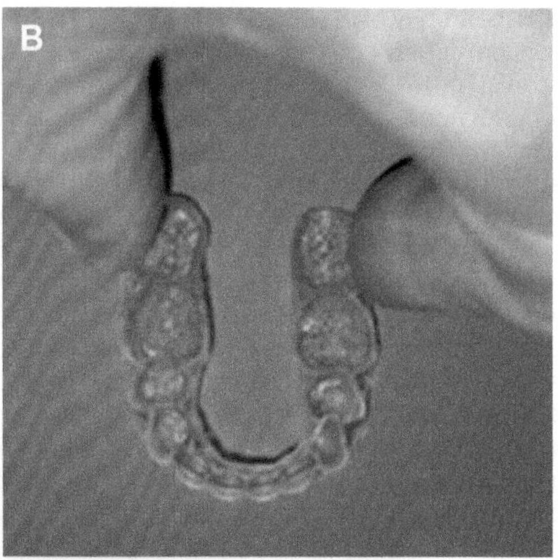

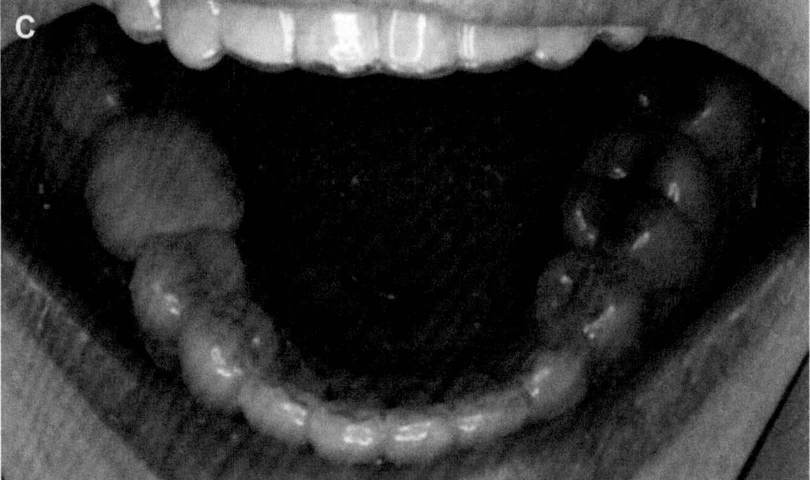

Fig. 8. (*A*) Occlusal coverage retainers are not recommended; because of the vertical separation between the maxillary and mandibular teeth, the splints may not interdigitate with each other. (*B*) The splints are usually flexible and do not provide transverse stability that can result in malocclusion, such as anterior or posterior open bites and posterior cross-bite relationships. (*C*) The retainers are more esthetic and easier to construct, but with significant liability to treatment outcomes.

Early Jaw and Occlusal Instability

Factors that contribute to skeletal and occlusal instability early in the postsurgical orthodontic treatment are usually evident within the first few days or weeks and include (1) TMJ edema, (2) inadequate surgical stabilization, (3) improper surgical positioning of the maxilla and/or mandible, (4) hypertrophy of the TMJ bilaminar tissues from presurgical long-term anterior repositioning splints, growth appliances, long-term class II mechanics (ie, Herbst appliance, class II elastics), or the chronic Sunday bite, (5) TMJ condylar displacement at surgery, and (6) orthodontic instability.

TMJ edema can occur when excessively traumatic orthognathic surgery has been performed causing swelling of the TMJ bilaminar tissues, intercapsular bleeding, or when simultaneous TMJ surgery has been performed along with the orthognathic surgery. Intraoperative TMJ edema that is present when the occlusion is set into the best fit cause the occlusion to shift toward a class II anterior open bite relationship as the edema resolves. Class II and anterior vertical elastics may help salvage the treatment results. TMJ edema that occurs immediately after surgery usually displaces the condyle and mandible forward 1 to 3 mm and creates a posterior open bite. The use of light force vertical and class III directional elastics helps to minimize and dissipate the edema. The condyles settle up and back with the mandible and occlusion following.

Hypertrophy of the bilaminar tissues can be present presurgery as a result of anterior repositioning splints, growth appliances, Herbst appliances, long-term class II mechanics, chronic Sunday bite, and specific TMJ pathologies. Orthognathic surgery, and particularly mandibular advancements, increase pressure on the TMJ, which slowly causes the bilaminar tissue to thin out, allowing the mandible to slowly retrude until the joints establish an equilibrium. This process may cause a shift of the occlusion toward a class II position and anterior open bite tendency, requiring extended orthodontics or additional surgery. When hypertrophy of the bilaminar tissues preexists the intended surgery, then class III mechanics can be used presurgery to decrease the tissue thickness to minimize the postsurgical relapse potential.

Inadequate stabilization of the maxilla and/or mandible could allow the jaws and occlusion to drift out of alignment, making it difficult to control the occlusion after surgery. This is usually due to inadequate rigid fixation, failure to bone graft when indicated, and/or clenching and bruxism. When the maxilla is involved, it tends to settle upward and/or posteriorly, creating a shift toward class III skeletal and occlusal relationship. This situation may result in a mobile maxilla, nonunion, facial imbalance, malocclusion, and requirements for further corrective surgery. When the mandible is inadequately stabilized, shifting of the mandible usually creates an anterior open bite and a shift toward class II or III occlusion, depending on the type and location of fixation that was initially used. These situations can be avoided by proper and adequate rigid fixation, appropriate grafting being applied at the time of surgery, and controlling clenching and bruxism.

Improper positioning of the maxilla and/or mandible at surgery can occur as a result of (1) unrecognized bony interferences, (2) poor positional placement of the maxilla and/or mandible, (3) poor adaptation of the bone plates and screws to the maxilla and/or mandible so that when the bone screws are tightened, the maxilla and/or mandible becomes displaced, (4) displacement of the mandibular condyles relative to the fossa and centric relation position, and (5) poorly fitting occlusal coverage splint (see **Fig. 2**). Any of these situations can result in malalignment of the jaws, functional and esthetic imbalances, and a malocclusion. This could result in the need for additional surgery if the orthodontist is unable to make dental compensations to achieve a reasonable result. These situations can be avoided by performing accurate surgery.

Orthodontic instability and relapse can also cause changes and is particularly related to transverse or vertical relapse of the orthodontically expanded maxilla or unstable dental extrusions or intrusions. Transverse collapse of the maxillary dentition will usually cause posterior cross-bites and dental interferences, as well as an anterior open bite. Transverse stability is paramount to provide predictable treatment outcomes. Also, inappropriate orthodontic closure of spaces created for correcting tooth size discrepancies is another orthodontic factor contributing to unwanted postsurgical occlusal changes. Performing careful stable orthodontics, providing good surgical results, no indiscriminate closing of spaces, and appropriate retention, should prevent these types of problems, providing that the TMJs are healthy and stable.

Late Jaw and Occlusal Instability

The factors commonly contributory to late (after 4–6 months) jaw and occlusal changes are usually related to (1) orthodontic instability or improper use of postsurgical orthodontic mechanics, (2) vertical, anteroposterior, and/or transverse maxillary surgical instability, (3) nonunion of the maxilla or mandible with continued shifting and settling, (4) failure to use proper postorthodontic retention, that is, rigid retainers, and/or (5) TMJ disorders and pathology.

Orthodontic and maxillary surgical instability have been discussed in previous sections of this article. These are major potential relapse factors. However, in cases treated with stable presurgery orthodontics, precise surgery, proper postsurgery patient management, and appropriate long-term retention, then these factors are usually nonissues. If instability is identified in the postsurgery stage of treatment, then using orthodontic mechanics, transpalatal bars, palatal retainers, heavy labial arch wires, elastics, or other devices may enable salvage of the case. The sooner the problems are identified and treated, the better the recovery. Proper postorthodontic retention is necessary using rigid retainers without occlusal coverage. Long-term retention will likely be necessary.

Nonunion of the maxilla or mandible can cause the jaws to keep shifting and create worsening occlusion with inability for the orthodontist to compensate and finalize the occlusion. These situations sometimes can be salvaged by quick action with appropriate mechanical forces and stabilization. Because clenching and bruxism can be contributory, control of these factors is paramount. Additional surgery may be necessary is some cases to correct the nonunion problem by repositioning the mandible and/or maxilla if indicated and applying appropriate rigid fixation and bone grafting.

Temporomandibular Joint Pathology

TMJ pathology or conditions are a common source for late skeletal and occlusal instability following orthognathic surgery as well as continued pain, headaches, and jaw dysfunction. The instabilities are usually a result of preexisting untreated TMJ pathology or TMJ conditions created by the orthognathic surgery such as excessively traumatic surgery that damages the joints or overloading the TMJs by intentionally creating posterior open bites at surgery. The most common TMJ-associated problem condylar resorption resulting with progressive shifting of the mandible and occlusion into a class II relationship with or without anterior open bite. Common condylar resorption conditions include adolescent internal condylar resorption (AICR), idiopathic condylar resorption, reactive arthritis, and connective tissue/autoimmune diseases such as juvenile idiopathic arthritis, rheumatoid arthritis, psoriatic arthritis, lupus, scleroderma, Sjogrens syndrome, ankylosing spondylitis, and other conditions.[10,11] Post Orthognathic surgical relapse in teenagers can often be attributed to the hormonally related condition of AICR with a 8:1 female to male occurrence ratio.[12,13] In this specific condition, the articular discs are always anteriorly dislocated, the condyles surrounded by hyperplastic synovial tissue, and the condyles slowly resorb. These patients initially present with a high occlusal plane angle facial morphology with retrusion of the mandible, commonly develop a class II open bite malocclusion, and the symptoms are usually mild to moderate, with 25% of patients having no symptoms; just slow condylar resorption. These patients, if treated within 4 years of onset, can be predictably treated with disc repositioning with Mitek anchors and orthognathic surgery. However, if orthognathic surgery only is performed on these patients, continued condylar resorption occurs with redevelopment of mandibular retrusion as seen in case 1 (**Fig. 9**A–D) with failed previous orthodontics two time and double jaw orthognathic surgery. In teenagers, this condition has a highly successful treatment protocol of surgically repositioning the articular discs and stabilizing with Mitek Anchors (Mitek Inc., Norwood, MA), if performed within 4 years of the TMJ onset, followed by orthognathic surgery performed at the same surgery or at a later surgery.[12–14] An adult patient who had this condition as a teenager, where it had gone into remission, will have a high risk of reinitiating further condylar resorption and increased pain after orthognathic surgery, particularly requiring mandibular advancement, if the TMJs are not properly treated. These adult patients and many of the other resorptive TMJ pathologies may have the most predictable treatment outcomes with custom-made total joint prostheses.[10,11,15,16]

Case 1

A 30-year old woman developed AICR of the TMJs beginning at the age of 12 years. She was treated orthodontically at age 14 to 16 with all 4 first bicuspids extracted, but developed an anterior open bite as well as TMJ pain, ear pain, and myofascial pain. She was in splint therapy (splints $\times$8) from age 20 to 30. Orthodontics were reinitiated at age 27. Double jaw orthognathic surgery was performed at age 28, which predictably relapsed (see **Fig. 9**A–D). The author initially saw the patient at 2 years after surgery. MRI and computed tomography scans showed severe condylar resorption and anterior displaced discs that were severely deformed and nonsalvageable. A cephalometric analysis (**Fig. 10**A) aided in the diagnosis and the prediction tracing (**Fig. 10**B) provided the blueprint for surgical correction that included counterclockwise rotation of the maxillomandibular complex with the mandible advancing 18 mm at pogonion. Virtual surgical planning was used for final planning and splint construction (**Fig. 11**). Bilateral patient-fitted TMJ total joint prostheses were manufactured for predictable outcome stability (**Fig. 12**). She was treatment planned for presurgical and postsurgical orthodontics and single-stage surgical intervention that included (1) bilateral TMJ reconstruction and counterclockwise mandibular advancement with patient-fitted total joint prostheses, (2) bilateral TMJ fat grafts, (3) bilateral coronoidectomies, (4) maxillary osteotomies, (5) bilateral partial turbinectomies, and (6) rhinoplasty. The patient is seen 2 years after surgery (**Fig. 9**E–H) demonstrating significantly improved function and esthetics as well as elimination of the pain factors.

The most common TMJ condition leading to class III skeletal and occlusal relapse is associated with unrecognized and untreated condylar hyperplasia (CH) type 1.[17,18] CH type 1 is a bilateral or unilateral TMJ condition where the normal condylar growth mechanism grows at an accelerated rate and extends beyond the normal growth years. It is initiated in the teenage years and the growth can continue into the early to mid 20s. This condition, when recognized, can be predictably treated with high condylectomies that stops

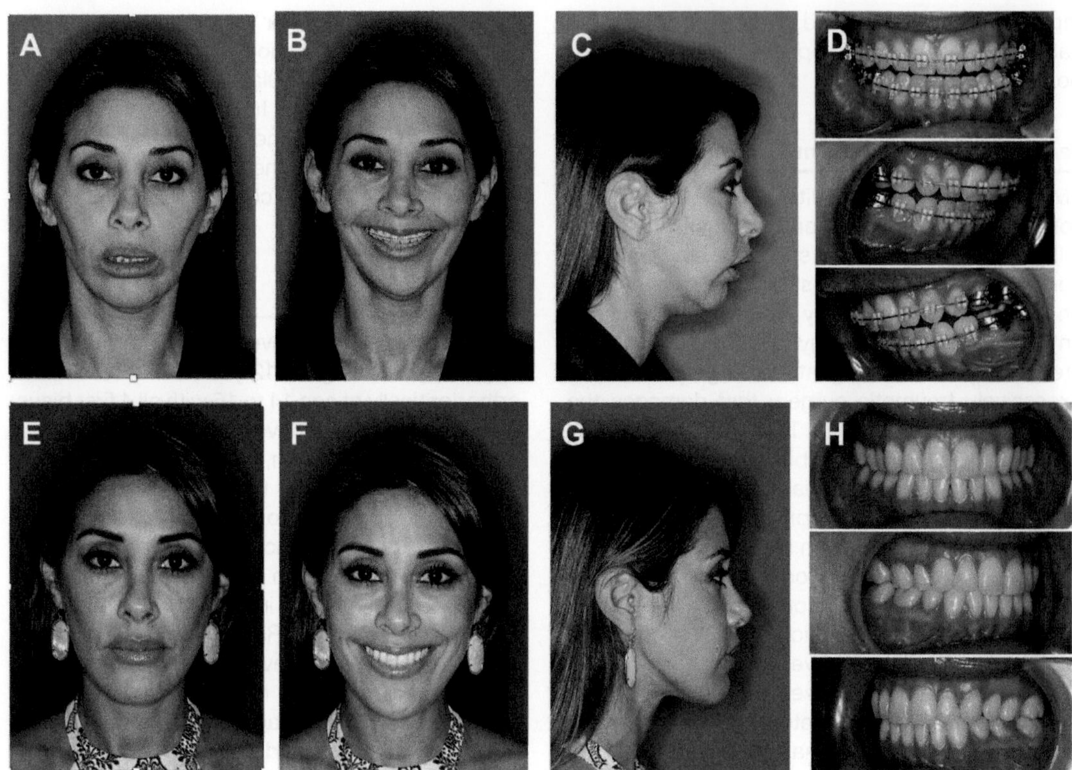

Fig. 9. Case 1. (*A–D*) A 30-year-old woman with AICR, nonsalvageable discs, condylar resorption, mandibular retrusion, and severe TMJ pain. She had previous orthodontics twice and failed double jaw orthognathic surgery. (*E–H*) Patient seen 2 years after surgery with a stable, pain-free outcome following TMJ reconstruction and mandibular advancement with TMJ patient-fitted total joint prostheses, maxillary osteotomies, and orthodontics.

the growth so orthognathic surgery can be performed predictably at the same operation[17,18] or at separate operations, but the high condylectomies must be done first.

Case 2

A 23-year-old woman was referred to the author after failed previous treatment. She was diagnosed with mandibular prognathism as a teenager but had unrecognized active CH type 1. She had orthodontics from age 11 to 16, orthodontics for another year at age 17, and again at age 20. She had orthognathic surgery for a mandibular setback at age 14 that relapsed into a class III relationship. She had double jaw orthognathic surgery at age 18, but the mandible relapsed into a class III relation again. She had a third orthognathic surgery at the age of 21 for a mandibular setback, but her mandible relapsed again. The author initially saw the patient at age 23 (2 years after the third failed

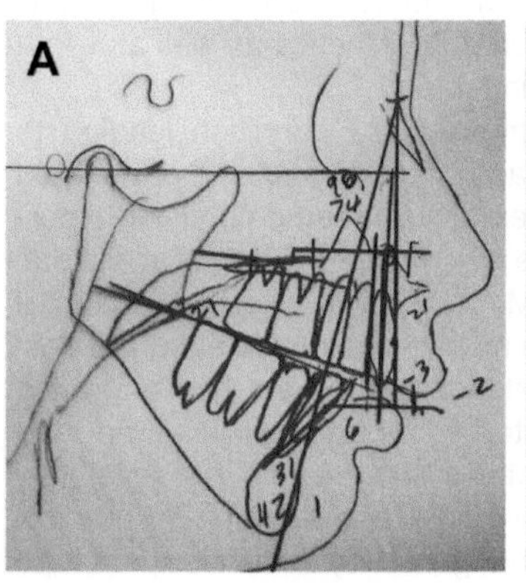

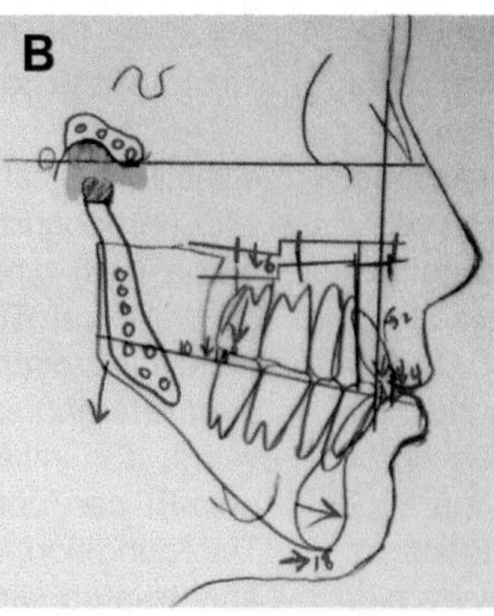

Fig. 10. Case 1. (*A*) Lateral cephalometric tracing showing jaw deformity with retruded mandible and high occlusal plane facial morphology. (*B*) Surgical prediction tracing with counterclockwise rotation of the maxillomandibular complex, bilateral TMJ reconstruction and advancement of the mandible, and maxillary osteotomies.

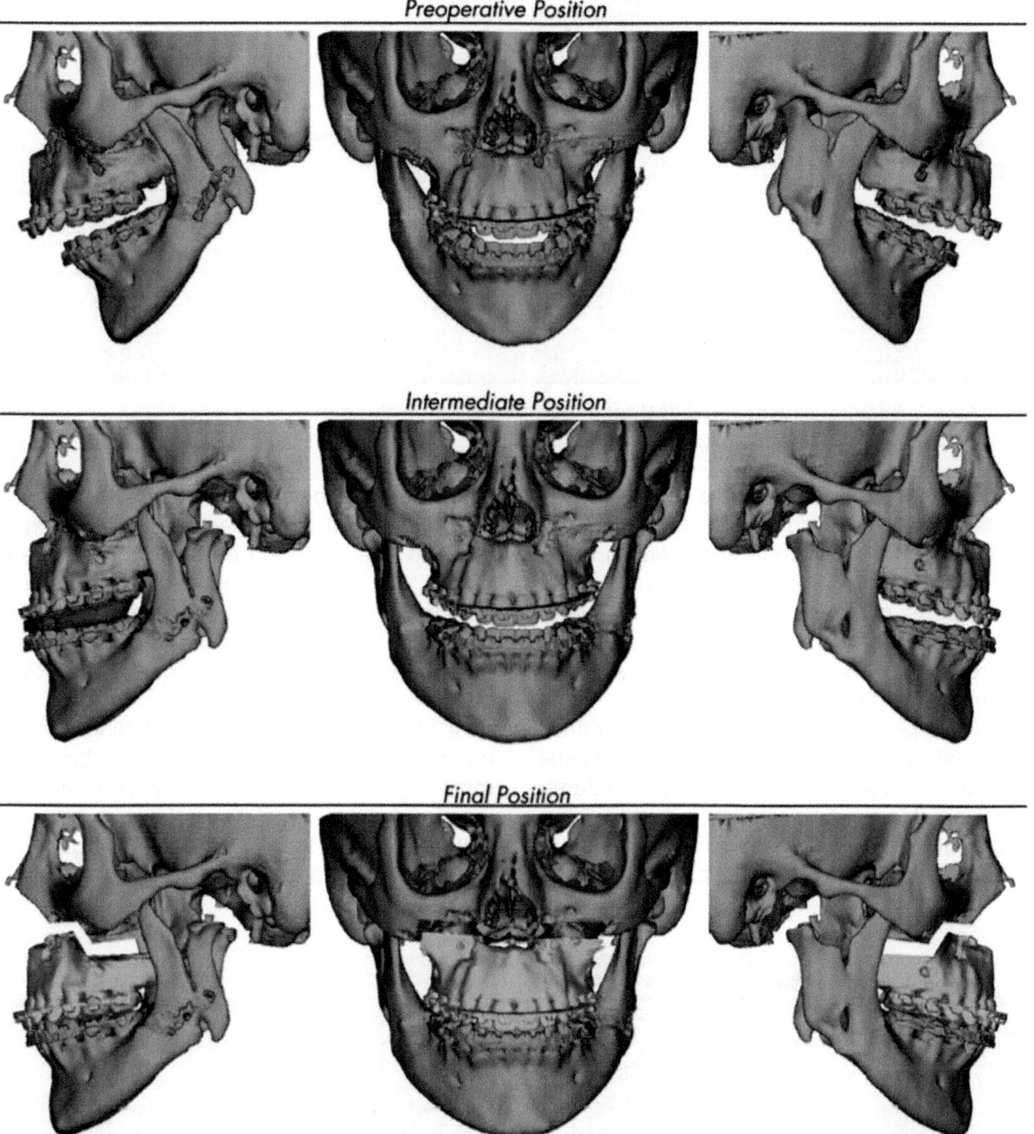

Fig. 11. Case 1. Virtual surgical planning with the initial relationship in the top row, repositioning the mandible with TMJ total joint prostheses in the middle row, and the final positioning of the maxilla to the mandible in the bottom row.

orthognathic surgery procedure) and diagnosed her with active CH type 1A (**Fig. 13**A–D). MRI showed she had bilateral posteriorly displaced articular discs (**Fig. 14**). The years of orthodontics caused severe root resorption of her teeth, and particularly the maxillary incisors (**Fig. 15**A). Presurgery lateral cephalogram showed the skeletal and occlusal class III relationship with anterior cross-bite and open bite (**Fig. 15**B). Because of the failed 3 previous surgical procedures, and severe root resorption, she refused the recommended double jaw surgery, so treatment was confined to presurgical orthodontics with segmentalization of the maxillary arch wire to decrease stress on the teeth to minimize further root resorption. Surgery included (1) bilateral TMJ high condylectomies to arrest the mandibular growth, (2) bilateral articular disc repositioning with Mitek anchors, (3) multiple maxillary osteotomies to reposition the maxilla by advancement and expansion as well as maximize the occlusal fit, and (4) anteroposterior reduction genioplasty. This procedure was followed by minimal postsurgery orthodontics. The patient was seen at 15 months after

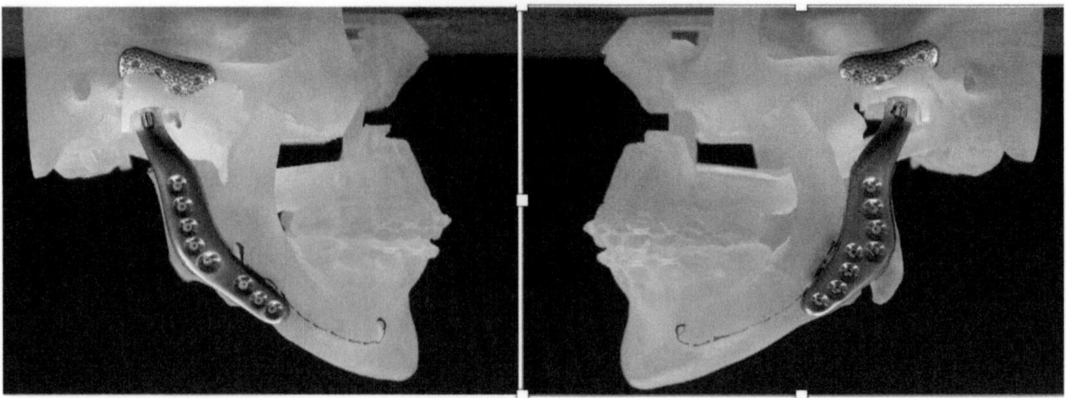

Fig. 12. Case 1. Bilateral patient-fitted TMJ total joint prosthesis on the stereolithic model.

surgery with a stable outcome (**Fig. 13**E–H; **Fig. 15**C, D). If the mandibular high condylectomies would have been done in the first orthognathic surgery procedure, the growth and relapse problem of the mandible would have been eliminated, avoiding the 3 additional orthognathic surgery procedures and the severe root resorption would have been avoided.

The development of transverse facial asymmetry in the late postsurgery phase of treatment usually means 1 condyle is resorbing (ie, unilateral, AICR, idiopathic condylar resorption, juvenile idiopathic arthritis, reactive arthritis, rheumatoid arthritis, psoriatic arthritis) or 1 condyle is growing (ie, osteochondroma, osteoma, unilateral CH type 1B, tumor). With a unilateral condylar resorption problem, the occlusion on the involved side will usually contact prematurely, the occlusion will shift toward a class II relationship, and a cross-bite may develop. The contralateral side may develop a slight open bite but can retain a class I occlusion with a buccal cross-bite tendency.[10,11,14] With a unilateral pathologic growing condyle, on the involved side, the occlusion may remain class I or shift into a class III and may develop an ipsilateral open bite. A cross-bite may develop on the contralateral side as well as development of a transverse cant to the occlusal

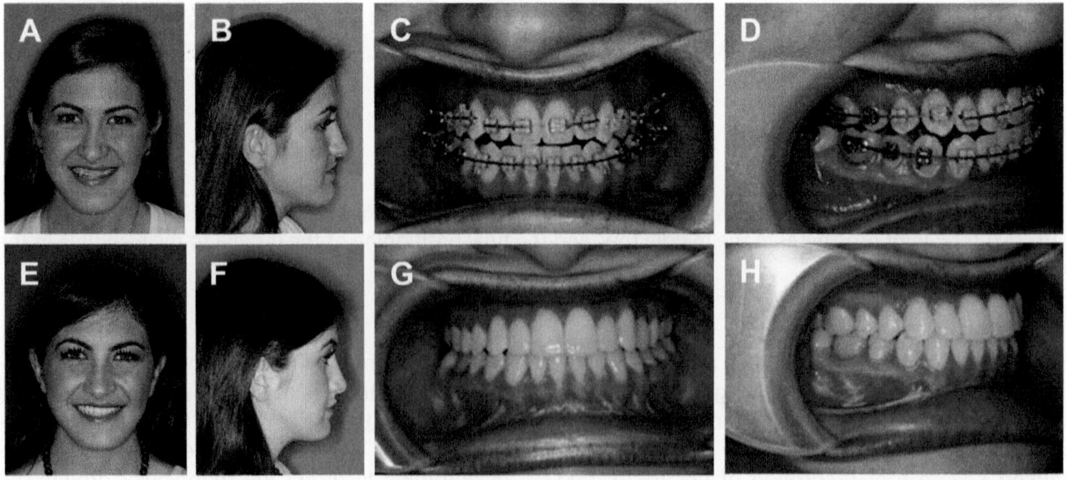

Fig. 13. Case 2. (*A, B*) A 23-year-old woman with bilateral CH type 1A, active since age 13 years. She had failed orthodontic treatment 3 times and relapsed orthognathic surgery procedures 3 times as a result of CH type 1A with repeated mandibular relapse into a class III skeletal and occlusal relation. (*C, D*) The extensive orthodontics have resulted in severe root resorption affecting all of her teeth. The maxillary arch wire was sectioned to minimize stress on the teeth. Surgery included (1) bilateral TMJ high condylectomies to arrest the abnormal mandibular growth, (2) repositioning of the bilateral posteriorly displaced articular discs, (3) maxillary osteotomies to advance and expand, and (4) anteroposterior reduction genioplasty. (*E–H*) The patient is seen 15 months after surgery with a stable result.

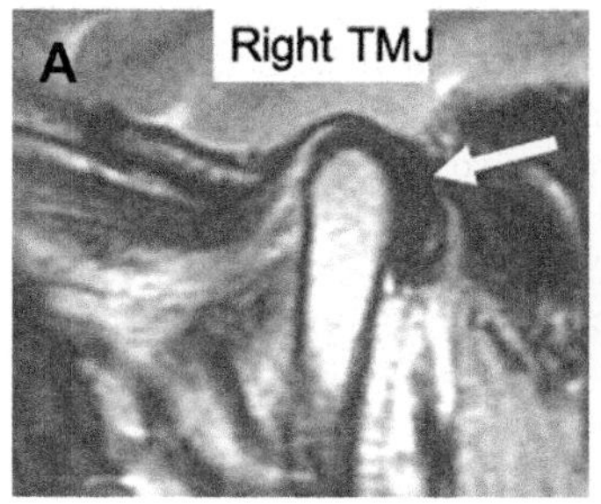

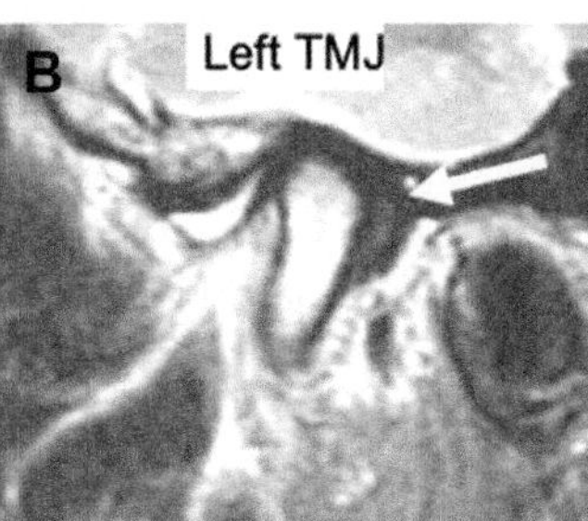

Fig. 14. Case 2. These MRIs clearly demonstrate the bilateral posterior displacement of the articular discs. (*A*) Right side, and (*B*) left side.

plane. If the mandibular shift is primarily a horizontal shift with a class III occlusion development on 1 side with the mandible shifting toward the opposite side where a cross-bite develops, then the diagnosis is likely unilateral CH type 1B, which can continue to grow into the mid 20s. This condition can be predictably treated with a mandibular high condylectomy on the involved side with repositioning of the articular disc, and the appropriate orthognathic surgery to obtain the best functional and esthetic outcomes.[17,18]

If the asymmetric growth is primarily in a vertical direction with the mandible and face unilaterally lengthening vertically, a lateral open bite developing on the same side, mandible shifting to the opposite side, and radiographic evidence of an ipsilateral enlarged and deformed condyle, then likely an osteochondroma or osteoma has developed in the condyle. This condition can be predictably treated with a low condylectomy, recontouring of the condylar neck, placing the articular disc over the remaining condylar neck, reposition the disc and new condyle in the fossa, and perform the necessary orthognathic surgery to achieve the best functional and esthetic results.[19–22] With class I or III facial and occlusal

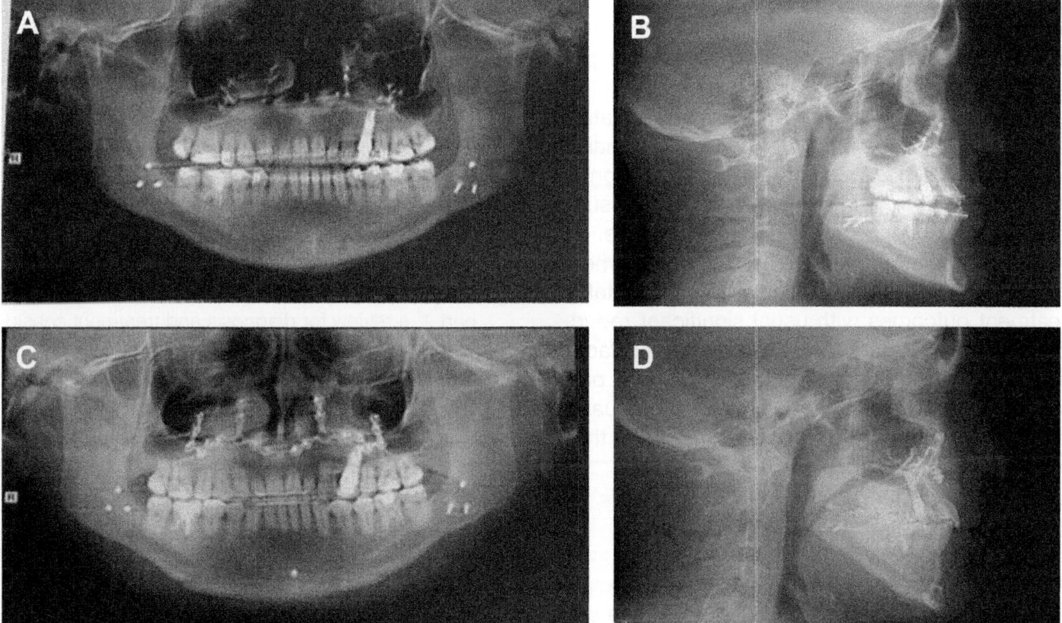

Fig. 15. Case 2. (*A*) Presurgery panogram shows evidence of previous surgery and the generalized severe root resorption, particularly noted on the maxillary incisors. (*B*) Presurgery lateral cephalogram shows the skeletal and occlusal class III relation, with an anterior cross-bite and anterior open bite. (*C*) The 15-month postsurgery panogram shows no worsening of the root resorption as a result of the minimal stresses placed on the teeth by using segmented arch wire and multiple maxillary segmentation to reposition the dentoalveolar structures and teeth into occlusion. (*D*) The 15-month lateral cephalogram shows establishment of a stable occlusal and skeletal class I relationship with a normal overbite.

asymmetry, the TMJ pathologic condition on the involved side increases the loading on the contralateral TMJ commonly causing articular disc dislocation and arthritis in that joint, which may indicate the necessity to perform disc repositioning or other indicated treatment to get the best treatment results.

TMJ pathology should be identified before the initial surgery and treated at the same time as the orthognathic surgery or at a separate operation before the orthognathic surgery. However, if the TMJ pathology is not identified until later, additional TMJ and orthognathic surgery may be necessary to correct and stabilize the TMJs, jaws, and occlusion.[7,8,10,11,16]

SUMMARY

Postsurgical patient management is a very important aspect of the treatment for providing optimal patient outcomes. Immediate postsurgical orthodontics should be approached aggressively if necessary to maximize high-quality occlusal results in the shortest time frame. It is important to understand orthodontic treatment protocols to facilitate good results and to be aware of those orthodontic mechanics that have a negative impact on outcomes. Early identification and proper management of postsurgical problems, such as infection, early relapses, and late relapses that may involve unrecognized and/or untreated TMJ pathology will improve treatment outcomes.

The TMJs are a vital component of orthognathic surgery, but are commonly ignored by clinicians. Failure to diagnose and properly treat TMJ conditions can result in relapse, unsatisfactory results relative to functional and esthetic outcomes, as well as pain and headaches. Proper management of TMJ pathology can provide highly predictable treatment outcomes with usual significant reduction in pain and improved jaw function and facial esthetics. Understanding the information presented in this article should improve the quality of postsurgical patient management and thus improve treatment outcomes.

REFERENCES

1. Wolford LM, Karras S, Mehra P. Concomitant temporomandibular joint and orthognathic surgery: a preliminary report. J Oral Maxillofac Surg 2002;60: 356–62.
2. Wolford LM. Concomitant temporomandibular joint and orthognathic surgery. J Oral Maxillofac Surg 2003;61:1198–204.
3. Ayers RA, Simske SJ, Nunes CR, et al. Long-term bone ingrowth and residual microhardness of porous block hydroxyapatite implants in humans. J Oral Maxillofac Surg 1998;56:1297–301.
4. Ayers RA, Wolford LM, Bateman TA, et al. Quantification of bone ingrowth into porous block hydroxyapatite in humans. J Biomed Mater Res 1999;47:54–9.
5. Pitta M, Castro V, Wolford LM. Stability of maxillary downgraft procedures using rigid fixation and porous block hydroxyapatite grafts. J Oral Maxillofac Surg 1999;57(Suppl 1):97–8.
6. Mehra P, Castro V, Freitas RZ, et al. Stability of the Le Fort I osteotomy for maxillary advancement using rigid fixation and porous block hydroxyapatite grafting. Oral Surg Oral Med Oral Pathol Oral Radiol Endod 2002;94:18–23.
7. Wolford LM, Reische-Fischel O, Mehra P. Changes in temporomandibular joint dysfunction after orthognathic surgery. J Oral Maxillofac Surg 2003;61: 655–60.
8. Fuselier C, Wolford LM, Pitta M, et al. Condylar changes after orthognathic surgery with untreated TMJ internal derangement. J Oral Maxillofac Surg 1998;56(Suppl 1):61.
9. Wolford LM, Alexander CM, Stevao ELL, et al. Orthodontics for orthognathic surgery. In: Miloro M, editor. Peterson's principles of oral and maxillofacial surgery. Lewiston (NY): BC Decker; 2004. p. 1111–34. Chapter 55.
10. Wolford LM, Goncalves JR. Surgical planning in orthognathic surgery and outcome stability. In: Brennan PA, Schliephake H, Ghali GE, et al, editors. Maxillofacial surgery. 3rd edition. St. Louis (MO): Elsevier Inc.; 2017. p. 1048–126.
11. Wolford LM, Movahed R. Concomitant TMJ and orthognathic surgery: diagnosis and treatment planning. Oral and Maxillofacial Surgery Knowledge Update. American Association of Oral and Maxillofacial Surgeons on line 2014.
12. Wolford LM, Galiano A. Adolescent internal condylar resorption (AICR) of the temporomandibular joint part 1: a review for diagnosis and treatment considerations. Cranio 2019;37(1):35–44.
13. Galiano A, Wolford LM. Adolescent Internal Condylar Resorption (AICR) of the Temporomandibular Joint Can Be Successfully Treated by Disc Repositioning and Orthognathic Surgery Part 2: Treatment Outcomes. CRANIO 2019;37:111–20.
14. Goncalves JR, Cassano DS, Rezende L, et al. Disc repositioning: does it really work? Oral Maxillofacial Surg Clin North America 2015; 27(1):85–107.
15. Wolford LM, Goncalves JR. Condylar resorption of the temporomandibular joint: how do we treat it? Oral Maxillofacial Surg Clin North America 2015; 27(1):47–67.
16. Al-Moraissi EA, Wolford LM. Does temporomandibular joint pathology with or without surgical management affect the stability of counterclockwise

rotation of the maxillo-mandibular complex in orthognathic surgery? A systematic review and meta-analysis. J Oral Maxillofac Surg 2017;75:805–21.

17. Wolford LM, Mehra P, Reiche-Fischel O, et al. Efficacy of high condylectomy for management of condylar hyperplasia. Am J Orthod Dentofacial Orthop 2002;121(2):136–51.
18. Wolford LM, Movahed R, Perez D. A classification system for conditions causing condylar hyperplasia. J Oral Maxillofac Surg 2014;72:567–95.
19. Wolford LM, Mehra P, Franco P. Use of conservative condylectomy for treatment of osteochondroma of the mandibular condyle. J Oral Maxillofac Surg 2002;60:262–8.
20. Wolford LM, Movahed R, Dhameja A, et al. Low condylectomy and orthognathic surgery to treat mandibular condylar osteochondroma: retrospective review of 37 cases. J Oral Maxillofac Surg 2014;72:1704–28.
21. Wolford LM. Facial asymmetry: diagnosis and treatment considerations. In: Fonseca, Marciani, Turvey, editors. Volume III, oral and maxillofacial surgery. 2nd edition. St. Louis: Saunders Elsevier; 2008. p. 272–315. Chapter 13.
22. Wolford LM. Mandibular asymmetry: temporomandibular joint degeneration. In: Bagheri SC, Bell RB, Khan HA, editors. Current therapy in oral and maxillofacial surgery. St. Louis (MO): Elsevier Saunders; 2012. p. 696–725.

Aesthetic Facial Surgery and Orthodontics

Common Goals

Petra Olivieri, MD, DMD[a], Flavio A. Uribe, DDS, MDentSc[b], Faisal A. Quereshy, MD, DDS[c,*]

KEYWORDS

- Facial aesthetics • Orthognathic surgery • Rhinoplasty • Genial enhancement • Malar augmentation • Liposuction • Soft tissue filler • Botox

KEY POINTS

- Oral and maxillofacial surgeons are facial experts uniquely qualified to address functional and structural facial components.
- The treatment sequence is unique for each individual patient, with simultaneous versus delayed procedures having their own unique pros and cons that are evaluated at the time of consultation.
- Many facial aesthetic procedures are minimally invasive and can be performed as an outpatient or same day surgery.
- Facial aesthetic procedures can be divided into bony alterations and soft tissue alterations.
- Bony alterations consist of rhinoplasty, genial enhancement, malar augmentation, and mandibular ramus, angle, and body alterations. Soft tissue alterations consist of: submental contouring, onabotulinum toxin type A, and soft tissue fillers.

ORAL AND MAXILLOFACIAL SURGEONS CAN DO AESTHETIC PROCEDURES

Oral and maxillofacial surgeons are the facial experts and are uniquely qualified to perform aesthetic procedures involving the functional and aesthetic aspects of the face, mouth, teeth, and jaws. Their surgical and dental background allow them to understand the relationship between hard and soft tissues and changes associated with movements. Extensive education and training in surgical procedures involving the skin, muscle, bone, and cartilage finely attune the oral and maxillofacial surgeon to the need for harmony between facial appearance and function. These aesthetic procedures can be performed simultaneously with orthognathic surgery or as a delayed treatment.

AESTHETIC AWARENESS

Patients may not comprehend the relationship between functional correction and structural outcome. It is the role of the oral and maxillofacial surgeon to educate the patient that changes in facial skeleton, muscles, and overlying soft tissue lead to significant change in the profile with minimal enhancements of any of these components.

Disclosure: The authors have nothing to disclose.

[a] Department of Oral and Maxillofacial Surgery, Case Western Reserve University, 9601 Chester Avenue, Cleveland, OH 44106, USA; [b] Division of Orthodontics, Craniofacial Sciences, UConn Health, 263 Farmington Avenue, Farmington, CT 06030-1725, USA; [c] Department of Oral and Maxillofacial Surgery, Case Western Reserve University, University Hospitals Cleveland Medical Center, 9601 Chester Avenue, Cleveland, OH 44106, USA

* Corresponding author.

E-mail address: faq@case.edu

Oral Maxillofacial Surg Clin N Am 32 (2020) 153–165
https://doi.org/10.1016/j.coms.2019.09.004
1042-3699/20/

THE CONSULTATION APPOINTMENT: WHAT TO EXPECT?

The consultation appointment generally consists of 1 to 2 appointments, in which the patient's chief complaint or concern is discussed, including their psychosocial motivation. Most important, educating the patient about realistic expectations is crucial to discuss at these appointments.

AESTHETIC FACIAL ANALYSIS

The clinical examination consists of the acquisition of facial measurements and the classification of these measurements. This process requires photo documentation of the frontal, profile, oblique, and submental facial positions, including face at rest, in smile, and activation of muscles of interest.

There are no absolute standards for what constitutes ideal facial aesthetics, but some parameters are useful for the clinician in the treatment planning process. Perhaps the most important element in the analysis of facial aesthetics is symmetry. Symmetry is quantifiable and has been considered as one of the most important characteristics in aesthetics. The second element to consider is the concept of averageness or the norm. This factor is also important in facial aesthetics and is typically applied to treatment planning for orthognathic surgery through cephalometric analysis and comparison of these measurements with normative values from a population of certain ethnicity. Related to normative values is another important aesthetic element, namely, proportions. Again, these can be evaluated in the different cephalometric analyses of the soft and hard tissues. The final important element in facial aesthetics is related to gender dysmorphism. For example, it is typically more accepted that males have a more prominent chin and forehead than females. In contrast, females have more prominent check bones and defined facial line angles.

MAXIMIZING FACIAL AESTHETICS WHILE CORRECTING THE MALOCCLUSION

Typically patients who undergo orthognathic surgery have an orthodontist on the team who is responsible to contribute with their expertise regarding the management of the occlusion. It is often found that the dysmorphology of the jaws closely matches the occlusion in all dimensions of space. For example, in the anteroposterior dimension, the majority of patients who have a class II malocclusion likely have a component of mandibular retrognathism, maxillary prognathism, or a combination of both situations.

Often the degree of maxillomandibular discrepancy is well-reflected in the occlusion. For example, a class II patient with 7 mm of anteroposterior maxillomandibular discrepancy will have a full cusp class II molar and canine occlusion and a similar amount of overjet. In these patients, the movement of the jaws (7 mm mandibular advancement) addresses the occlusal and facial aesthetics problems. However, this is not the case in many patients. Patients with more significant anteroposterior discrepancies may require adjunct procedures to maximize facial aesthetics within the constraints of correcting the malocclusion.

In the patients with class II malocclusion and significant facial convexity, genioplasties are common surgical adjuncts to enhance the mandibular projection. However, caution should be observed with this approach, because significant advancement genioplasties may increase the mentolabial fold depth with unfavorable aesthetic consequences. In contrast, patients with a class III malocclusion and facial concavity can benefit from malar implants, specifically if the paranasal area is deficient. Finally, in the short face patient, a lengthening genioplasty may favor facial proportions and decrease the depth of the mentolabial fold.

TREATMENT SEQUENCE

Deciding on the treatment sequence is unique to each individual patient and takes into consideration the anatomic areas, the recovery time, the patient's financial considerations, and whether it is a delayed or immediate correction at the time of orthognathic surgery. The dilemma becomes, how do we decide to perform a simultaneous versus delayed adjunctive aesthetic procedure with orthognathic surgery? To answer this, we must look at the predictability of the outcome, as well as the pros and cons of simultaneous versus delayed surgery.

The benefits of simultaneous surgery includes that it is a single day procedure, which maximizes the productivity and acceptance to the patient. However, one consideration is that intraoperative facial edema during orthognathic surgery can cause a loss of landmarks and altered anatomy, which increases the chance of an undesirable outcome after surgery. This leads to a longer intraoperative surgical time and postoperative healing period.

Staged surgery allows for a shorter initial surgery time, allows for minor corrections after the main surgery, and yields a more predictable outcome after waiting the appropriate time period to allow for a more stable soft tissue state.

However, there is an increased overall cumulative recovery time, increased cost to the patient (including the possibility of refusing a second surgery in the future), and loss of income.

With the development of advanced medical devices and biomaterials, many facial aesthetic procedures are minimally invasive and can be performed in an office setting using local and/or intravenous anesthesia. Some procedures may require use of an outpatient or same day surgery center or hospital.

The available procedures can be divided into bony alterations and soft tissue alterations. Bony alterations consist of rhinoplasty (nasal reshaping), genial enhancement, malar augmentation, and mandibular ramus, angle, and body alterations. Soft tissue alterations consist of submental contouring, onabotulinum toxin type A (Botox), and soft tissue fillers.

RHINOPLASTY

Preexisting nasal deformities are one of the primary indications for a rhinoplasty procedure. These deformities include a bulbous or widened nasal tip, nasal dorsal convexities, widened nasal bridge, and alar base widening. The second indication for a rhinoplasty procedure is postoperative orthognathic surgery nasal changes, which include nasal tip asymmetry, widened alar base, nasal septal deviation (also leading to tip deviation), and nasal dorsal profile alterations.

Nasal and jaw deformities are intricately linked, and orthognathic surgery can significantly impact the nasolabial envelope, and at times requires an adjunctive rhinoplasty.[1] Whether to perform the rhinoplasty as a simultaneous or staged procedure with orthognathic surgery must then be assessed. Single-stage orthognathic surgery and rhinoplasty have been found to be an effective method for the full rehabilitation of patients with malocclusion[2] (**Fig. 1**). However, certain patters of nasal morphology in orthognathic patients can have predictive values in the timing of rhinoplasty. Some authors have even proposed an algorithm to treat the nasomaxillofacial relationship using orthognathic surgery alone, orthognathic surgery in concert with rhinoplasty, or orthognathic surgery followed by staged rhinoplasty.[1] Complex and extreme maxillary movements can render the rhinoplasty unpredictable, and there is always a potential need for revision surgery. Simultaneous rhinoplasty with mandibular osteotomies has greater stability and predictability, because the mandibular movements do not directly affect the nasomaxillary complex.

GENIAL ENHANCEMENTS

The chin is an important component of facial aesthetics, and along with the nose, is one of the major determinants of facial profile balance. When it is appropriate in size, shape, and position, the chin can enhance the normal harmony and symmetry of the face, even camouflaging less than ideal jaw relationships.[3]

Correction of the lower face and neck is accomplished through multiple surgical interventions, performed alone or in combination. Determination of the appropriate procedures is based on individual anatomy, including skeletal structure, soft tissue distribution, muscular anatomy, and skin quality. Genial enhancement procedures encompass a large portion of these interventions. Genial enhancements include procedures, such as genial augmentation (genioplasty via an osteotomy, and genial implants or fillers) and genial reduction.

Indications for genial enhancements include hyperactive chin musculature, the presence of labial incompetence and lip strain, the failure of previous

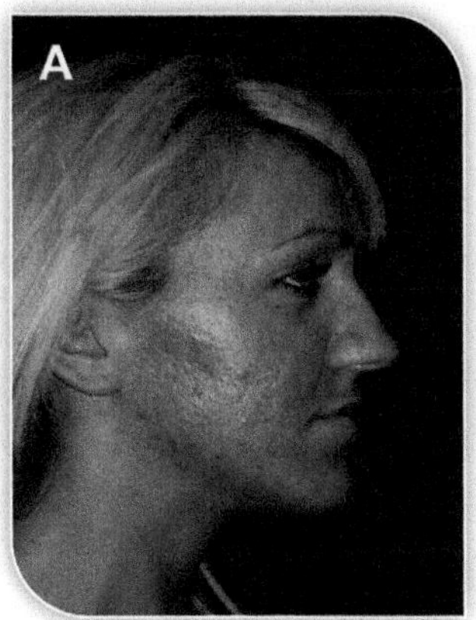

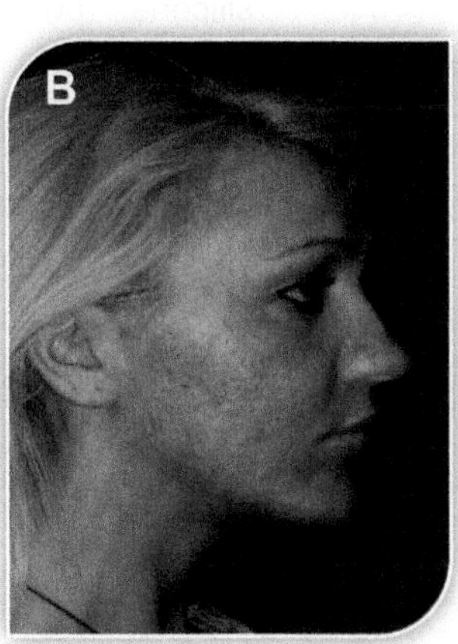

Fig. 1. Profile view of preoperative (*A*) versus postoperative (*B*) orthognathic surgery with simultaneous rhinoplasty.

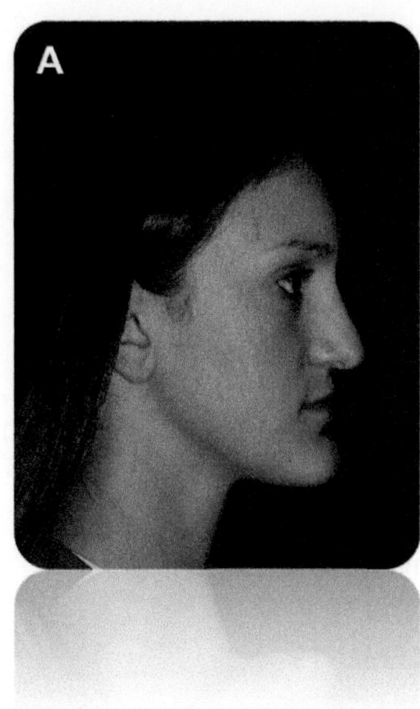

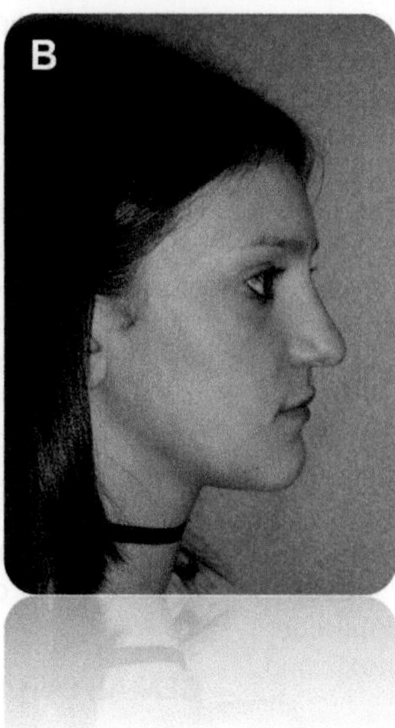

Fig. 2. Profile view of preoperative (*A*) versus postoperative (*B*) genial reduction surgery.

alloplastic implant owing to infection, and to provide an obstructive sleep apnea functional benefit. It is also generally accepted, and it is this author's practice, that if augmentation requires more than 4 to 6 mm, a genial enhancement is warranted.

Whether desirable or undesirable, when the chin is too long in the vertical or horizontal planes, the profile can convey masculinity and strength, whereas when it is deficient, it can convey weakness and femininity. The patient or the surgeon should not minimize the effects of the chin on facial proportions and aesthetics (**Fig. 2**).

Genial augmentation via an advancement osteotomy has been shown to have greater patient satisfaction (93.3% vs 87.5%), as well as a 100% soft tissue change predictability[3] (**Fig. 3**). In addition, there is less bony resorption, lower infection rates compared with implants, and greater versatility for those with greater facial asymmetry (**Fig. 4**).

The versatility of the genioplasty is generally unquestioned; however, there are certain circumstances in which alloplastic augmentation through the use of implants could be considered as the treatment of choice for a genial deficiency (**Fig. 5**). When comparing genioplasty with alloplastic augmentation, it is important to consider that the genioplasty is more invasive, causes more postoperative swelling, a longer postoperative recovery time, and rarely can result in a fracture of the mandible.[4] Owing to the proximity of the mandibular anterior teeth and mental nerve to the required osteotomy site in a genioplasty, it is possible to experience postoperative paresthesias to the anterior teeth, lip, and chin.[4] A study performed by Lindquist and Obeid[5] found that 72.5% of their patients had inferior border notching evidenced radiographically, but the aesthetic results satisfied 93.6% of the patients.

The alloplastic chin can be performed simultaneously with orthognathic surgery. Some of the alloplasts used include: porous polyethylene, silicone, polytetrafluoroethylene, high-density polyethylene (all are approved and acceptable materials and depends on surgeon preference).

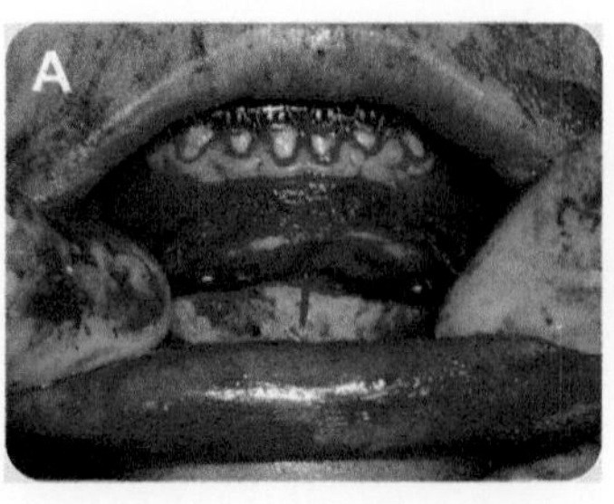

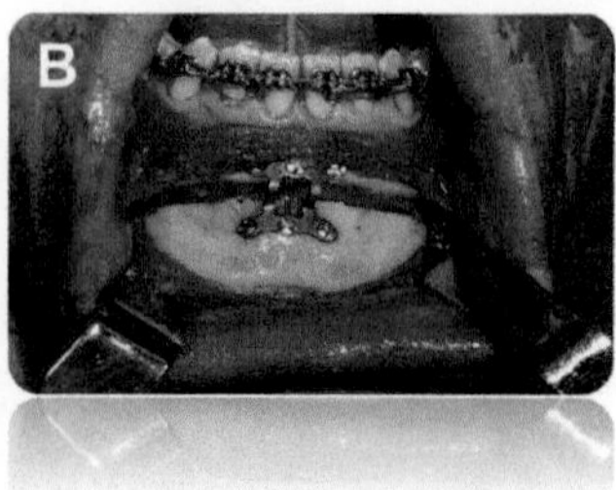

Fig. 3. Genial advancement osteotomy. Intraoral approach to a horizontal osteotomy (*A*), fixated with titanium plate and screws (*B*).

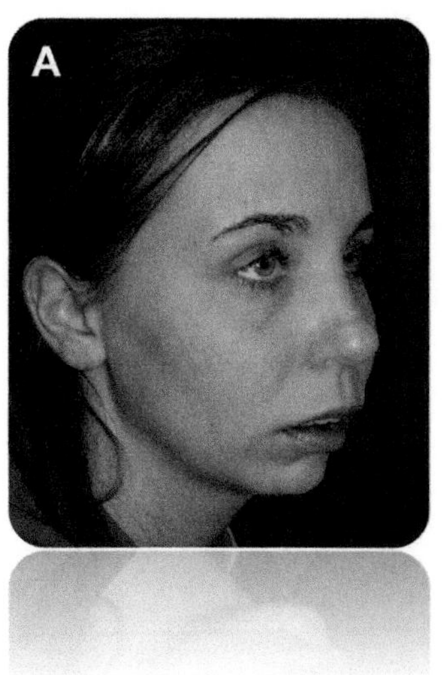

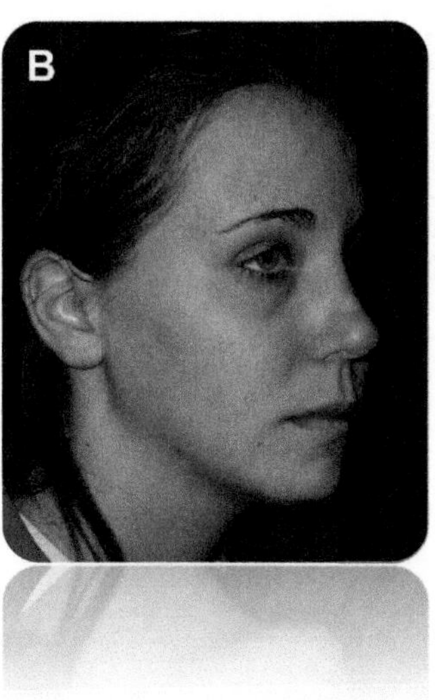

Fig. 4. Genial advancement osteotomy. Preoperative (*A*) versus postoperative (*B*) soft tissue changes.

A commonly associated unfavorable result with implants has been underlying bone resorption.[6] The resorption is universal among implants; however, it is of a minimal amount and stabilizes after time without loss of aesthetic result. Binder[7] (2011) reported on more than 500 alloplastic implants that resorption did not cause a significant problem aesthetically. Similarly, Flowers[8] (1991) reported on more than 1000 alloplastic implants and also noted that resorption did not cause significantly problems aesthetically. Other common complications include implant displacement, extrusion, and infection. Stabilization is the most important for alloplastic implants; most displacements, extrusions, and infections are due to inadequate stabilization at the time of implant placement.

The main indications for the alloplastic chin are very thin patients where a genioplasty procedure poses concerns for notching, and those patients with low mental foramens that may make the osteotomy for a genioplasty difficult (**Fig. 6**)

Surgical approaches for the chin implant are typically via a submental crease incision (**Fig. 7**). However, although many facial surgeons use an external approach, the intraoral method (midline intraoral incision approach) affords excellent aesthetic outcomes while avoiding an external scar.[9] The size of the required implant plays a major role in determining which approach should be considered (ie, if a very large implant is required, then the external approach should be considered). The chin implant can often be combined with other aesthetic neck procedures, such as liposuction, which would also require an extraoral approach. Rigid fixation during placement is recommended for stabilization of the implant. Secure implant fixation allows for less opportunity of motion at the interface, thus reducing wound inflammation. Chronic inflammation over the long term leads to formation of an avascular fibrous capsule.[6] Contraction of this fibrous capsule can lead to aesthetic deformation, and if infected it must be removed.

Currently, Medpor (Stryker, Kalamazoo, MI) is the best alloplastic material available. It is a high-density polyethylene implant material that is also biocompatible. It is long lasting, has a low

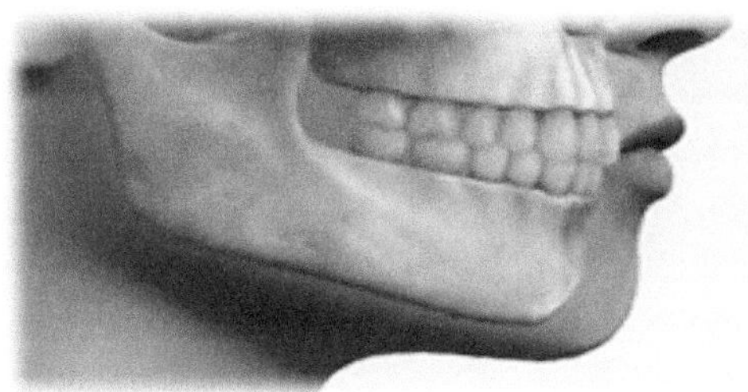

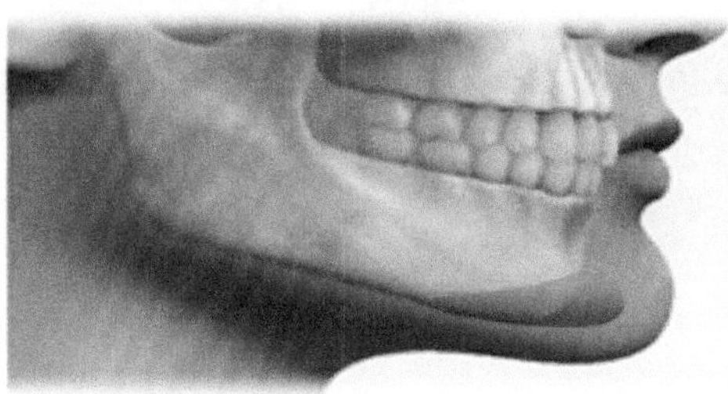

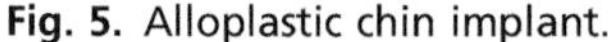
Fig. 5. Alloplastic chin implant.

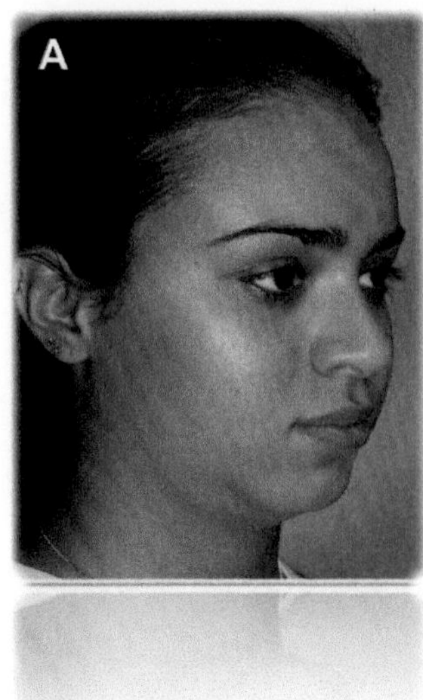

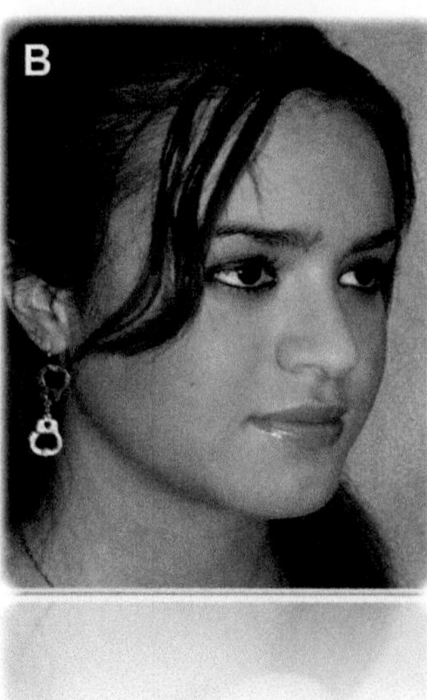

Fig. 6. Three-quarter view of preoperative (*A*) versus postoperative (*B*) alloplastic chin insertion.

frequency of complications, and high overall patient satisfaction as it had a bony feel.[10] Niechajev[10] (2012) performed a prospective study evaluating the long-term host tissue tolerance of Medpor, and found that Medpor implants had soft tissue ingrowths and collagen deposition, with subsequent vascularization.

MALAR AUGMENTATION

Indications for cheek or midface augmentation include poor lateral cheek projection in relation to bigonial and bitemporal widths, midface hypoplasia or congenital deformities, and infraorbital hallowing or increased scleral show. The options that exist to correct these aesthetic deformities include alloplastic material or autogenous bone grafting (such as calvarial parietal bone and anterior iliac crest graft). Unfortunately, autogenous grafts result in a second site morbidity.

Cheek implants can be performed with orthognathic surgery or as a delayed procedure. However, if performed simultaneously with orthognathic surgery the risk of infection is increased as a result of multiple intraoral surgical incisions. Alternatively, if indicated, cheek implants can be placed to correct an isolated midface deficiency (**Fig. 8**).

Robiony and colleagues[11] (1998) evaluated 17 patients with maxillomandibular malrelationships and deficient cheekbone contour who were treated by malar augmentation with porous high-density polyethylene in association with maxillary advancement and mandibular setback. The authors found excellent aesthetic results in

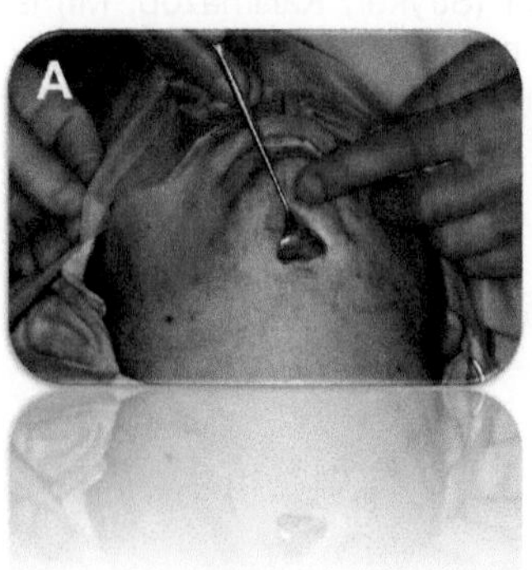

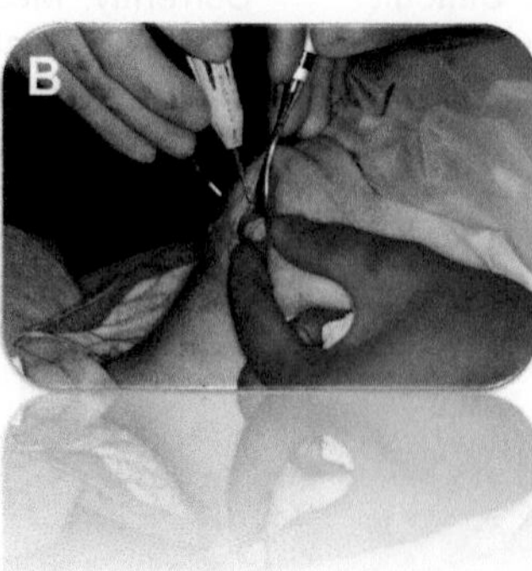

Fig. 7. Alloplastic chin implant via a submental crease incision (*A, B*).

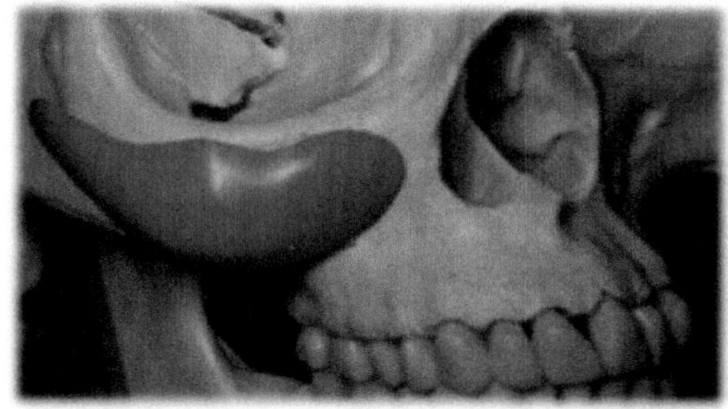

Fig. 8. Alloplastic cheek implant for malar augmentation.

all patients and that malaroplasty in association with bimaxillary orthognathic surgery seems to be an effective procedure for treating midface skeletal deficiencies (**Fig. 9**).

The pedicled buccal fat pad technique is a reasonable alternative for malar augmentation during simultaneous orthognathic surgery. Hernández-Alfaro[12] (2015) found that the pedicled buccal fat pad provides satisfactory soft-tissue augmentation, avoids the use of foreign materials, and has minimal morbidity, high patient satisfaction, and adequate stability at 12 months of follow-up.

Some patients may even have facial aesthetic improvement with the simple removal of the buccal fat pad (**Fig. 10**). The buccal fat pad is a single fatty structure between the facial muscles, and its removal may enhance the zygomatic prominences creating a more youthful and aesthetic facial profile (**Fig. 11**). Studies have examined the long-term effects of this approach; however, it has been concluded that more controlled clinical

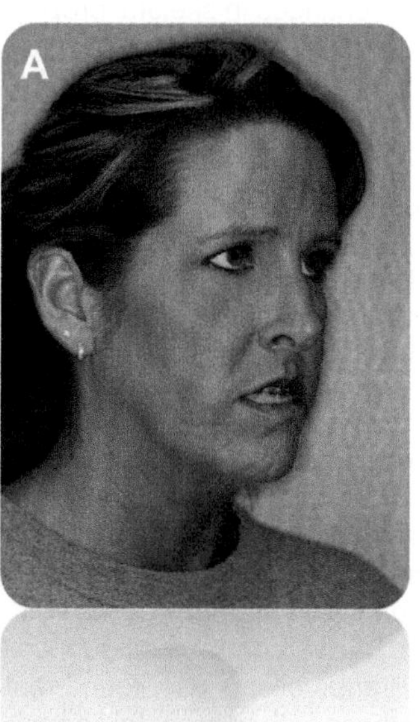

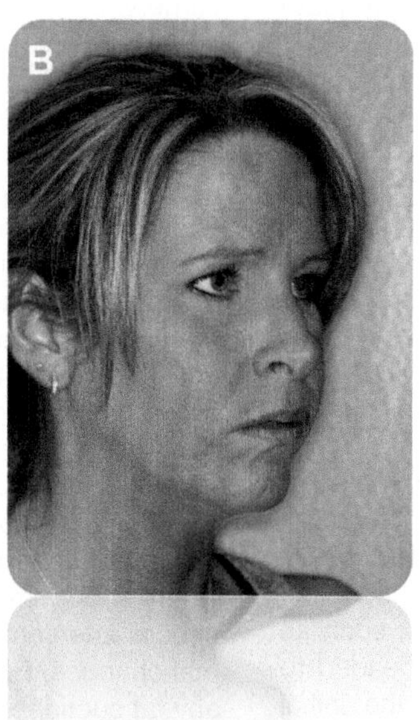

Fig. 9. Malaroplasty in association with bimaxillary orthognathic surgery for correction of midface deficiency, preoperative (*A*) versus postoperative (*B*).

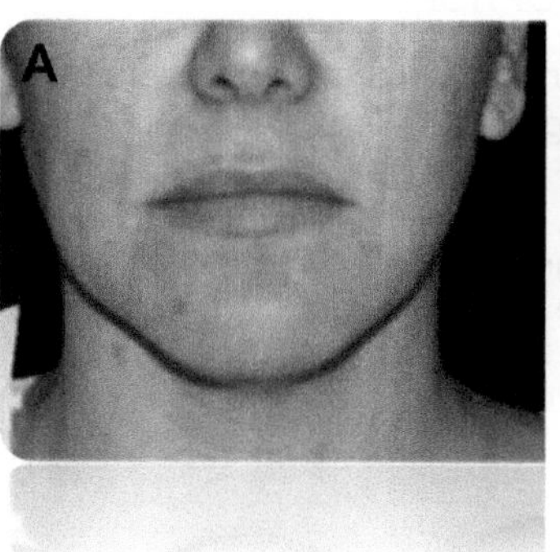

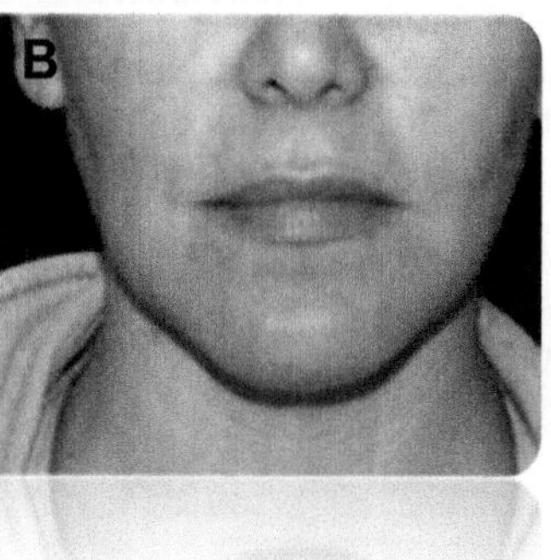

Fig. 10. Preoperative (*A*) versus postoperative (*B*) surgical removal of the buccal fat pad.

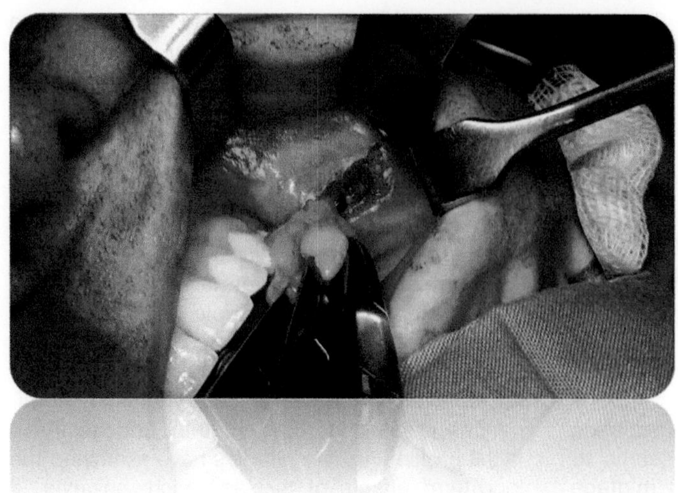

Fig. 11. Intraoral approach to the buccal fat pad.

studies should be performed to achieve adequate clinical evidence for this technique[13]

MANDIBULAR ANGLE DEFINITION AND RAMUS AUGMENTATION

Mandibular angle and ramus augmentation is more frequently requested by men to gain a more masculine face (**Fig. 12**). It is also used to improve facial asymmetries and to improve facial proportions, such as the bigonial dimension (**Fig. 13**). Similarly to the alloplastic materials discussed elsewhere in this article: silicone, porous polyethylene materials, and allograft are all examples of materials used to perform these augmentations.

Angle and ramus augmentations can also be performed simultaneously at the time of orthognathic surgery. However, complex deficiencies, such as 3-dimensional asymmetries, are recommended to be treated in stages 6 months after the initial surgery.

FACIAL LIPOCONTOURING

Orthognathic surgery can either improve or worsen the submental region and cervicomental angle (**Fig. 14**). However, submental liposuction can be performed simultaneously with orthognathic surgery, only after the changes in skeletal proportions of the submental profile are made. If the procedures are lengthy or complicated, the amount of edema that ensues distorts normal contours, and submental liposuction should be delayed. Liposuction serves as an adjunct where orthognathics is limited in aesthetic improvement. It removes fat accumulation, permits tissue redraping, and improves overall contour (**Fig. 15**). Submental liposuction has been found to be the most common aesthetic procedure in conjunction with orthognathic surgery, and that 71% of patients reported to be very satisfied with liposuction aesthetic results.[14]

Although orthognathic surgery improves the soft tissue profile in many cases, there are situations where suboptimal soft tissue changes necessitate special intervention. To overcome these suboptimal changes, Bohluli and colleagues[15] found that any fat suctioned in those with submental lipomatosis can be transferred to other areas of need, such as the lips and paranasal region, instead of discarding it (**Fig. 16**).

NONSURGICAL OPTIONS

In exploring adjunctive aesthetic procedures with orthognathic surgery, it is important to take into

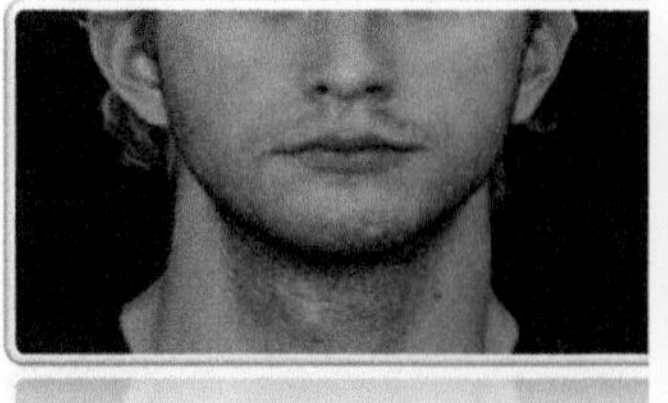

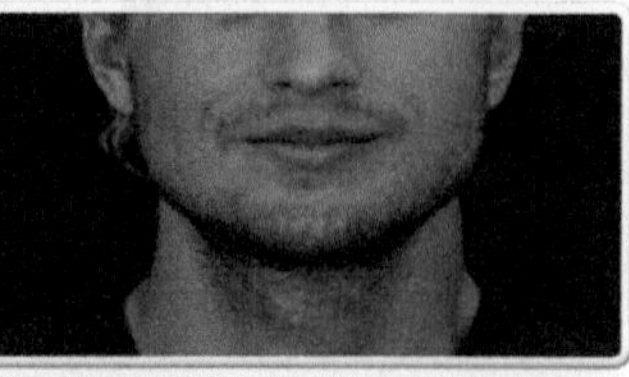

Fig. 12. Mandibular angle and ramus augmentation to gain a more masculine face.

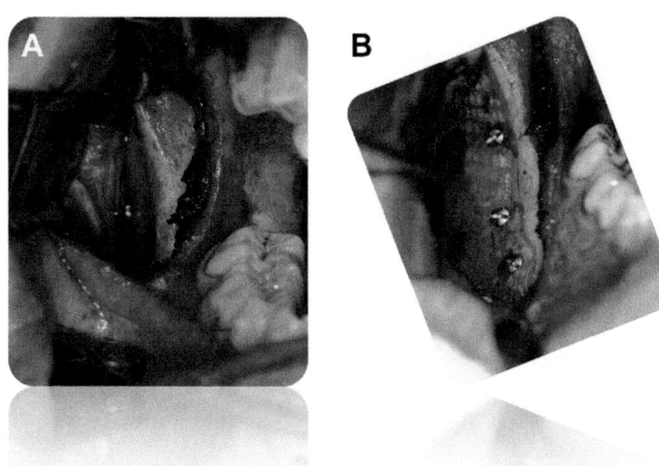

Fig. 13. Intraoral approach (*A*) for the placement of bigonial angle alloplastic implants (*B*).

account nonsurgical treatment options. These include soft tissue fillers, lipodissolving agents, and onabotulinum toxin type A.

Soft Tissue Filler Injectable

Hyaluronic acid has become the new gold standard in the last few years. This is mostly due to the fact that it is nonimmunogenic. There are 2 main categories: animal derived (Hylaform, and no longer on the market) and bacteria derived (Restylane and Juvederm). Radiesse was approved for use as a soft tissue filler by the US Food and Drug Administration in 2006. It consists of 30% calcium hydroxyapatite aqueous gel and stimulates cutaneous cells to induce neocollagenesis by fibroblast activation. The substance is radiopaque with a slow rate of degradation, similar to human bone. These soft tissue filler injectables can be used for adjunctive procedures, such as chin augmentation (**Fig. 17**) and nonsurgical rhinoplasty (**Fig. 18**).

Onabotulinum Toxin Type A

Onabotulinum toxin type A is a useful tool for the aesthetic reduction and narrowing of the width of the lower face. This goal can be accomplished by its ability to reduce the bulk and volume of hypertrophic masseteric muscles and enlarged parotid glands.[16] Onabotulinum toxin type A can be administered in such a way that degree of reduction and exact location in the muscle to be reduced is controlled. Consequently, the jawline becomes better defined and the cheekbones take on a sculpted appearance with relative, aesthetic cheek hollowing under the zygomatic arch.[16] It has even been successful for the neuromuscular correction

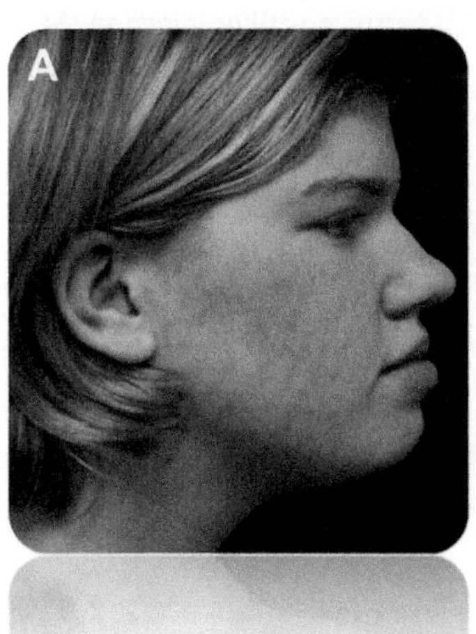

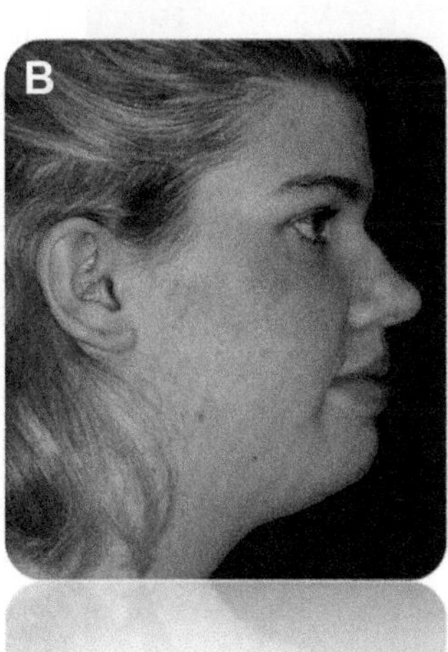

Fig. 14. Worsening of the submental lipomatosis and cervicomental angle after orthognathic surgery. Preoperative (*A*) versus postorthognathic surgery (*B*).

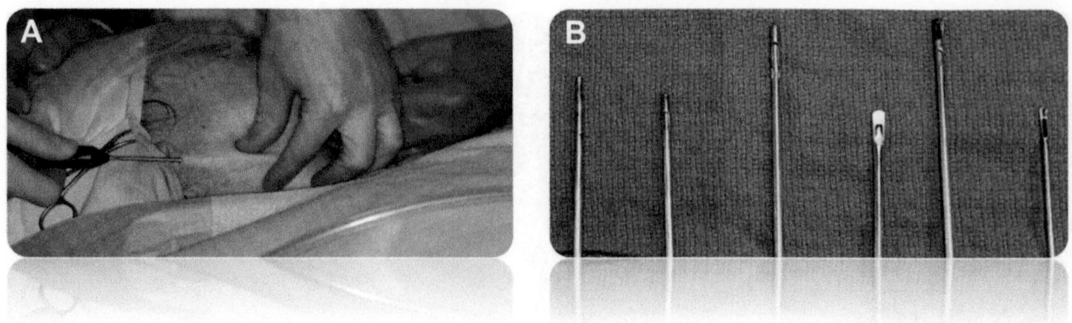

Fig. 15. Intraoperative photo of submental and cervicomental liposuction (*A*). Variety of liposuction cannulas (*B*).

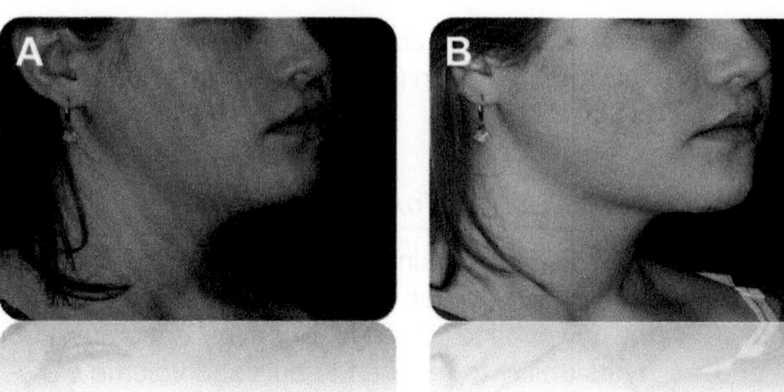

Fig. 16. Submental fat transfer to the upper lip in a patient with submental lipomatosis. Preoperative (*A*) versus postoperative (*B*).

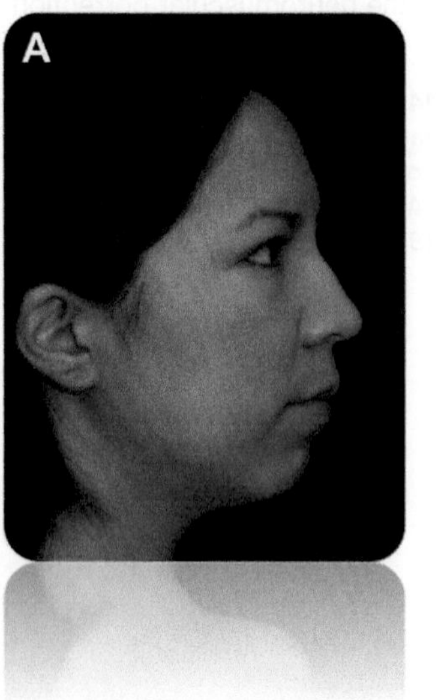

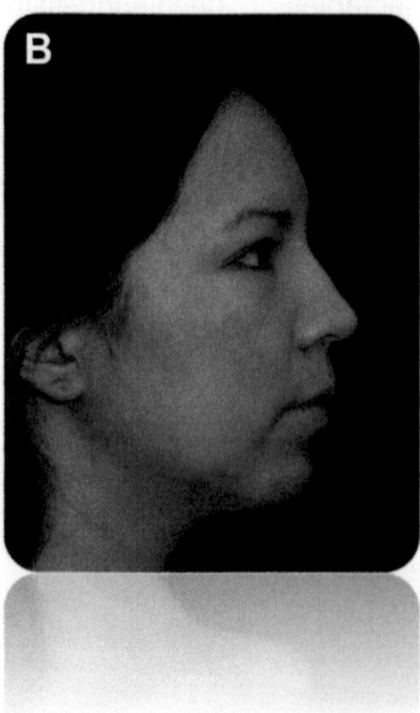

Fig. 17. Soft tissue filler injectables used for chin augmentation. Preoperative (*A*) versus postfiller injection (*B*).

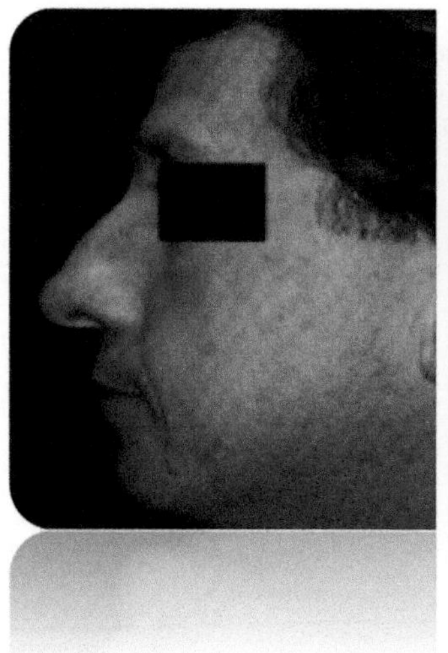
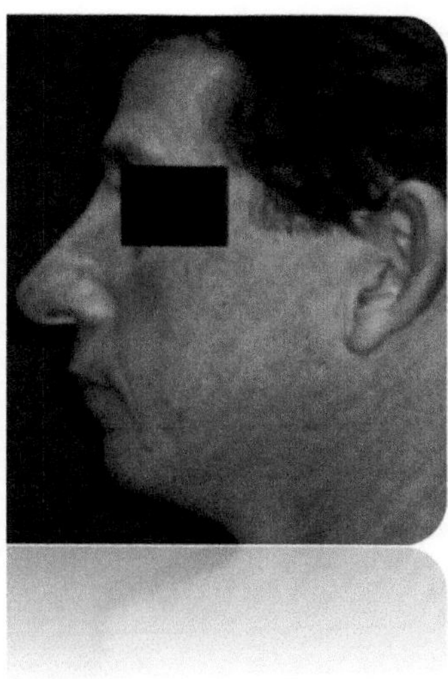

Fig. 18. Soft tissue filler injectables used for nonsurgical rhinoplasty.

of excessive gingival display on smiling, or commonly referred to as a gummy smile.[17] Various surgical and nonsurgical modalities have been described in the treatment of gummy smile, which includes Lefort I osteotomy, crown lengthening procedures, maxillary incisor intrusion, microimplants, headgears, self-curing silicone implant injected at Anterior Nasal Spine with myectomy and partial resection of levator labii superioris with muscle repositioning.[18] However, these procedures do not help in reducing the hyperactivity of the muscles and, therefore, nonsurgical treatment with onabotulinum toxin type A may be a desirable option[19] (**Fig. 19**).

Klybella is the only lipodissolving injectable agent approved by the US Food and Drug Administration in 2015 for the treatment of submental fullness (**Fig. 20**). It is a deocycholic acid, a naturally occurring molecule in the body, which aids in the breakdown of dietary fat. Additionally, it is a cytolytic agent that causes permanent destruction of adipocytes via cell lysis. Klybella can safely and effectively be performed in combination with orthognathic surgery.

Orthodontics, Temporary Anchorage Devices, and Soft Tissue adjuncts, in lieu of Conventional Orthognathic Surgery

The application of temporary anchorage devices (TADs) has significantly altered the orthodontic field by facilitating dental movements that previously were only achievable by means of orthognathic surgery. Conventionally, the osteotomies performed during orthognathic surgery are able to obtain close to ideal occlusal relationships with minimal orthodontic movement after surgery. The bone movements are responsible for the aesthetic changes and at the same time achieving an occlusion close to an ideal standard. With TADs, the osteotomies are not necessary to achieve ideal occlusion. The range of orthodontic movements have been expanded extensively by means of TADs.

In this manner, complex malocclusions can be resolved through orthodontic treatment with mini-implant or miniplates driving the more complicated movements that were not possible in the past, such as molar intrusion, distalization,

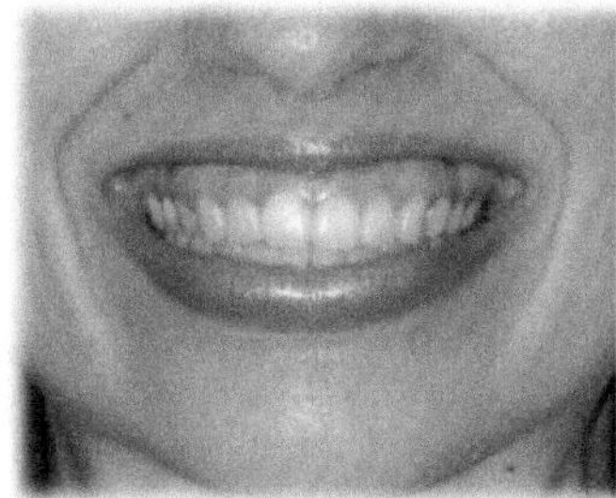
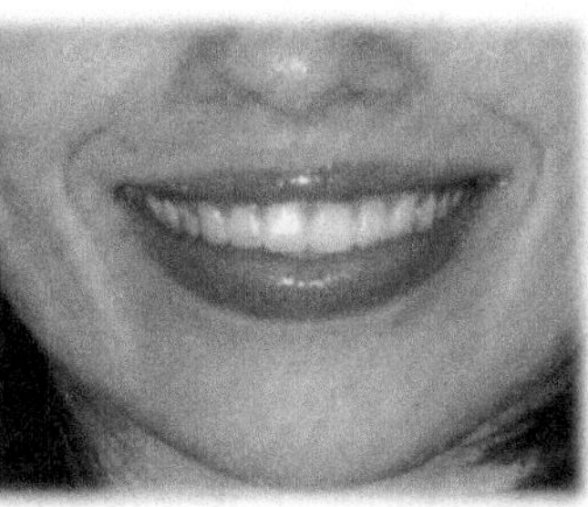

Fig. 19. Onabotulinum toxin type A injections for the neuromuscular correction of excessive gingival display on smiling.

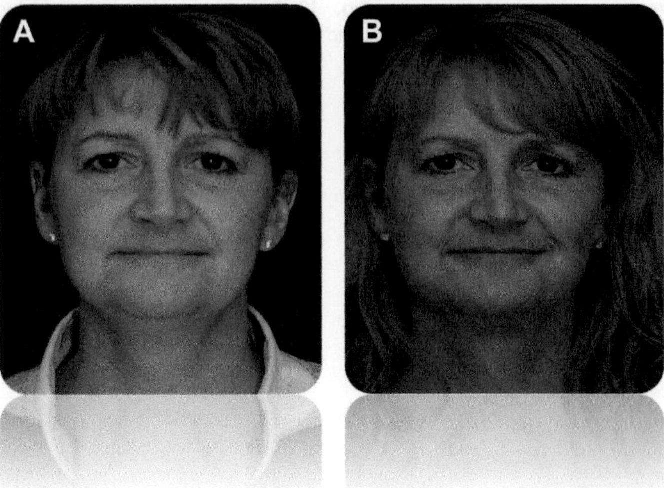

Fig. 20. Klybella injections for the reduction of submental fullness. Preoperative (*A*) versus post-Klybella injections to the submental region (*B*).

and molar protraction. The desired occlusal outcomes can be obtained without the need for conventional bimaxillary surgery; however, the facial aesthetic enhancements are still necessary in areas such as the chin, cheek, angle of the mandible, and lips. All the techniques described in this article can be combined with orthodontics using skeletal anchorage to refine the aesthetic outcome, in an approach that can be considered as minimally invasive surgery.

For example, the patient in **Fig. 21** presented with a significant skeletal anterior open bite, slight mandibular prognathism, and paranasal deficiency. Dentally, the patient was missing the lower right second premolar and the lower left first molar. Conventionally, this patient would had been treated with bimaxillary surgery with or without genioplasty. The specific goal would had been posterior maxillary impaction, expecting that the mandible would autorotate to then proceed to

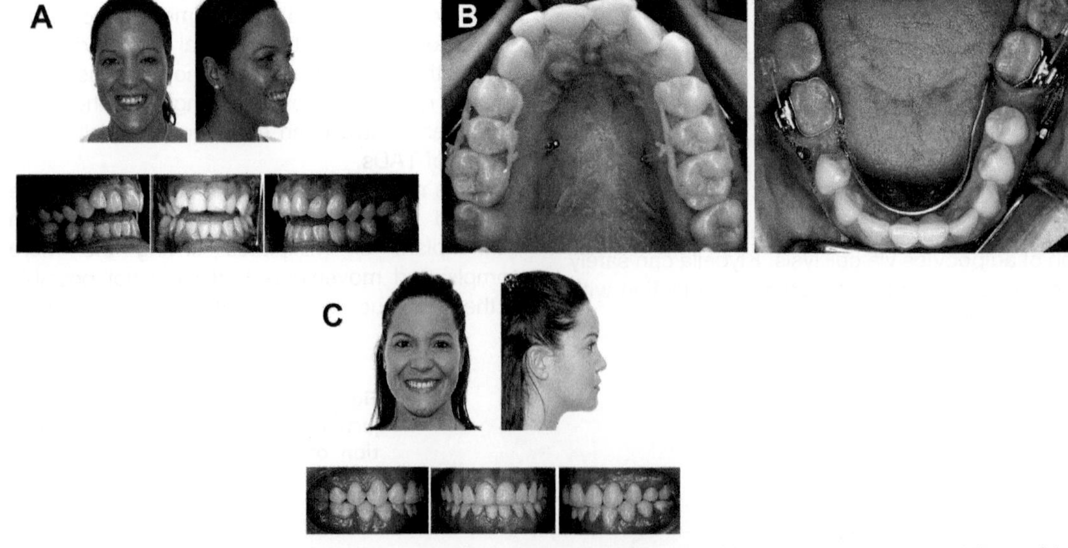

Fig. 21. Orthodontic treatment with TADs to address the malocclusion in addition to genioplasty and fat grafting to address soft tissue aesthetics. Pretreatment extraoral and intraoral photos showing the vertical maxillary excess and anterior open bite malocclusion (*A*). TADs used to intrude maxillary molars and to protract mandibular molars in the mandible (*B*). Posttreatment extraoral and intraoral photos after shortening genioplasty and malar and lip fat grafting (*C*). (*From* Uribe F, Azami N, Steinbacher D. Skeletal open-bite correction with mini-implant anchorage and minimally invasive surgery. J Clin Orthod. 2018;52(9):485–92; with permission.)

perform a setback, which would normalize the anteroposterior relationship. However, it was decided to treat the malocclusion orthodontically, and the facial aesthetics were refined by means of a shortening genioplasty and fat grafting of the cheeks and lips. This procedure could be considered minimally invasive surgery, which addressed the major aesthetic problems, while the orthodontics with TADs targeted the occlusal discrepancy.

SUMMARY

Many of the aesthetic facial procedures can be performed simultaneously at the time of initial orthognathic surgery. Any residual deformities after surgery, such as mandibular notching, malar asymmetry, labiomental crease, and any camouflage treatment should be performed as a delayed procedure when the outcome is predictable. Additionally, all these procedures could be used to enhance the orthodontic result, without the need of osteotomies to reposition the bones.

REFERENCES

1. Sun AH, Steinbacher DM. Orthognathic surgery and rhinoplasty: simultaneous or staged? Plast Reconstr Surg 2018;141(2):322–9.
2. Glushko A, Dobyshev A, Dobysheva N, et al. Effectiveness of the one-stage orthognathic surgery and rhinoplasty. Int J Oral Maxillofac Surg 2017;46:156.
3. Strauss RA, Abubaker AO. Genioplasty: a case for advancement osteotomy. J Oral Maxillofac Surg 2000;58(7):783–7.
4. Reed EH, Smith G. Genioplasty: a case for alloplastic chin augmentation. J Oral Maxillofac Surg 2000; 58(7):788–93.
5. Lindquist CC, Obeid G. Complications of genioplasty done alone or in combination with sagittal split-ramus osteotomy. Oral Surg Oral Med Oral Pathol 1998;66(1):13–6.
6. Freidman CD, Constantino PD. Alloplastic materials for facial skeletal augmentation. Facial Plast Surg Clin North Am 2002;10(3):325–33.
7. Binder WJ. Facial rejuvenation and volumization using implants. Facial Plast Surg 2011;27(1):086–97.
8. Flowers RS. Alloplastic augmentation of the anterior mandible. Clin Plast Surg 1991;18(1):107–38.
9. Aynehchi BB, Burstein DH, Parhiscar A, et al. Vertical incision intraoral silicone chin augmentation. Otolaryngol Head Neck Surg 2012;146(4):553–9.
10. Niechajev I. Facial reconstruction using porous high-density polyethylene (Medpor): long-term results. Aesthetic Plast Surg 2012;36(4):917–27.
11. Robiony M, Costa F, Demitri V, et al. Simultaneous malaroplasty with porous polyethylene implants and orthognathic surgery for correction of malar deficiency. J Oral Maxillofac Surg 1998;56(6): 734–41.
12. Hernández-Alfaro F, Valls-Ontañón A, Blasco-Palacio JC, et al. Malar augmentation with pedicled buccal fat pad in orthognathic surgery: three-dimensional evaluation. Plast Reconstr Surg 2015; 136(5):1063–7.
13. Moura LB, Spin JR, Spin-Neto R, et al. Buccal fat pad removal to improve facial aesthetics: an established technique? Med Oral Patol Oral Cir Bucal 2018;23(4):e478–84.
14. Bach DE, Newhouse RF, Boice GW. Simultaneous orthognathic surgery and cervicomental liposuction. Clinical and survey results. Oral Surg Oral Med Oral Pathol 1991;71(3):262–6.
15. Bohluli B, Varedi P, Bayat M, et al. Submental fat transfer: an approach to enhance soft tissue conditions in patients with submental lipomatosis after orthognathic surgery. J Oral Maxillofac Surg 2014; 72(1):164.e1-7.
16. Wu WT. Botox facial slimming/facial sculpting: the role of botulinum toxin-A in the treatment of hypertrophic masseteric muscle and parotid enlargement to narrow the lower facial width. Facial Plast Surg Clin North Am 2010;18(1):133–40.
17. Polo M. Botulinum toxin type A (Botox) for the neuromuscular correction of excessive gingival display on smiling (gummy smile). Am J Orthod Dentofacial Orthop 2008;133(2):195–203.
18. Indra AS, Biswas PP, Vineet VT, et al. Botox as an adjunct to orthognathic surgery for a case of severe vertical maxillary excess. J Maxillofac Oral Surg 2011;10(3):266–70.
19. Sandler PJ, Alsayer F, Davies SJ. Botox: a possible new treatment for gummy smile. Virtual J Orthod 2007;20:30–4.

Moving?

Make sure your subscription moves with you!

To notify us of your new address, find your **Clinics Account Number** (located on your mailing label above your name), and contact customer service at:

Email: journalscustomerservice-usa@elsevier.com

800-654-2452 (subscribers in the U.S. & Canada)
314-447-8871 (subscribers outside of the U.S. & Canada)

Fax number: 314-447-8029

Elsevier Health Sciences Division
Subscription Customer Service
3251 Riverport Lane
Maryland Heights, MO 63043

*To ensure uninterrupted delivery of your subscription, please notify us at least 4 weeks in advance of move.

Printed and bound by CPI Group (UK) Ltd, Croydon, CR0 4YY
08/05/2025
01864691-0017